THE HOSPITAL MEDICAL STAFF

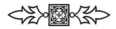

THE HOSPITAL MEDICAL STAFF

Charles H. White, Ph.D.

Emeritus, Medical Staff Executive
Grossmont Hospital, La Mesa, CA

Director, Health Professions Education
Sharp Healthcare, San Diego, CA

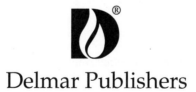

Delmar Publishers

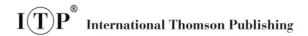 International Thomson Publishing

Albany • Bonn • Boston • Cincinnati • Detroit • London • Madrid
Melbourne • Mexico City • New York • Pacific Grove • Paris • San Francisco
Singapore • Tokyo • Toronto • Washington

Notice to the Reader

Publisher does not warrant or guarantee any of the products described herein or perform any independent analysis in connection with any of the product information contained herein. Publisher does not assume, and expressly disclaims, any obligation to obtain and include information other than that provided to it by the manufacturer.

The reader is expressly warned to consider and adopt all safety precautions that might be indicated by the activities herein and to avoid all potential hazards. By following the instructions contained herein, the reader willingly assumes all risks in connection with such instructions.

The publisher makes no representation or warranties of any kind, including but not limited to, the warranties of fitness for particular purpose or merchantability, nor are any such representations implied with respect to the material set forth herein, and the publisher takes no responsibility with respect to such material. The publisher shall not be liable for any special, consequential, or exemplary damages resulting, in whole or part, from the readers' use of, or reliance upon, this material.

Cover Design: *Carol D. Keohane*
Delmar Staff
Publisher: *William Brottmiller*
Acquisitions Editor: *Bill Burgower*
Assistant Editor: *Hilary Schrauf*
Production Coordinator: *James Zayicek*
Art and Design Coordinator: *Carol D. Keohane*
Editorial Assistant: *Diane Biondi*

COPYRIGHT © 1997
By Delmar Publishers, Inc.
an International Thomson Publishing Company

The ITP logo is a trademark under license.

Printed in the United States of America

For more information, contact:

Delmar Publishers, Inc.
3 Columbia Circle, Box 15015
Albany, New York 12212-5015

International Thomson Publishing
Berkshire House
168-173 High Holborn
London, WC1V7AA
England

Thomas Nelson Australia
102 Dodds Street
South Melbourne 3205
Victoria, Australia

Nelson Canada
1120 Birchmont Road
Scarborough, Ontario
M1K 5G4, Canada

International Thomson Editores
Campos Eliseos 385, Piso 7
Col Polanco
11560 Mexico D F Mexico

International Thomson Publishing GmbH
Konigswinterer Stasse. 418
53227 Bonn
Germany

International Thomson Publishing Asia
221 Henderson Road
#05-10 Henderson Building
Singapore 0315

International Thomson Publishing—Japan
Kyowa Building, 3F
2-2-1 Hirakawa-cho
Chiyoda-ku, Tokyo 102
Japan

1 2 3 4 5 6 7 8 9 10 XXX 01 00 99 98 97 96

Library of Congress Cataloging-in-Publication Data

White, Charles H.
   The hospital medical staff / by Charles H. White.
      p.   cm. — (Delmar series in health services administration)
   Includes bibliographical references and index.
   ISBN 0-8273-7166-7
   1. Hospitals—Medical staff. 2. Hospitals—Physician leadership.
   I. Title. II. Series.
   [DNLM: 1. Medical Staff, Hospital—organization & administration.
   2. Models. Organizational.   WX 203 W583h 1996]
RA972.W48 1996
362.1'1'0683—dc20
DNLM/DLC
for Library of Congress   96-11483
                                                       CIP

INTRODUCTION TO THE SERIES

This Series in Health Services is now in its second decade of providing top quality teaching materials to the health administration/public health field. Each year has witnessed further strengthening of the market position of each of the principal books in the Series, also reflecting the continued excellence of the products. Each author, book editor, and contributor to the Series has helped build what is widely recognized as the top textbook and issue collection of books available in this field today.

But we have achieved only a beginning. Everyone involved in the Series is committed to further expansion of the scope, technical excellence, and usability of the Series. Our goal is to do more for you, the reader. We will add new books in important areas, seek out more excellent authors, and increase the physical attributes of the books to make them easier for you to use.

We thank everyone, the authors and users in particular, who have made this Series so successful and so widely used. And we promise that this second decade will be dedicated to further expansion of the Series and to enhancement of the books it contains to provide still greater value to you, our constituency.

Stephen J. Williams
Series Editor

DELMAR SERIES IN HEALTH SERVICES ADMINISTRATION

Stephen J. Williams, Sc.D., Series Editor

Ambulatory Care Management, second edition
Austin Ross, Stephen J. Williams, and Eldon L. Schafer, Editors

The Continuum of Long-Term Care
Connie J. Evashwick, Editor

Health Care Economics, fourth edition
Paul J. Feldstein

Health Care Management: Organization Design and Behavior, third edition
Stephen M. Shortell and Arnold D. Kaluzny, Editors

Health Politics and Policy, second edition
Theodor J. Litman and Leonard S. Robins, Editors

Introduction to Health Services, fourth edition
Stephen J. Williams and Paul R. Torrens, Editors

Motivating Health Behavior
John P. Elder, E. Scott Geller, Melbourne F. Hovell, and Joni A. Mayer, Editors

Really Governing: How Health System and Hospital Boards Can Make More of a Difference
Dennis D. Pointer and Charles M. Ewell

Strategic Management of Human Resources in Health Services Organizations,
second edition
Myron D. Fottler, S. Robert Hernandez, and Charles L. Joiner, Editors

Financial Management in Health Care Organizations
Robert A. McLean

Principles of Public Health Practice
F. Douglas Scutchfield and C. William Keck

The Hospital Medical Staff
Charles H. White

Essentials of Health Services
Stephen J. Williams

Essentials of Health Care Management
Stephen M. Shortell and Arnold D. Kaluzny, Editors

Health Services Research Methods
Leiyu Shi

SUPPLEMENTAL READER:

Contemporary Issues in Health Services
Stephen J. Williams

CONTENTS

PART TWO
MOVING AWAY FROM THE JOINT
COMMISSION MODEL

ACKNOWLEDGMENTS

Thanks most of all to Jo, who tolerated all those hours when I could not tell her what it was I had been doing that took so long. To Cheryl and Michael, who brought us Elizabeth and Joshua; Leslie, who bailed me out of all my computer mistakes; and Nancy. Some notable colleagues include Ed Smith, who made sense out of the RMP; Ralph Ingersoll, who started the whole thing; Gerald McManis, always the greatest. No one could ask for better coworkers than Ted Fourkas, Larkin Morse, Steve Lewis, Mike Vaida, Cindy Arstein, and Molly Ariey. For nearly 20 years, I benefited from the wise and helpful support of Lee Short and Natalie Stenen.

Thanks also to the help and support of Mike Long, who brought me to Grossmont; Basil Maloney, my friend for 25 years; Emily Friedman, who adopted us; Paul Ward, Curt Kelly, Eleanor Langpaap, Henry Dunlap, Pete Lehmann, who created and appointed the Strategic Planning Committee; Ron Johnson; Joe Leonard; Andy Alongi; Rokay Kamyar; Maynard Olson; Brad Kesling; David Gibson; Neil Andrews; and many others, some of whom have been named in the text.

No reference to Grossmont Hospital during its rich period of experimentation and a willingness to try new and different ideas would be complete without thanking Trudi Ferenchak, who always knew what I was trying to say in correspondence and presentations; Mari Thompson, who managed the Office of the Chief of Staff with such skill and class; and Kathy Downs, who managed well the functions of Medical Staff Services and still made time to help advance her profession by teaching at state and national training programs.

The administration at Grossmont supported the idea and the implementation of the medical staff executive organizational structure and deserve much credit for their efforts to move toward self-directed work teams and quality improvement programs. Unfortunately, such humane and enlightened management styles are the first to go in the days of managed care. Thanks for all of their efforts to Michael Erne, Pam Parmelee, Marian Furlong, Linda Ollis, and Robin Eskow.

I include also in these credits my favorite attorneys, John Whitney in La Jolla, Charles "Chuck" Forbes in Los Angeles, and Linda Haddad in Pittsburgh. This entire book-writing project was suggested by Stuart Marylander, with local support from Steve Williams and Dennis Pointer at San Diego State University.

PREFACE

This work is intended as a textbook, primarily for the use of those practicing physicians who become medical staff leaders. Each year, new people ascend to the chairs of leadership in the hospital medical staff. Most of them mean well but are unprepared for the culture shock that awaits them. This book hopes to be of some help with learning how to do those new duties and how to anticipate and understand the inevitable stresses that go with the territory.

The book is intended to be of assistance also to graduate students in health care administration. The graduate students in administration may be more likely to read the whole thing but will never participate in most of the activities described. Doctors are not told about the medical staff self-governance process that lies ahead of them, and neither are would-be administrators. Now they both can know.

Many friends and coworkers have aided my career, but this book is not their fault. Rather, in sitting through some 20,000 hours of medical staff meetings and uncounted others, both administrative and board, it is inescapable that some of the better parts will stick as good examples, and, then there are also those unlovable but real testing situations that seem to bring out both the best and the worst in some physicians. So many examples of good leadership, good citizenship, and intelligent attention to the job are always around us during the internal life of the hospital medical staff. Then, there are those others. Why did they go to medical school, and why are they practicing medicine when they are so filled with hate and disgust for almost everything? Those men and women are truly the cross to bear for well-meaning chiefs of staff, medical executives, VPMAs, and medical staff coordinators who keep the world turning.

The book is dedicated to the medical staff of Grossmont Hospital, who accepted me warmly, were unfailingly helpful and willing to learn, at the same time they were teaching me.

INTRODUCTION

Physicians function in society with a number of roles, understood more or less well by their patients, their families, and themselves. The more obvious or apparent of these roles is as health care professional who sees patients and performs examinations and procedures.

To his or her employees, the modern day physician in office practice may be a small businessman or woman who pays taxes and struggles with office management, a science for which many medical care experts are spectacularly unprepared. The worst part of that process is the never-ending hassle with private and public third parties who pay (or refuse to pay) bills and claims for treatments already provided to patients.

Or, a very modern day physician may be a member of a group practice that services contracts or health plans. The doctor sees an endless parade of patients who have been sorted and classified according to coverages or criteria set by the group. Office management and bills may not a part of this practice setting, but more regular (though long) hours may be.

To the family, the physician can be a loving spouse and model parent deeply involved in family life in many personal roles. In the business and professional roles, a physician may also be a person with practically unlimited credit ratings for buying large houses, luxury cars, club memberships, and tuition to private schools. Sometimes, this money machine is also charged with paying alimony to previous spouses who want to continue the financial good times brought on by society's willingness to pay well for health care. At the intersection of business and family roles, that physician may be a person who is gone from home most of the time, is always late for every promised commitment, and gets phone calls at all hours. They are not dependable in being able to stay on their time schedule, probably because there were too many patients that day who were sicker than expected for the time intervals scheduled for appointments, or because someone seriously ill took a turn for the worse and had to be hospitalized. But modern day physicians, mostly specialists who join hospital medical staffs, also join a professional responsibility that no one warned them about and that has remained largely unexplained after literally decades of the existence of that duty.

At no time in any medical school or residency curriculum is there a discussion or explanation of the obligation to be accountable as a profession to society in lieu of governmental regulation. This professional obligation is to carry out a governance function, that of joining with all other members of the hospital medical staff to perform as an unincorporated association for self-governance. The unincorporated association collectively performs the assigned tasks of a Joint Commission model of a hospital medical staff.

There are a number of specific assignments presented as standards by the Joint Commission on Accreditation of Hospitals and Healthcare Organizations (JCAHO), the accrediting body for U.S. hospitals. The lack of previous information during the training era in a physician's career sometimes leads to a resentment of these JCAHO standards or a refusal to recognize their legitimacy by some doctors. There are also obligations imposed by federal law (Healthcare Quality Improvement Act of 1986) and by state law or regulation (Health and Safety Code in California or the equivalent in other states). There are further obligations formed in increments over time by precedent court decisions. In addition, there are the obligations formed by local hospital boards of directors or trustees. Boards are the legally responsible bodies in hospitals, and it is their hospital, and sometimes the board, who gets sued when a hospital is accused of causing or permitting unacceptable quality of care by doctors, nurses, or any other caregiver.

Boards delegate to medical staffs the crucial responsibilities and duties to safe guard patient care and safety and it is that delegation that is the subject of this volume. The hospital medical staff is a collection of individual practitioners who studied alone, took tests alone, performed science experiments alone, made good grades alone, make innumerable patient care decisions alone, are alone in their individual liability for their actions. Now they are asked to join together as a team to subjugate that individuality in order to collectively carry out the assigned duties of a medical staff that has been delegated responsibilities for quality of care and patient safety by the governing board of the hospital.

Those duties cannot be escaped by the entire collective body of physicians, although only a small minority of staff members do the large part of the work. The remainder of the staff are governed or affected by the work of this minority, whether or not they are fully aware of it. Some realize and appreciate the work of their more willing colleagues. Some understand what needs to be done and that someone needs to do it (but not them). A few others do not know and do not care.

The modern day hospital medical staff—who it is, what it does, along with some suggested ways of doing it better—is the subject of this discussion, written from the point of view of an insider who took part in the process, who helped and admired the chiefs of staff in the performance of their burdens of office, and who believes that no matter what is reformed about the health care system, certain functions will remain that only physicians can and should do:

- *Credentialing:* Is the physician qualified?
- *Privileges:* What care is to be provided?
- *Peer Review:* How well is it being done?
- *Reappointment:* Should appointment be continued?

Most of the speakers and consultants who advise medical staff behavior have never been in a confidential peer review meeting where a leading, well-known physician faces loss of privileges and the possible end of a long and honorable career because of a mistake in judgment or skill. After some 10,000 hours of peer review, let me assure you that those dramatic moments are charged with the tension and dread by each committee member that "this could be happening to me."

It is a loss to the profession, and those leaders that will come after, that most of the physicians who took part in those meetings had not published accounts and descriptions of the process in terms that will help less-experienced colleagues learn how to perform their duties during their term of office. There will be continued turnover of medical staff leaders. There will continue to be a need for realistic, plain-language assistance and guidance for chiefs, VPMAs, medical directors, department chairs, and medical staff services professionals. This is the goal of this believer in the process of self-governance: to be useful and helpful.

It is curious that in the midst of the highest levels of medical science and complex technology, with every form of electronic assistance and communication immediately at hand, conducting the affairs of the medical staff is such an unscientific trial-and-error procedure. But it is.

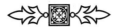

PART ONE

MOVING TOWARD THE JOINT
COMMISSION MODEL

CHAPTER

Hospitals:
Pesthouses to Systems

The modern hospital is the key resource and organizational hub of the American health care delivery system. It is central to the delivery of patient care, the training of health personnel, and the conduct and dissemination of health-related research. The hospital represents the community's collective investment in health care resources, presumably available for the benefit of all, and it is often the first place people think of when they need medical care. Since the turn of the century, hospitals, the indispensable workshop of the physician, have become even more the economic and professional heart of the medical practice of physicians as the accelerating pace of advances in medical knowledge and technology continues. In recent years, hospitals and their management have expanded further beyond their inpatient role in an effort to become comprehensive, vertically integrated community health systems. As highly advanced, scientific institutions, hospitals manifest the complexity and detached efficiency of a clinical laboratory. As human service organizations, they are charged with the emotions of life and death, of triumphs and tragedies. Hospitals are frequently the caregivers of last resort for many of the nation's poor, the uninsured and underinsured, who have nowhere else to turn for health care.

Hospitals are also big business. Collectively, they are among the largest industries in the United States in terms of the number of people they employ. In many localities, the local hospital is the town or county's leading employer. By far the largest part of the health care system, hospitals employ about three-fourths of all health care personnel and consume 38 percent of the nation's health expenditures. About 53 percent of all federal health expenditures and about 40 percent of all state and local government health expenditures are for inpatient hospital care (Haglund & Dowling, 1993). Although the focus of attention and emphasis is usually centered on their inpatient role, hospitals now play an increasingly important role in the provision of outpatient care and are evolving toward a new role as providers of a comprehensive and integrated continuum of health services.

It is ironic that the magnitude of the hospital sector, its success as an industry, and the central role hospitals play in the delivery of health services now place hospitals, their boards, administrations, and medical staff at the root of many of the health care system's most pressing problems. These confounding issues include apparently unrestrainable cost increases, duplication of services, bed surpluses, overemphasis on specialized services versus primary care, depersonalization of care, arguments about withholding or withdrawing of care, and so forth. While each of these individually, and all of them collectively, seem to affect most directly administration and the board, there are also accompanying impacts on individual physicians and the organized medical staff. There should be no implication that physicians are not involved with rising costs in their own fee structures, as well as being responsible for driving 75 percent to 80 percent of spending in hospitals.

Furthermore, as community institutions, sometimes public, sometimes quasi-public, hospitals have been heavily dependent on public dollars through philanthropy, direct subsidy, receipt of tax funds, state and local revenue bonds, and payment for services by publicly financed health care services programs. These multiple roles and public images have made hospitals, more than most other businesses, subject to influences from outside forces and, therefore, susceptible to the efforts of community groups, political partisans of all stripes, external agencies (both public and private), business coalitions, and insurance carriers to use them as instruments of social change and health system reform (Shortell, 1977).

FROM TENDING TO HEALING

The history of hospitals in this country can be traced back to the almshouses and pesthouses that existed in some form in almost all cities of moderate size by the mid-

1700s. Almshouses, also called poorhouses or workhouses, were established by city governments to provide food and shelter for the homeless poor, including many aged, chronically ill, disabled, mentally ill, and orphaned people. Medical care was a secondary function of the poorhouse; however, in some facilities, those who became ill were isolated in infirmaries where care, such as it was before the advent of modern medicine, was provided, typically, by other residents. Not until the late 1800s did the infirmaries or hospital departments of city poorhouses break away to become medical care institutions on their own—the first public hospitals.

The first pesthouses were operated by local governments as isolation or quarantine stations in seaports where it was necessary to isolate people who contracted contagious diseases aboard ship. During epidemics, these institutions were used to isolate victims of cholera, smallpox, typhus, and yellow fever. Their primary purpose was to control the spread of infectious diseases by removing infected individuals from the community. As in almshouses, medical care was a secondary function—in this case, secondary to protecting the community from outbreaks of contagious disease. Pesthouses were often established during epidemics and discontinued or closed down when the threat of disease subsided. These institutions were the predecessors of the contagious disease and tuberculosis hospitals that later emerged. Almshouses and pesthouses were maintained for the poor and the homeless and were avoided by everyone else. These institutions were dismal places: crowded, unsanitary, and poorly heated and ventilated. Nutrition was often inadequate, nursing care was incompetent, and separation of different types of patients was minimal. The contagious, the disabled, the dying, and the mentally ill were often crowded together. Cross infection was rampant and mortality high. All those who could be were cared for at home or in the homes of neighbors.

The first community-owned or voluntary hospitals in this country were established in the late 1700s and early 1800s, often at the urging of influential physicians trained in Europe who needed facilities to practice obstetrics and surgery in the manner in which they had been taught and to provide preceptor-type instruction for medical students. These early hospitals depended upon philanthropy, and contributions were solicited from both private citizens and the local government. Voluntary hospitals generally preceded both religious and public hospitals in the United States, representing a departure from the patterns in England and Europe. These early voluntary hospitals admitted both indigent and paying patients and were supported by community contributions and philanthropy, rather by a church or the state. Except in the largest cities, where the concentration of poor was too great, the early voluntary hospitals cared on a charitable basis for people in their communities who were unable to pay, drawing on philanthropy and donations of time by members of the medical staff.

These early voluntary hospitals cared for patients with acute illnesses and injuries but did not care for or admit persons with contagious diseases or mental illness. Isolation of these unfortunates from the rest of the community was seen as a government responsibility. Although voluntary hospitals provided better accommodations and care for the sick than had the poorhouses that preceded them, the efficacy of care improved little, and it was not until the late 1800s that hospitals became accepted by persons of all economic strata as the best setting for the care of illness and injury.

During the last quarter of the nineteenth century and the first quarter of the twentieth century in the United States, there was an increase in the number of hospitals from 178 to 6,665, with a corresponding increase in the number of beds from 35,604 to 907,133. Such rapid growth was brought about by advances in medical science, which rapidly transformed the hospital's role from a custodial institution in which to isolate and shelter the poor to a curative institution in which communities concentrated their health care resources in support of the practicing physician for the benefit of all (Haglund & Dowling, 1993). This redefinition of the voluntary hospital has been characterized as a transformation from a social welfare facility to an institution of medical science, from a charitable organization to a business, and from an orientation toward patrons and the poor to a focus on professionals and patients (Starr, 1982).

FORCES AFFECTING DEVELOPMENT OF HOSPITALS

Six major developments in health care were particularly significant in transforming hospitals into the institutions of today. They were:

- advances in medical science that increased the efficacy and safety of hospitals
- the development of technological sophistication and specialization that necessitated the institutionalization of care
- the development of professional nursing that brought about more humane treatment of patients
- advances in medical education that added teaching and research to the hospital's role
- the growth of the health insurance industry
- the greatly increased role of government in the financing of health care.

Advances in Medical Science

Most noticeable in terms of their impact on hospitals were the discovery of anesthesia and the rapid advances in surgery that followed, and the development of the germ theory of disease and the subsequent discovery of antiseptic and sterilization techniques. By the early 1800s, enough was known about anatomy and physiology that surgeons were able to perform a variety of fairly complex surgical procedures; however, the inability to deaden pain meant that surgery had to be carried out with extreme speed.

Before the formulation of the germ theory of disease, a few scientists had observed and reported that fever, infection, and mortality could be reduced through cleanliness.

Holmes in the United States and Semmelweiss in Vienna both concluded that childbed fever, which was the cause of high maternal mortality, was an infection transmitted by physicians, midwives, and medical students to women in labor. In 1861 Pasteur proved that bacteria were living, reproducing microorganisms that could be carried by air or on clothing or hands. It became clear that germs were the cause rather than the result of infection and could be destroyed by chemicals and heat. Lister's work built on Pasteur's and, in 1867, introduced carbolic acid spray in operating rooms as an antiseptic to keep air and incisions clean. In 1886 steam sterilization was introduced, providing a means of freeing medical equipment from microorganisms. Surgical infection rates fell. Advances in surgery led to the need for skilled preoperative and postoperative care and operating room facilities, which could only be provided in hospitals. By 1900, 40 percent of all hospitalizations were for surgery (Haglund & Dowling, 1993).

Development of Specialized Technology

By the late 1800s medical technology began to proliferate. The first hospital laboratory opened in 1889, and x-ray films were first used for diagnosis in 1896. These developments greatly increased the diagnostic effectiveness of hospitals. Further progress included the discovery of blood types, which made transfusions safer, and the development of the electrocardiogram and the electroencephalogram, which increased the efficiency of medical care. But they also affected the sight and organization of care for the next century. Since the tools of the new technology could no longer be carried around in the physician's black bag, hospitals became the central resource where the equipment, facilities, and personnel required by modern medicine were housed. In addition, since one person could no longer be competent in all areas of medical practice, specialization began to occur within medicine, and new professional and technical occupations began to emerge. Again, the hospital became the place where physicians and support personnel came together to provide patient care.

Development of Professional Nursing

Humane treatment of patients awaited the development of professional nursing. Before the late 1800s humane nursing care was provided primarily by Catholic sisters and Protestant deaconesses, who were dedicated to caring for patients. Some religious orders established their own hospitals, and occasionally they were called upon by city officials to provide nursing services in public institutions. Almshouses used untrained female residents to provide nursing care, and hospitals relied on poorly paid, unskilled labor.

The transformation of nursing into a profession is credited to Florence Nightingale, who completed four months of nurses' training in a deaconess school in Germany. In 1854, Nightingale and 38 nurses were sent by the British government to the Crimea to take charge of nursing care for wounded soldiers. The nurses found conditions deplorable and instituted cleanliness and sanitation, dietary reforms, simple but humane care, discipline, and organization. As a result, mortality dropped dramatically. On her return to England, Nightingale wrote of her experiences in the Crimea and on the contributions of sanitation to the recovery of wounded and ill patients.

In the United States, President Abraham Lincoln called on Catholic religious communities to provide nursing care for the wounded during the Civil War, but more nurses were needed. Dorothea Dix was appointed superintendent of nursing for the Union Army. She began recruiting and encouraged a one-month hospital training program for new nurses. By the end of the war, there were 2,000 lay nurses in the United States. Although there was some initial reluctance on the part of hospital administrators and trustees to establish nursing schools, the benefits of good nursing soon became apparent. In addition, student nurses provided better care and were less expensive than the untrained women previously employed to do this work.

Advances in nursing contributed to the growth of hospitals in two ways. Increased efficacy of treatment, cleanliness, nutritious diets, and formal treatment routines all contributed to patient recovery, while considerate, skilled patient care made hospitals acceptable to all people, not just the poor. The public's well-deserved fear of hospitals began to give way to an attitude of confidence and respect.

Advances in Medical Education

Changes in medical education brought about by the Flexner report in 1910 had a major impact on the development of hospitals (Flexner, 1910). Before 1900 there was a great variation in the nature and quality of medical education. A large number of small, poorly staffed, freestanding medical colleges existed throughout the country. There were no standards of academic training for physicians. Most medical schools were proprietary and were not connected with universities. They were dominated by influential practitioners, and most instruction was through didactic (often unscientific) lectures. Apprenticeship practices varied widely. There was little clinical or laboratory instruction and little research.

In 1910 Abraham Flexner undertook a study of medical education for the Carnegie Foundation for the Advancement of Teaching and, in his report, *Medical Education in the United States and Canada,* recommended that medical education in this country undergo radical reform. In particular, he recommended that the training of physicians be made a university function and that it be based on a firm scientific foundation. On the basis of Flexner's recommendations and with the support of the Rockefeller Foundation, many of the small, unaffiliated medical schools began to close and many of the remaining ones became part of universities, with the important result that physicians began to be trained as scientists as well as practitioners (Torrens, 1993).

The Flexner report led to changes in the content and methods of instruction to emphasize the scientific basis of medicine by changing the standards of education. These standards of education were widely accepted by both the profession and the public. As a result, schools that did not meet the standards were forced to close. State laws were established requiring graduation from a medical school accredited by the American Medical Association as the basis for a license to practice medicine. A four-year course of study at a medical school based in a university became standard, as did clinical training in the wards of a hospital.

These changes expanded the role of the hospital to include education and research as well as patient care. The hospital's role in education became even more prominent as specialization in medicine led to a proliferation of internships and residencies in the 1920s and 1930s. The requirements of medical education necessitated the expansion of hospital facilities and services and the addition of equipment and personnel. Hospitals were called on to assume a greater responsibility for coordinating and organizing these resources. Quality of care improved through advances in medical education, especially for patients with complex and serious illnesses. On the other hand, specialization led to fragmentation of care among different physician specialists and ancillary personnel and a lack of interest in chronic, routine, and other "uninteresting" medical conditions.

Although the growth of hospitals was a direct result of advances in medical science that made those institutions effective and safe, hospitals have not been quick to respond to the chronic health care problems of an aging population. The concentrated, highly technical, and increasingly expensive resources of modern tertiary care hospitals have tended to concentrate on curable, short-term illnesses that respond quickly to medical treatment, rather than on chronic, long-term illnesses that must be managed over long periods of time. Hospitals are just now beginning to expand their role to include extended or skilled nursing care units, inpatient or outpatient rehabilitation programs, day care, home care, and other services that are nontraditional behavior for the inpatient setting (Coile, 1986).

Growth of Health Insurance

Another factor that has significantly affected the development of hospitals is the growth of the health insurance industry. Private insurance for hospital care grew rapidly, especially between 1940 and 1960, increasing both the proportion of the population with insurance and the adequacy and scope of coverage. In recent years, the out-of-pocket cost of hospital care at the time of use has been relatively modest for most people, because most of the bill has been covered by some third-party purchaser—either government or private health insurance.

A variety of factors led to the growth of hospital insurance. From the consumer's perspective, of course, a hospital stay is sufficiently expensive to warrant the purchase of insurance protection. The hospital industry's interest in insurance began with the Great Depression of the 1930s, when the number of patients who could not pay their bill increased markedly and hospital use declined, threatening the financial solvency of a number of hospitals. As a result, acting through the American Hospital Association, hospitals took the initiative in actively encouraging the development of hospital insurance plans, primarily Blue Cross (Haglund & Dowling, 1993).

The growth of health insurance has had a substantial impact on hospitals. The most important impact was to ensure the financial stability of hospitals, providing the flow of funds that made possible the great expansion of facilities and services and the prompt implementation of new medical technology that have characterized the hospital industry since the end of World War II. Insurance also contributed to the increased demand for health services. Historically, services in the hospital have been better covered by insurance than services provided outside the hospital, so patients have been reluctant to substitute less expensive out-of-hospital care. This attitude resulted in a bias toward hospital use rather than the use of ambulatory care services, home care programs, or nursing care facilities as sources of care as well as a general overuse of expensive hospital services (Feldstein, 1971). In recent years, however, concern over the rising costs of hospital care and inappropriate hospital admissions has reversed this trend. Insurance carriers are now actively promoting nonhospital alternatives for medical care and stringent control over inpatient admissions.

Another problem in the hospital industry can be traced at least partially to cost-based reimbursement, the method of payment used until recently, by Medicare, Medicaid, Blue Cross, and most other private carriers. Cost reimbursement does not provide hospitals with an incentive to control costs. The result has been inefficiency, duplication of services, and overbuilding. To stem rising hospital costs, public and private payers have experimented with a number of regulatory and competitive approaches to cost containment. All purchasers, both public and private, have taken actions to replace payment systems based on retrospective costs with those based on competitive prices and prospective rates.

The Medicare program converted reimbursement to a prospective, per-case system based on diagnosis related groups (DRG). In turn, several states have revised their Medicaid programs and now pay hospitals on a prospective basis. In addition, managed care programs, including health maintenance organizations (HMOs) and preferred provider organizations (PPOs), which feature stricter utilization review controls over hospital admissions, have proliferated in the private health insurance sector. Hospitals now find themselves competing on the basis of prices and discount for patients covered by health insurance plans. While cost reimbursement is widely blamed as the root cause of runaway hospital costs, it nevertheless has allowed hospitals to keep up to date with advances in medical technology and demands from their communities and physicians for access to a broad range of services. A key public policy issue yet unresolved is how to guarantee access by the poor and disadvantaged to a decent standard of care in a system driven by competitive forces.

Role of Government

Government's role in the hospital industry has changed substantially in both form and level. During colonial times, government involvement was mainly at the local level through ownership of almshouses and pesthouses and grants to help construct and support voluntary hospitals. State government limited its role to running hospitals for merchant seamen, military personnel, and veterans. Gradually, the forms of involvement have multiplied and the balance has shifted to the federal level.

The initial thrust of federal involvement began in 1935, with federal categorical grants-in-aid to state and local governments to assist in the establishment of traditional public health programs: public health departments, communicable disease programs, maternal and child health programs, and public assistance for specific groups, such as crippled children, the aged, the blind, the disabled, and poor families with dependent children. These programs were part of the general social reform movement that developed during the Depression with the recognition that state and local governments and voluntary efforts were not sufficient to meet social needs.

Direct federal involvement in the hospital industry began in 1946 with the Hill-Burton (Hospital Survey and Construction) Act. Few hospitals had been constructed during the Depression and World War II, and by the end of the war, a severe shortage of hospitals existed, in proportion to population growth and distribution. The Hill-Burton program was enacted to help states and communities plan for and construct hospitals and other health facilities by providing federal grants on a matching basis to supplement funds raised at the community level. Although the initial emphasis of the program was to provide funds for the construction of new hospitals, priorities changed over time from construction to modernization and from inpatient to outpatient. Funds were available through the program for the construction of nursing homes as well.

The Hill-Burton program assisted in the construction of nearly 40 percent of the beds in the nation's short-term general hospitals and was the greatest single factor in the increase in the nation's bed supply during the 1950s and 1960s. Another positive impact of the program is that hospital facilities are more evenly distributed across rural and urban areas and high-and-low income states than they would have been without the program. However, the program also contributed to the overbuilding of hospitals and to the preponderance of small rural hospitals that still exist today.

From assisting with the financing of hospital construction, the federal government's involvement in the hospital industry has expanded to financing the provision of care and regulating the construction, operation, and use of hospitals. Fifty-three percent of hospital expenditures are now made by government programs, primarily Medicare and

Medicaid, which puts the federal government in a strong position to exercise a great amount of control over the operations of hospitals.

Patterns of hospital financing and ownership differ from country to country. Most nations recognize health care as an essential service in which government should have a major role. In Great Britain and other industrialized European nations, the government owns and operates the hospitals and employs the physicians who work in them. In other countries, the government limits its role to financing care provided by private doctors and hospitals. In countries such as Canada, where comprehensive health insurance is in effect, hospitals operate primarily on public funds and hence are essentially controlled by the national or provincial government even though many are not government-owned.

In the United States, by contrast, the government's role has generally been limited to financing care for needy groups, such as the aged, the poor, and the disabled. Even though short-term community hospitals in this country receive the majority of their income from government sources (Medicare and Medicaid), the United States has a pluralistic public-private financing system with largely privately-owned hospitals. However, as an inevitable result of the increase in the portion of hospital income financed by government has come an accompanying increase in regulation of the private sector.

The limited role of government in the ownership of hospitals in the United States has been shaped by several major forces that reflect the cultural values and beliefs about the role of government and the private sector.

Government was still relatively weak in the 1800s, when the short-term hospital as it exists today was evolving as a result of advances in medical, nursing, and management science. Innovations and progress have generally come from the private sector. At that time, poverty was not perceived as so severe that the needy could not be cared for through charity and philanthropy in private hospitals, with the unpaid assistance of small groups of hospital-related physicians.

It was generally believed that the private sector could provide care for the poor as well as those who could pay. The exception was in major cities, where there were large concentrations of the poor. There, public hospitals were established to care for that population of the needy.

Government responsibility for the public's health was viewed narrowly before the Depression of the 1930s and was limited mainly to public safety, such as protecting citizens from persons with communicable diseases and mental illness; providing care for special groups such as merchant seamen, military personnel, and veterans: and assisting the needy. State governments operated hospitals for their beneficiary groups, and city and county governments in large urban areas operated hospitals for the poor.

The strong social ethic of reliance on the private sector should mean that government becomes involved only when the private sector fails to provide a critical service. For example, chronic disease, mental illness, and tuberculosis hospital care would have been difficult to finance privately. The long stays that previously prevailed would have been expensive and not readily insurable. Hospitalization generally meant loss of job and income, especially since the incidence of hospitalization for these conditions was greatest among the poor. As a result, these areas of care have traditionally fallen to the public sector. The private sector proved better able to finance short-term hospital care through direct patient payments and private health insurance, and so the government's role has been supplementary for providing that care.

Government involvement has been resisted by both the medical profession and the hospital industry. Both special-interest groups, acting through their national and state lobbying associations, have represented particularly powerful political forces in the United States and have been long concerned, with good reason, that government involvement in the health care system would compromise their economic and professional interests (Haglund & Dowling, 1993).

CHARACTERISTICS OF THE HOSPITAL SYSTEM

The hospital industry is complex, diverse, and difficult to describe simply. Hospitals can be classified generally in one of three ways: length of stay, predominant type of service provided, and ownership. In terms of length of stay, the most common type of hospital is the short-stay or short-term hospital, in which most patients suffer from acute conditions requiring hospital stays of less than 30 days.

The second method of classification is by type of service. Predominant is the general hospital that offers a wide range of medical, surgical, obstetric, and pediatric services. Specialty hospitals, on the other hand, provide care for a specific disease or population group. Examples of such specialty hospitals include children's hospitals, maternity hospitals, chronic disease hospitals, psychiatric hospitals, and tuberculosis hospitals. During the first part of the twentieth century, a number of specialty hospitals were established as a result of philanthropists responding to the initiative of prestigious physician specialists who wanted to develop their own hospitals. Because of financial difficulties and advances in medical science that make general hospitals more appropriate and efficient, specialty hospitals dwindled in number. Most have either closed down or converted to general hospitals.

The third method of classifying hospitals is according to the form of ownership: government or public, private for-profit (proprietary), and private nonprofit (religious or voluntary). A more complete description of each type of ownership is necessary to trace evolution of the modern American community hospital and how physicians came to practice there.

Public Hospitals

Public hospitals are owned by agencies of federal, state, or local governments. Federally owned hospitals are maintained primarily for special groups of federal beneficiaries: Native Americans, merchant seamen, military personnel, and veterans. State governments have generally limited themselves to the operation of mental and tuberculosis hospitals, reflecting government's early role of protecting the healthy by isolating the mentally ill and persons with contagious disease from the rest of society. Most local city or county hospitals are short-term general hospitals of two different types.

The first is city, county, or hospital district institutions, mostly of small or moderate size, with medical staffs consisting of private physicians, and serving both indigent and paying patients. For all practical purposes they resemble and function the same as community-owned hospitals.

The second type is large city or county hospitals in major urban areas. These hospitals serve mostly the poor, near-poor, and minorities. These are generally staffed by salaried physicians, mostly residents studying medical specialties. Most are affiliated with medical schools. Their costs generally exceed patient revenues, and so their inevitable deficits must be made up through tax subsidies from one source or another.

Large urban hospitals play an important role in the health care system. They are the place of last resort for the poor, both because they care for all patients regardless of ability to pay and because they provide services that private hospitals cannot finance or do not wish to offer, such as burn and trauma care, alcohol and drug abuse treatment, psychiatric services, care for persons with chronic and communicable diseases, treatment of persons with AIDS, abortion and family planning services, and so forth. They are usually located in areas where health resources, especially private physicians, are in short supply, and their outpatient departments are often the only accessible source of ambulatory care for many inner-city residents. In addition, these large public hospitals play a major role in medical education. Most are affiliated with a medical school and offer residency training programs. More than one-half of all practicing physicians receive at least some of their training in public hospitals.

For-Profit Hospitals

For-profit, investor-owned, or proprietary hospitals are operated for the financial benefit of the individual, partnership, or corporation that owns the institution. Around the turn of the century, more than one-half of the nation's hospitals were proprietary. Most of these hospitals had been established by one or a small group of physicians who wanted a place to hospitalize their own patients, and most were quite small. Gradually these facilities were closed or sold to community organizations (*Hospital Statistics*, 1991). The most significant trend over the past few years related to investor-owned hospitals is the virtual disappearance of individual doctor-owned facilities and the formation of national and international systems. These investor-owned corporations have increasingly affiliated and merged into fewer and much larger ownership structures with less local control.

Not-for-Profit Hospitals

Nearly 60 percent of the nation's short-term hospitals are nonprofit or voluntary institutions owned and operated by community associations or religious organizations. These hospitals accommodate more than two-thirds of all short-term hospital admissions and outpatient visits. The term *not-for-profit* refers to the tax status of the hospital and its classification as a charitable organization. The promotion of health is considered to be a charitable purpose. A hospital whose purpose and activity are providing not-for-profit hospital care is promoting health and may, therefore, qualify as organized and operated for a charitable purpose (IRC Section 501 (c)(3); Rev. Rul. 69-545).

For-profit hospitals pay local, state, and federal taxes, while non-profits usually do not pay any of these taxes on the patient care operations of the facility. Sometimes members of the public and some physicians interpret nonprofit to mean that the hospital should produce just enough revenue to break even, or even lose a little. They may not understand that the difference between for-profit and nonprofit is that in the one instance, profit margins can be returned to investors; while in the other, profits must be plowed back into the institution in the form of buildings and equipment and cannot inure to any "insiders" or benefit any private individuals.

Community Hospitals

Taken together, nonfederal short-term hospitals, whether for-profit, nonprofit, or public, are commonly referred to as "community hospitals," because they are typically available to the entire community and meet most of the public's needs for hospital services. Community hospitals represent more than 80 percent of the nation's hospitals. They provide care for more than 90 percent of all patients admitted to hospitals each year and accommodate more than 80 percent of all outpatient visits. There has been a steady decline in the length of stay in community hospitals over the past decade, due to changing styles of medical practice, the emphasis placed on utilization review in hospitals, and the shift to prospective per-case payment by Medicare and other payers.

The major role of community hospitals is to provide short-term inpatient care for patients with acute illnesses and injuries. However, their outpatient role has been growing in importance and number and now accounts for more than the 20 percent of gross hospital revenues that was common in 1980 (Starr, 1982). Community hospitals are experiencing pressures to expand their roles even more to become true community health systems or networks. The fundamental rationale is that these hospitals represent their community's collective investment in health resources, assembled in one place and financially supported by all. Hence, access to these resources should not be limited to patients who happen to need inpatient hospitalization. Now, in the 1990s, diversification is being undertaken for competitive and economic reasons.

Many of these community hospitals are now seeking to be the base or nucleus for playing a more central and substantial role in planning and coordinating the entire continuum of community health services. Their role as only an inpatient provider is changing rapidly, as their leaders are motivated to search for new and diversified services to offer. Just as the for-profit community hospitals have moved toward national, state, or regional chain status, so the nonprofit community hospitals are moving through merger or consolidation into multihospital systems. A different form of administrative or executive skill is required for such restructuring of the individual facility and for the industry as a whole. Some hospital administrators who have been very good and successful managers at the facility level do not appear to be the right types for multihospital systems.

Two fundamental motives underlie the multihospital system movement that is so dramatically changing the character of the hospital sector. Those motives are very clear: organizational survival and organizational growth to add strength. Survival applies to the freestanding, single-ownership institution and explains why such a hospital decides to relinquish its autonomy and become part of a system. Organizational growth, on the other hand, applies to the system itself and explains why it seeks to build, buy, lease, or manage additional hospitals.

For the single stand-alone institution, today's increasingly complex, fast-changing, demanding, and even hostile health care environment has made survival of the fittest a stark reality. Competition, financial pressures, regulation, and other external forces so weaken or threaten solo institutions that they turn to systems for the strength to survive, albeit under different ownership. For the established systems, acquisition of additional hospitals is a means to grow. Growth is intended to produce new services, enter new markets, establish new referral patterns, or build more financial and political power.

Another associated trend is the recent proliferation of hospital alliances, which are defined as formally organized groups of hospitals or hospital systems that have come together for specific purposes, have specific membership criteria, and are controlled by independent and autonomous member institutions. These hospital alliances differ from multihospital systems in that they are generally voluntary affiliations of hospitals that have joined together to reap the benefits of joint activities such as group purchasing and shared product development. The members of the alliance have not relinquished their independent identity and autonomy as have the members of the systems or networks. Alliances thus lack the corporate control found in multihospital systems and are prohibited from undertaking some health plan contracting behaviors by the provisions of the federal antitrust statutes.

Small and Rural Hospitals

These trends present special problems for small and rural hospitals whose difficulties in attracting resources, keeping up to date with advances in medical technology, and maintaining financial viability raise questions about their future survival and how they should relate to larger institutions offering the specialized services they are not able to provide. In part because Hill-Burton priorities in the early years channeled funds to thinly populated areas, the United States is a nation of many small hospitals. Nearly half of all community hospitals have fewer than 100 beds (*Hospital Statistics,* 1991). These hospitals have a number of problems that threaten their future viability, such as losing patients and declining census figures. Labor requirements are high in small hospitals for the services offered, and small hospitals tend to operate at less efficient levels of occupancy than larger institutions. These efficiency limitations, coupled with the limited financial means of some rural populations, have caused many small hospitals to incur substantial operating losses. Small hospitals offer a more limited range of services than larger institutions, because they have neither the patient volume nor the physicians or specialized personnel to support much beyond the basic essential services. Small hospitals are often located in areas that have a hard time attracting qualified personnel. All of these problems may lead to difficulty in achieving accreditation and in meeting hospital certification and licensing standards. In a growing number of instances during the past decade, the combination of these forces has proven fatal to the survival of some small and rural hospitals.

Small hospitals also find it especially difficult to keep up with the increasingly complex and demanding regulatory environment without the range of management specialists common to larger institutions. As a result, many are contracting with regional hospital systems or larger hospitals to take over their management. It would appear that the future of small and rural hospitals will depend upon adapting their mission and the services they offer to fit the available financial support within the constraints of location, regulation, and the encroaching market that threatens to gobble them up. They will undoubtedly need to seek relationships with other institutions and seek new resources to support more programs so as to broaden their role in health care delivery in the communities they serve (*Hospital Statistics,* 1991). Otherwise, the competitive world will overwhelm them because they are almost defenseless in resisting the onslaught of managed care.

COMPETITION AND PROSPECTIVE PAYMENT

The high and persistently climbing cost of hospital care, combined with increasing disenchantment with regulatory efforts to reduce those costs, has led to a new emphasis on marketplace competition for hospitals. Although the overall rate of inflation for hospitals has declined from a high point of nearly 15 percent in 1982, health care costs in general, and hospital costs in particular, have continued to increase at a rate far in excess of the consumer price index (CPI) or any other measure of growth in the economy. The obvious conclusion is that while inflationary pressures have been controlled for the general economy, hospitals have not been as successful in containing their costs. There are several reasons for this, including prior commitments to expensive building and construction projects by many hospitals, the growing role of sophisticated technology in hospital care, the greatly increased role of computer information systems, the power of unions, and, most of all, the hospital's limited ability to control the variability in practice patterns of physicians on the medical staff. As a result of their continuing high costs, hospitals tend to be the prime target of the cost-containment efforts of both public and private payers.

The mid-1980s witnessed dramatic changes in hospital utilization patterns—changes strongly influenced by the introduction of prospective payment methodologies by Medicare and other payers; and by the explosive growth in managed care health plans such as HMOs and PPOs. Average hospital occupancy rates declined by nearly 11 percent between 1980 and 1990 (Bisbee, 1982). Lower occupancy has led to a widespread perception that hospitals are a mature, if not declining, industry. Declining occupancy combined with pressure to contain costs has resulted in a new competitive mind-set for hospitals that are actively pursuing diversification strategies, product-line management, marketing, and advertising. The long-term effects of this competitive approach to health care delivery continue to be debated, with many people deeply concerned about the impact it may have on what remains of hospitals' public service commitment to the poor.

It appears clear that the continuing high rate of inflation in hospital costs cannot be explained by increases in utilization or volume, since occupancy has declined steadily for more than a decade. Instead, hospital cost increases are more likely attributable to changes in the nature of hospital output, which means the intensity, scope, sophistication, and quality of hospital care. All of these demands have forced hospitals to employ more and better labor and nonlabor inputs. Hospital services are continuously increasing in intensity, scope, and sophistication as a result of advances in medical science coupled with community and physician demands for the widest range of the most up-to-date services. Both physicians and patients want to take advantage of all that modern medicine has to offer.

The prices that hospitals charge what few private-pay patients remain have increased even faster than total costs because of the difference between what hospitals charge to meet their full financial needs and what Medicare and Medicaid actually pay. These allowances, or discounts, along with the charity care and bad debts that hospitals incur and the public programs do not reimburse, are passed on to private-pay patients and their insurance carriers in the form of higher prices. This "cost shifting" explains why hospital charges or prices have been increasing at a considerably faster rate than actual hospital costs. Private insurance carriers in recent years, however, have taken steps to limit the amount of cost shifting they have traditionally absorbed. Seizing the initiative inherent in HMOs and PPOs, carriers negotiated selective contracts with hospitals that grant them discounts or preferred rates. Individual patients insured under such plans are given financial incentives for using the "preferred" hospitals and doctors. The dilemma faced by hospital management in that scenario is to either offer discounted rates to carriers or face ruinously lower volume. Since hospital admissions were declining anyway, for several reasons, most hospitals became willing to compete for patients through competitive bidding on selective contracts.

Adapting to the New Environment

Hospitals across the United States are adapting in various ways to the new competitive environment, as described more fully in Chapter 24. Prospective payment, price competition, and the move toward managed care are creating strong incentives for hospitals to achieve efficient staffing levels since labor represents much more than 50 percent of the average hospital's costs. Approaches being tried in an attempt to respond to lower inpatient census include:

- more efficient utilization of nurses
- substitution of vocational or practical nurses for registered nurses
- moving to an all registered nurse staff
- increasing productivity standards
- using cross-training to fill positions

Hospitals are investigating other methods of increasing their profitability, including product-line (also called service-line) management. The practice of analyzing hospital programs and services as strategic business units in order to identify and enhance profitable services and turn around or eliminate unprofitable services is being advocated by many as a more businesslike approach to hospital management. As more hospitals merge or consolidate into local or regional systems or networks, there must be a change of thinking away from the old-fashioned profession called hospital administration. From hospitals to systems: That is the way of the 1990s.

There can be a concern that service-or product-line management may lead to hospitals discontinuing services that may be unprofitable but that are needed by the community. Many argue that continuing the marketplace approach of defining health care as a commodity and rationing it on the basis of ability to pay is unacceptable if society holds that health care is a basic right. That argument continues to unfold while some hospitals are caught in the middle between the need to remain viable and even survive in a competitive world that is not listening to the philosophy of a basic right to free or unpaid health care. The market is deaf to moral or philosophical arguments.

Still, a positive aspect of service-line management is the development and organization of services to meet the special needs of certain segments of the population. Examples include women's health centers, sports medicine, cancer centers, and others. It can be argued that competition is forcing hospitals to be much more sensitive to the needs and desires of people for convenient, specially tailored services. In the case of regional systems or networks, it also forces corporate (not just hospital) management to think about whether there should be a cardiac surgery program in each institution, and how many transplant programs one system really needs?

Under the Medicare prospective payment system, there is a strong incentive to discharge inpatients as soon as medically warranted. Therefore, Medicare DRGs have done a great deal to foster the effectiveness of discharge planning. The role of the discharge planner is critical in ensuring that patients receive the proper level of care after leaving the hospital. For elderly patients in particular, rapid rehospitalization may result unless proper discharge instructions and support services are received. In many instances, the elderly patient cannot be discharged from the hospital until placement in a nursing home is secured or arrangements are made for home care. The necessity of ensuring that patients will receive proper postdischarge treatment has heightened the interest of many hospitals in operating their own skilled nursing units and home care programs (Haglund & Dowling, 1993).

One major concern of the Medicare program and its Professional Review Organizations (PROs) has been that doctors and hospitals may be discharging patients too soon in some instances. Physicians and the hospitals where they practice have been under great pressure for a decade to deliver exactly the right amount of care to Medicare patients, since too much care may result in reimbursement denials and too little care can result in penalty assessments or lawsuits. One of the results of this pressure has been the placing of more emphasis on the complete and timely documentation of patient treatment records.

Utilization Review

Another result of the pressure placed by payment systems and more stringent scrutiny of hospital practices has been the growth of attempts to control utilization. Medicare first required that hospitals and extended-care facilities establish utilization review programs as a condition of participation. Another federal control tied to Medicare and Medicaid as a condition for participation or payment is certification by the designated state agency, to ensure that services of the public programs are purchased only from institutions that can meet minimum quality standards. However, it would appear to the casual observer that since virtually all community hospitals are certified, the administration of this program by the state health departments is not very stringent and almost no hospitals have been sanctioned by noncertification.

In order to carry out the utilization review requirement that was placed on hospitals so that they could be paid for services rendered, physician committees were established to review the medical records of discharged Medicare patients to determine the necessity of the hospital care provided. This requirement was seen as a way to discourage inappropriate admissions and unnecessarily long lengths of stay. In theory, then, this practice would keep down expenditures in the Medicare and Medicaid programs. However, utilization review has raised a number of sensitive issues, because establishing standards and monitoring physician practices with regard to their hospital care has been widely regarded by them as an infringement on their professional judgment regarding patient care.

As the decade of the 1980s passed, other payers adopted the utilization review approach, and many health plans went even further in their regulatory efforts than had Medicare with its first-generation review organizations, Professional Standards Review Organizations (PSROs), and the following program, Professional Review Organizations (PROs). Both programs became expensive for hospitals, as did the efforts by the private payers. Additional staff had to be hired, additional physician committees needed to be appointed and staffed, and the entire structure added to costs of care as well as offering a major irritant to practicing physicians. The global cost-benefit issue of regulatory requirements has been discussed many times without definitive resolution. A number of experts have opined that the forces currently moving the health care delivery system toward a more competitive approach will eventually make extensive regulation unnecessary.

Vertical Integration

The increasingly stringent economic environment has also spurred the interest of hospitals and their boards and administrations toward the possibilities of merger, consolidation, and formation of local or regional vertically integrated systems or networks. Vertical integration represents a response by hospitals to try to capture and control more of the factors that lead to inpatient hospitalization. The ultimate goals of vertical integration include:

- increasing an individual hospital's market and financial position
- enhancing the hospital's overall cost effectiveness
- improving continuity of care
- responding to changing consumer preferences

Vertical integration in a health enterprise involves linking together different levels of care and assembling the human resources needed to deliver that care. Vertical integration may be distinguished from diversification efforts in that vertical integration involves the development of new nonhospital services to support and enhance the hospital base while diversification involves the development of distinct new business lines that are independent from the hospital and have profit as their primary objective (Placella,

1986). Vertical integration has historically proceeded in two directions. As industrial firms integrated forward toward the ultimate consumer of the firm's products, they either bought out the distributors of their goods or created their own distribution systems to bring their goods to market. As they integrated backwards toward the supply of raw materials, they purchased either raw materials or the primary producers of the goods needed to manufacture their products (Goldsmith, 1981).

Backward integration involves all of the activities in which a firm engages to secure an adequate supply of the raw materials needed to produce its particular product. In the health care setting, the product is a human service, health care. Therefore, backward integration involves the equipment, supplies, and human resources needed to care for patients. The most critically scarce resources of a hospital are its professional caregivers: physicians, nurses, technicians, and other health personnel.

Efforts to secure adequate supplies of these individuals are essential to a health care provider's ability to function. Many hospitals have therefore developed linkages with educational institutions, providing a source of new recruits by serving as training sites. Some hospitals have considered integrating backwards into medical supplies and other goods needed to operate; however, these organizations may be entering very competitive markets dominated by large firms. Chances are, also, that these large firms are experienced at succeeding in their field of endeavor while the hospital, as a neophyte in that field, does not bring with it any experience at owning or managing anything but hospital inpatient care, much of which is delivered by doctors who are not part of the new venture.

Because the hospital is the most highly organized form of production of health services, efforts by the hospital to provide those forms of care rendered to the patient prior to hospitalization can be considered forward integration, or reaching out toward the patient. A major form of forward integration for a hospital involves development of ambulatory care systems as part of the complete continuum of care that stretches all the way from wellness and health promotion through acute care past skilled nursing units, home care, and hospice. In health care, a distribution or feeder system is the set of pathways that result in bringing the patient to the hospital. The feeder system of a hospital includes all of those settings in which the potential patient receives ambulatory services, or diagnosis, as well as the transportation systems and physician referral relationships that ultimately lead to hospitalization (Goldsmith, 1981).

Physicians Bringing Patients

The principal feeder system for most hospitals is a network of private physician offices and group practices, composed of members of the hospital medical staff. One way hospitals have moved to integrate physician practices is by providing office space on the hospital campus, assisting new physicians in starting practices, and helping market physician services. Physician support services, such as office training, management, billing, and referral services, are also activities that build a feeder system and further develop forward integration.

Arrangements between hospitals and physicians must clear a number of legal and regulatory hurdles that should be addressed before any financial moves are made. Among these is the requirement that such financial arrangements satisfy private inurement, private benefit, and unreasonable compensation tests so as not to jeopardize the hospital's tax-exempt status and furtherance of the charitable purpose of the hospital (*IRS Audit Guidelines for Hospitals,* March 27, 1992).

As well, there are restrictions on referrals, such as the Medicare Fraud and Abuse statute and regulations prohibiting the payment or receipt of any remuneration to induce referrals [Social Security Act, Section 1128 (B) (b); the various state antireferral statutes, such as the California Business and Professions Code Section 650]. Also noteworthy are the state and federal prohibitions of physician referrals to certain providers in which the physician has a financial interest [California Business and Professions Code Section 650.1; Title XVIII of Social Security Act, Section 1877 (a) (1)].

Many physicians may not understand that any financial inducement extended by a hospital or system, even if it is not in cash, might violate portions of the regulations dealing with unrelated trade or business taxable income (IRC Section 513; Rev. Rul. 69-463). Finally, in this list of horribles, there are the prohibitions in some states against the corporate practice of medicine which a hospital/physician relationship might violate (Calif. Business and Professions Code, Sections 650 and 2400; 55 Ops. Cal. Atty. Gen. 108).

Advertising and Marketing

Many hospitals have recognized the importance of a feeder system in building the name recognition of the facility and promoting patient accessibility. As a result, hospitals are engaging in more marketing and advertising activities that increase the visibility of their institutions, including direct-mail advertising, use of billboards, and broadcasting on radio and television. There are three channels through which advertising may assist hospitals or vertically integrated health systems in increasing their market share.

Advertising that features hospital image or name recognition may influence the choice of patients who are admitted through emergency departments or outpatient clinics. That is, the patients may exercise a choice (if the health plan of which they are a member will allow them to make that choice).

Familiarity with the name or image of a particular hospital may enable patients to influence the choice of physicians with admitting privileges at multiple institutions (but only if the particular physician is on the panel of the patient's health plan). Patients may actually choose a physician affiliated with a particular hospital, especially if they use a hospital referral service, and if the hospital and doctor belong to the plan (Folland, 1985).

Vertical Integration Strategies

Vertical integration strategies for hospitals experiencing declines in census include several options for changing the array and uses of facilities as well as changing the governance or ownership structure.

Convert Facilities

Underused acute inpatient facilities can be converted to long-term care, substance abuse, mental health, or other services or even closed altogether.

Develop Systems

Hospitals or their health care systems can focus on developing coordinated and integrated delivery systems whereby local residents can obtain the services they need through the programs, services, and facilities in the most appropriate and effective setting.

Joint Venture

Physicians' office buildings and ambulatory surgery, diagnostic, and primary care centers have been developed by many institutions through joint ventures with individuals or groups of physicians on their medical staff in order to improve their market penetration.

Contracting

Hospitals or networks that are able to contract directly with HMOs, PPOs, third-party payers, and major corporate employers to provide a full range of preacute, acute, and postacute services at a highly competitive price will place themselves in an excellent market position.

Success of Integration Strategies

The movement toward vertical integration presents the viewer with a mixed bag of findings so far. There is relatively little assessment by empirical research to prove the impact on hospital performance. But there is widespread perception in the hospital industry that integration is both right and necessary. There have been barriers and slowdowns in the integration process because of difficulties such as loss of institutional identity and autonomy, fear of domination by the larger players in the integrated system, uncertainty of roles within the umbrella corporation, and possible imbalances in political power at the governing board, medical staff, or management level.

Many of these fears are well founded, and many hospital executives will lose their jobs as a result of integration. Some of the doctors may lose their practices or find themselves aligned in new and different ways, but most physicians will find themselves staying in the same office and trying to learn how to deal with new administrators or new corporate hotshots. Vertical integration presents additional problems for the hospital members of the system, such as controlling the flow of patients within the network, acquiring the requisite expertise to manage new ventures, and maintaining traditional values and character. Yet integration may represent the only available pathway toward salvation and financial viability in a competitive world.

Paying Attention to Patient Satisfaction

As a result of growing competition, the satisfaction of hospital patients has become more salient to hospital administration in recent years. In the past, hospital boards and administrators considered physicians to be their customers and concentrated on satisfying members of their medical staffs in order to increase their market share. Now, conceding that patients and their health plans are also prime customers, more attention is being given to the patient and patient preferences for care. A strong trend has developed toward continuous quality improvement approaches to providing services that actively consider the opinions of patients as customers (Lathrop, 1991). As a measurable indicator of the success of these approaches, many hospitals are now routinely administering patient satisfaction surveys while others have initiated programs based on techniques used in hotels and other consumer-oriented service organizations. In many respects, observers could wonder where these programs have been for so long and why hospitals have paid so little attention to patient satisfaction in the past.

It is a widely accepted truism that the hospital environment can be unpleasant and that patients and their families are often fraught with apprehension and anxiety. Studies show that negative aspects of hospital care have been linked with poor compliance with medical treatment protocols and even delayed physical recovery (Wartman, Morlock, Malitz, 1983). Thus, it is desirable to identify and, within reasonable limits, alter those factors that contribute to negative experiences within the hospital. Evaluation of patient and family satisfaction provides important information on the patients' perception of the quality of care and allows the patient as a customer and consumer to have a greater voice in the design and delivery of personal health services.

BIOMEDICAL ETHICS ISSUES FOR HOSPITALS

Increasingly, hospital decision making is affected by issues of biomedical ethics. Within the hospital setting, these ethical concerns touch on a variety of administrative and patient care duties, including respect for patient privacy and confidentiality, informed consent, continuation of life-support services to terminally ill patients, resource allocation decisions, and care for the poor (Darr, Longest, & Rakich, 1986). Many hospitals and their medical staffs have constituted institutional ethics committees to provide ethical guidance on both clinical and administrative problems. Because they are the focal point of the most complex applications of modern medicine, hospitals are naturally at the center of many of the most difficult and painful bioethical decisions of this generation. One of the most critical of these decisions relates to patient competency and the right to refuse treatment. While the right of competent patients to refuse medical care is well established, the desires of incompetent or comatose patients presents a great ethical dilemma. Treatment decisions for terminally ill patients who are not able to express their own wishes are often shared among family members, legal guardians, and/or health care providers.

Understandably, these health care providers are often reluctant to discontinue medical intervention because it violates their own personal ethical commitment to sustain life and because they fear legal repercussions. No less challenging is the ethical issue surrounding the definition of extraordinary or artificial intervention for the purpose of sustaining life. For example, medical and legal experts differ on the controversial issue of withdrawing nutrition and hydration supplied through artificial means to a dying patient. No less difficult are treatment decisions for severely handicapped newborns, as illustrated by the federal government's "Baby Doe regulations," which attempted to establish procedures and guidelines for the care of such infants and to assure that they receive equal protection under the law (Bresnohan & Drane, 1986; Reiser, 1986). The challenge for hospitals is to ensure that such decisions are made in a responsible manner, that family and physician viewpoints are exchanged, and that legal guidelines are understood and upheld. Frequently, it is the role of a medical staff ethics committee to serve as a facilitator in the ethical decision-making process—a role that requires extreme sensitivity to the interests of all parties. Sometimes that leadership role is laid at the door of administration by default.

Patient Rights to Make Decisions

The Patient Self-Determination Act applies to all health care facilities receiving public funds from Medicare or Medicaid and requires them to provide all patients on admission with written information that describes the patient's rights to make decisions regarding medical care, to refuse treatment, and to formulate advance directives. Advance directives refer to the patient's wishes regarding continuation of treatment directives, such as living wills stating treatment preferences and durable power of attorney appointments indicating proxy decision makers.

The intent of this statute is to establish a procedure that ensures increased clarity about the patient's wishes while creating an environment that makes it more likely that health care professionals will honor the patient's directives. Concern about the law and its provisions on the part of health care providers include:

- possible insensitivity in the process of requiring patients to indicate advance directives, thereby inducing unnecessary patient anxiety;
- patients may lack sufficient information about treatment options;
- the statute requires special training for health care workers;
- advance directives may overrule other actions in the patient's best interest;
- the patient may change his or her mind at a later point in the care process.

Hospitals in the United States are part of a dynamic and changing health care system. They face significant challenges in their multiple and often competing roles as health care providers caring for the sick, as charitable institutions to serve the poor, and as businesses functioning within a difficult financial environment. They also play important roles in community and professional education. At present, hospitals face new challenges as they expand beyond their traditional boundaries as providers of short-term, acute care to assume growing responsibilities for the delivery of a wide range of health services that correspond to community needs. Current trends in health care, including the need to provide humane and respectful treatment for AIDS patients, care for the growing elderly population, the health needs of unsponsored and unpaid patients, and the application of new technological breakthroughs, particularly in the area of genetic engineering, can only increase the central role of the community hospital and its medical staff in ethical decision making for health care in the years ahead.

On the broader question of ethics, the American Medical Association has adopted the position that

> a just society has the duty to offer its members reasonable protection against general threats including diseases, and to ensure that its members have a fair opportunity to pursue their goals in life. Given that health care resources are finite, determination of what should be included as adequate health care benefits needs to take into account the degree of benefit, meaning differences in outcome with and without treatment, the likelihood of its provision, its duration, its costs, and the number of people who will benefit from the particular procedure or treatment. A just outcome requires a fair process for implementing these ethical criteria. ("Ethical Issues," 1994)

INTERNAL ORGANIZATION OF HOSPITALS

From the outside, the prevalent view of the organization of a community hospital would be one possessing a clear goal of providing high-quality health care to which the efforts of the professional and technical groups working there are dedicated. From the inside, it is apparent that there are at least two different organizations with two distinct sets of goals. The administrative organization has a responsibility for the efficient management and operation of the institution as a whole. The medical staff organization has a responsibility for the patient care provided by individual physicians.

The Traditional Structure

Within the traditional structure of a typical community not-for-profit hospital, there are three loci of authority: the governing board, the administration, and the medical staff. Stating this generalization serves to obscure somewhat the differences, which could be major, among for-profit corporate structures, religious hospitals, individual or chain organizations with their various sponsoring orders, and the several approaches to governance by academic medical centers. Some would say that this view serves to perpetuate the outdated concept that the administration, governing board, and medical staff are operationally separate components of a hospital. Barry Bader, (private communication, 1996) says that while this was historically true, the limitations of this concept have been recognized since the mid-to late 1980s.

Nevertheless, in the most frequent and more easily observable structure of local hospitals, much balancing goes on between and among the three groups with authority as they practice practical politics. Each authority group has a distinct responsibility. The board is ultimately responsible for everything that goes on in the hospital, both administratively and professionally. It oversees the operation of the hospital and carries out its responsibility by

- adopting policies and plans to guide the hospital's operation,
- selecting and delegating responsibility for the day-to-day management of the hospital to the administrator and supervising that person's performance,
- appointing physicians to the medical staff, approving the medical staff's organization for governing itself and for supervising the professional activities of its members, and delegating responsibility to the medical staff for the provision of high-quality patient care.

In actual practice, the three areas of authority are not as clear or distinct as they might appear to be. For example, it might seem that there is a clear distinction between governance and the medical staff's responsibility for patient care. Court decisions have made it clear that the hospital as an institution has a corporate responsibility or legal liability for ensuring that patients receive high-quality patient care. Therefore, the governing board must make sure that only qualified physicians are permitted to practice medicine in the hospital and that quality review mechanisms are established and working. However, only the medical staff has the expertise to assess the qualifications and care provided by physicians. Although the medical staff is clearly subordinate to the governing board in terms of authority for the overall affairs of the institution, physicians are independent of strict control over their medical practices because the board does not share their expert knowledge and special skill.

Employees of the hospital working in clinical areas often find themselves caught in the middle when physicians' actions conflict with hospital policy. Legally, the employees should follow hospital policy and could be found liable for failing to do that. However, professionally they are expected to follow the physicians' orders regarding patient care, and their day-to-day working relationships are with the medical staff. A substantial degree of physician independence from the hospital exists because most are in private practice and are not employed by the institution. On the other hand, physicians must have access to a hospital in order to practice modern medicine, and only the governing board has the power to grant them privileges to practice there (Perkins, 1975). This unique relationship between physicians and hospitals is not without stresses and strains, and it makes the governance and management of hospitals a challenging responsibility and sometimes a real adventure, as shall be seen during the remainder of this text. That relationship can also produce some real human successes, notably in the saving of lives and the conquering of disease and injury. It is this relationship in all its color, glory, despair, and, sometimes, almost a lack of relationship that is the subject of this volume.

The distinction between adopting policies to guide hospital operations and managing operations on a day-to-day basis is not always clear either. Problems arise when the governing board becomes involved in administrative matters, such as acting directly on employee grievances that come to their attention rather than referring them to the administration. On the other hand, in running a complex enterprise, the administrator must make many decisions that the board, in adopting policies, has not explicitly voted on. Thus the community hospital is not a united front, as it might appear. Nor is it a hierarchial structure, as it might also appear, with a corporate or military top-down flow of authority. Rather, it is an organization with at least two separate lines of authority—administrative and medical—and with some ambiguity among what is governance, what is management, and what is medical staff self-governance. Power at the top is shared, not hierarchial, both because the board depends on the expertise of the medical staff and because of the independent contractor status of physicians. Administrators have also become influential because of their expertise in dealing with the increasingly complex operational and regulatory issues confronting the modern hospital in this country. Since the internal powers do not always agree among themselves on priorities and programs, hospitals often experience internal tensions and find it difficult to respond in a timely, appropriate, and systematic way to external environmental conditions and changing community needs. Sometimes, it seems impossible to make any decision at all.

The Governing Board

The governing board of the community hospital has evolved in function and structure as the hospital itself has developed new roles. During the late 1800s and early 1900s, when advances in medical science were transforming hospitals from custodial institutions for the sick poor to sources of effective and safe care for the entire community, board members were mostly wealthy benefactors who made substantial donations to establish and equip the hospital and meet its deficits. The primary function of the board at that time was trusteeship, that is, preserving the assets that they and others like them had donated. The trustees' job was seen as providing the facilities that the medical staff needed to care for their patients. There was little trustee involvement in medical matters. The administrator was essentially a clerk, and administrative duties were divided among the board members (Haglund & Dowling, 1993).

After World War I, the complexity and size of hospitals grew to the point where board members could no longer administer and financially support the hospital. Business managers were hired to handle administrative and financial matters. The business manager, along with the superintendent of nurses, reported to the board, and the board coordinated the two. As the complexity of the hospital and the competence of managers increased, the business manager gradually assumed responsibility for overseeing nursing and all other departments as well, so that only one person then reported to the board. The manager's title became "superintendent." The board of trustees moved into an oversight role, relinquishing day-to-day management matters to the superintendent (Johnson, 1970).

The governing board's role changed further as hospitals continued to grow, as management decisions took on greater complexity and significance, and as philanthropy yielded to patient revenue as the primary source of financial support. The board's role became one of overall policymaking and planning, and board membership was used to augment and supplement the skills of the administrative staff. Boards began to be composed of fewer philanthropists and more individuals with specific management skills, such as business executives, attorneys, bankers, architects, and contractors (Johnson, 1970). Even so, community hospital boards remained relatively closed to external scrutiny, with their membership consisting essentially of self-perpetuating groups of community influentials (Blankenship & Elling, 1962; Burling & Wilson, 1956). Board decisions were mostly in areas of finance, personnel, physical plant, and their areas of expertise, and boards typically deferred to medical staffs on medical and patient care matters, delegating fully the responsibility for the qualifications and quality of care provided by the medical staff.

During the 1960s, four major factors caused further changes in the governing board's role (*Darling*, 1965; Totten, Orlikoff, & Ewell, 1990). Continuing advances in medical science, the proliferation of medical technology, and the rapid growth in the size and sophistication of hospitals gave rise to public concern about the cost of hospital care, all the while making the hospital even more central in the delivery of health care and even more valuable to the public.

Public expectations regarding the hospital's responsibility to the community changed, so that hospitals began to be viewed as community resources with a definite obligation to respond to community needs.

State and federal regulation of hospital construction, costs, quality, and use, as well as labor relations, became more and more stringent, particularly following the establishment of Medicare and Medicaid. Not the least of these factors were the precedent court decisions that established the concept of corporate or institutional responsibility for ensuring the quality of patient care.

As a result of these forces, the governing board's role broadened and became even more demanding. Boards grew active in environmental surveillance, becoming knowledgeable about community concerns and external trends and interpreting their significance for the hospital (Guest, 1972). External pressures forced hospitals to reexamine their priorities and programs, and boards found it necessary to provide clearer direction and stronger leadership in strategic planning. Boards have also assumed an active role in seeing that community concerns and interests are brought into hospital decision making, and many have expanded community representation within their membership. The board now finds itself in the role of balancing and mediating between the demands and pressures on the hospital from the community and external agencies, on the one hand, and from the medical staff, employees, and other internal groups, on the other hand.

As a result of the changing environment of payment system changes as well as precedent court cases, governing boards have been forced to take a more active role in quality control, rather than abdicating this responsibility entirely to the medical staff. Although the professional work and the function of quality monitoring is still delegated to the medical staff, the board is now being held responsible for how well this function is carried out. The board is responsible for ensuring that the mechanisms for evaluating the credentials of physicians and monitoring the care they provide are established and working. Courts have held the hospital responsible in malpractice cases in which reasonable precautions were not taken to ensure:

- careful selection of the medical staff
- establishment of high standards of care
- monitoring and supervision of care
- enforcement of policies, rules, and regulations

In practice, board control over medical staff performance remains limited and depends more on the commitment of the medical staff, the character of hospital-medical staff relations, and legal sanctions, such as suspending or terminating a physician's privileges, an action that is rare.

As governing boards become more actively involved in medical and patient care matters, in both determining the hospital's role and relationships with other institutions and overseeing quality assurance mechanisms, physicians have begun to seek more involvement in hospital planning and policymaking. At the same time, boards felt a greater need for more direct physician participation in their deliberations to address issues related to quality, medical staff privileges, and changing medical technology and practice patterns (Haglund & Dowling, 1993). The product of these expectations has been the addition of physicians to an increasing number of boards. More than half of all community hospitals now include physicians. Also emerging and becoming more frequent is the tendency for the administrator to serve on the board, generally with a title change to "president," "CEO," or "executive vice president" in a corporate type of structure (Blues, 1987).

Today, governing boards are being challenged and scrutinized as never before. They are being called upon to demonstrate their effectiveness in ensuring that the hospitals they govern meet community needs and provide high-quality care while at the same time function effectively within a complex structure of guidelines and regulations, all in an environment of constant change. Not all boards all capable of performing this task. Boards have been criticized as too inward-looking, passive, uninformed, reluctant to become involved in medical matters, and unwilling to change the status quo. Recent legal decisions have found hospital board members personally liable for making hasty, ill-informed decisions (Umdenstock, 1987).

Under ordinary circumstances, a board member does not incur personal liability simply by reason of holding office. However, a board member, who may be a physician, can become personally liable if he or she directs or participates in a tortius act. Many states have enacted legislation granting various degrees of immunity to persons serving on not-for-profit boards (*Hospital Law Manual,* 1995). Conditions of immunity often require a board member to have acted within the scope of the member's duties and not recklessly or with gross negligence (California Corporations Code, Section 5239).

It appears, however, that the pressures discussed here are causing boards to take active steps to broaden and strengthen their membership, educate themselves more fully, and streamline their structure so that they will be better equipped to provide the strong leadership that will be required for the future (Bader, 1986; Schulz & Johnson, 1976).

Hospital Administration

Hospital administration has grown in importance and status as hospitals have grown in size and sophistication. The job of implementing board policy and responsibility for the day-to-day management and supervision of the hospital is delegated by the board to the hospital administrator, whether called that or CEO or executive vice president. Referring to the on-site manager of the hospital as an "administrator" may serve to deny that person's rightful position as an executive leader, yet to the eyes and ears of the doctors on the medical staff, it is all the same. Using the title of CEO looks and sounds pretentious to those physicians who really only want someone who will give them what they want with a minimum of trouble and delay. For the remainder of this volume, if the term *administrator* is used, it refers to that person who is available to the organized medical staff leadership on a daily and ongoing basis. Many system or corporate CEOs are located in another office in another part of the city while each hospital facility offers a building administrator.

The administrator has responsibility for managing the hospital's finances, acquiring and maintaining equipment and facilities, hiring and supervising hospital personnel, and coordinating hospital activities. A key aspect of the administrator's job is to coordinate and serve as the channel of communication among the governing board, medical staff, and hospital departments. Another is strategic planning for the future development of the hospital's services. Large hospitals have may have a number of assistant administrators who are responsible for nursing, professional services, support services, and hospital finance.

In addition to financial, personnel, and physical plant matters, the administration plays an important role in patient care. For example, the administration is responsible for coordinating the patient care departments with each other and with the support departments, ensuring that they are adequately equipped and staffed and technically up to date, and ensuring that they function smoothly.

The administration must also make sure that physician orders for the treatment of patients are carried out correctly and promptly by hospital personnel and that orders do not conflict with governing board policies or hospital rules. The administration is also actively engaged in planning for new patient care services and in ensuring that the hospital meets accreditation, licensing, and other standards. Because the medical staff is not employed by the hospital, the administration must establish and maintain a cooperative working relationship with the members in order to effectively handle the many tasks that involve both the administrators and doctors.

As if that were not enough, the administration acts as the liaison with the community and with external agencies, bringing information from these sources into hospital decision making and planning as well as representing the hospital to these outside parties and giving information about the hopes and aspirations the hospital family offers regarding patient care for the citizens and their families. Because of the increasing impact of external and regulatory pressures on hospitals, this boundary-spanning role has become one of the most important aspects of the administrator's job.

SUMMARY

Hospital administration has advanced rapidly as a profession, in a transition from business manager to coordinator and now to corporate chief with full authority for directing all aspects of the hospital's operation and management and promoting participative decision making by board, medical staff, nursing staff, and administrative representatives ("Ethical Issues," 1994). From those early and humble beginnings, administrators have become full participants and even leaders in the development of policies and plans, as well as in their implementation and in the internal and external affairs of the hospital. The next generation in the evolution of hospital management will probably see more physicians move on to those positions, but by whomever, doctor or lay person, the future challenges encountered by hospitals in the competitive environment and in dealing with managed care will require the development of new skills and priorities.

This book focuses on the modern American community acute care hospital and the self-governance roles of the medical staff who practice in those facilities, describing how the hospital is the key resource, the organizational hub, and the central site of patient care in the American health care delivery system. A historical perspective has been used to show the evolution and development of the hospital as a place for caring, for curing, and, inevitably, as a business that needs to do well in order to do good.

A number of main themes are presented, including how hospitals changed from almshouses established by city government for providing food and shelter for the home-less poor and sick to highly advanced scientific institutions delivering short-term services financed by mixes of public and private dollars. An essential ingredient of hospital devel-opment has been the advent and evolution of professional nurses employed in hospitals. As well, the ethic of devotion to caring and sympathy toward sick people that remains strong today in many portions of the health care sector grew.

As hospitals moved more toward accumulation of community resources and increas-ing technology, the need for patient care revenues became the primary focus. Previous trustees, whose charitable intent and philanthropy included day-by-day management, gave way to trained administrators who became legally responsible for governance. The roles of hospital financing and ownership are discussed, as is the role of government within a system that has reflected the American ethic of reliance on the private sector.

Persisting rises in costs of hospital care have brought about a number of efforts to con-tain the high rate of inflation. In-depth discussions of those efforts are presented in later chapters.

REFERENCES

Bader, B. S. (1986). *Three Waves of Change: Hospital Board Responsibilities in the New Health Care Environment.* Rockville, MD: Bader & Associates.

Bisbee, G. H. Jr. (Ed.). (1982). *Management of Rural Primary Care: Concepts and Cases.* Chicago: The Hospital Research and Educational Trust.

Blankenship, L. V., & Elling, R. H. (1962). Organizational support and community power struc-ture: The hospital. *Journal of Health and Human Behavior, 3,* 257–369.

Blues, S. M. (1987). New legal standards for trustee performance. *Health Progress, 68,* 60–63, 95.

Bresnohan, J. F., & Drane, J. F. (1986). A challenge to understand the meaning of living and dying. *Health Progress, 67,* 32–37, 98.

Burling, T., & Wilson, R. N. (1956). The board of trustees. In *The Give and Take in Hospitals.* New York: G. P. Putnam's Sons.

Coile, R. C. Jr. (1986). *The New Hospital: Future Strategies for a Changing Industry.* Rockville, MD: Aspen Publishers.

Darling v. Charleston Community Memorial Hospital. (1965). 33 Illinois, 2nd. 236 211 ME 2nd. 253.

Darr, K., Longest, B. B. Jr., & Rakich, J. S. (1986). The ethical imperative in health services governance and management. *Hospital and Health Services Administration, 31,* 53–66.

Ethical issues in health care system reform—the provision of adequate health care. (1994). *Journal of the American Medical Association, 272(13),* 1056–1062. Council on Ethical and Judicial Affairs. Reprinted in *Healthcare Trends Report, 8(11, November),* 1994.

Feldstein, M. (1971). The Rising Cost of Hospital Care. Washington, DC: Information Resource Press.

Flexner, A. (1910). *Medical Education in the United States and Canada.* (Bulletin No. 4). New York: Carnegie Foundation for the Advancement of Teaching.

Folland, S. T. (1985). The effects of health care advertising. *Journal of Health Politics, Policy and Law, 10,* 329-345.

Goldsmith, J. C. (1981). *Can Hospitals Survive?* Homewood, IL: Dow Jones-Irwin.

Guest, R. (1972). The role of a doctor in institutional management. In Georgeopolis, B. (Ed.), *Organizational Research in Health Institutions.* Ann Arbor: University of Michigan Press.

Haglund, C. L., & Dowling, W. L. (1993). The hospital. In Williams, S. J., & Torrens, P. R. (Eds.), *Introduction to Health Services (4th ed.).* Albany: Delmar Publishers.

The Hospital Law Manual, Attorney's Volume (1995). Gaithersburg, MD: Aspen Publishers.

Hospital Statistics. (1991). Chicago: American Hospital Association.

Johnson, E. L. (1970). Changing role of the hospital's chief executive officer. *Hospital Administration, 15,* 21–34.

Lathrop, P. J. (1991). The patient-focused hospital. *Healthcare Forum Journal, July/August,* 17–20.

Perkins, R. (1975). The physician's view of the hospital: A love-hate relationship. Parts 1 and 2. *Hospital Medical Staff, 4,* 1–7, 10–14.

Placella, L. E. (1986). Choosing a growth strategy: diversification vs. vertical integration. *Trustee, 39,* 26–28.

Reiser, S. J. (1986). Survival at what cost? Origins and effects of the modern controversy on treating severely handicapped newborns. *Journal of Health Politics, Policy and Law, 11,* 199–214.

Schulz, R., & Johnson, A. C. (1976). *Management of Hospitals.* New York: McGraw-Hill.

Shortell, S. M. (1977). Organization of hospital resources. *Hospitals in the 1980s.* Chicago: American Hospital Association.

Starr, P. (1982). *The Social Transformation of American Medicine.* New York: Basic Books. Copyright (c) 1982 by Paul Starr. Reprinted by permission of Basic Books, a division of Harper Collins Publishers, Inc.

Torrens, P. R. (1993). Historical evolution and overview of health services in the United States. In Williams, S. J., & Torrens, P. R. (Eds.), *Introduction to Health Services (4th ed.).* Albany: Delmar Publishers.

Totten, M. K., Orlikoff, J. E., & Ewell, C. M. (1990). *The Guide to Governance for Hospital Trustees.* Chicago: The Hospital Research and Educational Trust.

Umdenstock, R. J. (1987). Refinement of board's role required. *Health Progress, 68,* 44–49.

Wartman, S. A., Morlock, L. L., Malitz, F. E., et al. (1983). Patient understanding and satisfaction, and predictors of compliance. *Medical Care, 21,* 886–891.

CHAPTER

Doctors: Slavery to Specialties

Physicians have not always occupied the same positions of honor and comfort as they enjoy today. Under the Romans, physicians were primarily slaves, though some were freedmen and foreigners; medicine was considered a low-class occupation. Under managed care, there are, undoubtedly, some physicians who will say they are still slaves in a low-class occupation.

The dream of the philosophers after the Enlightenment was that the Age of Reason, in the form of the arts and sciences, would be powerful enough to liberate humanity. There could then be freedom from scarcity and the caprices of nature, ignorance and superstition, tyranny, and the diseases of the body and spirit. Rigid adherence to the religious dogma of the Middle Ages could be abandoned or at least lessened in its control over thought and action. There was also the possibility of relief from the arbitrary behavior of kings and nobles. Humankind could therefore exert more control over the physical and social environment in a steady growth toward perfection.

Modern medicine is one of those extraordinary works of reason. It is composed of an elaborate system of specialized knowledge, technical procedures, and rules of behavior.

Medicine has realized much of the philosophers' dream by liberating humanity from much of the burden of disease. But medicine is also, unmistakably, a world of power and position, where some practitioners are more likely to receive the rewards of reason than are others. From a relatively weak, traditional profession of minor economic significance, the practice of medicine and the medical profession has become a sprawling system of hospitals, clinics, health plans, insurance companies, and myriad other organizations employing a vast labor force (Starr, 1982).

GROWTH AND ACCEPTANCE OF PHYSICIAN AUTHORITY

The medical profession and the physicians who form it have had an especially persuasive claim to the justification of their authority, because humans are dependent upon the knowledge and competence of doctors. When professionals claim to be authoritative about the nature of the world, lay citizens generally defer to their judgment. The interpretations of professionals often govern lay people's understanding of the world and helps explain their experience. Unlike law and religion medicine enjoys close bonds with modern science, and, at least for the past century, scientific knowledge has held a privileged status. Even among the physical and social sciences, medicine occupies a special position. Its practitioners come into direct and intimate contact with people in their daily lives; they are present at the critical moments of existence. For many people, doctors are the only contact with a world that otherwise stands at a forbidding distance. Physicians offer to patients a kind of individualized objectivity, bringing to bear in personal relationships the science and art of medicine as well as authoritative counsel. The very circumstances of sickness promote more ready acceptance of the physician's judgment. The power of medicine is avowedly enlisted solely in the interests of health—a value of usually unambiguous importance to its clients and society. On this basis, physicians exercise authority over patients, their fellow workers in health care, and even the public at large in matters within, and sometimes outside, their jurisdiction (Starr, 1982).

May (1993) aptly defines the concepts of illness and disease in a way that will assist in further exploration of this unique authority that physicians have been allowed to accumulate and exercise on others' behalf, while they allow fitting and appropriate rewards of money and social status to the profession in return. Illness is a lay experience that connotes both a physical and a social state. It is an individual's reaction to a biologic alteration and is defined differently by different people according to their state of mind and cultural beliefs. It is, therefore, an imprecise term that represents an individual response by the ill person or patient to a set of physiologic and psychological stimuli.

By contrast, disease is a professional construct. It is perceived as being precise and reflecting the highest state of professional knowledge, particularly that of the physician. The definition of disease is used as the vehicle for informing the patient of the presence of pathology, as a means for deciding on a course of treatment, and as a basis for comparing the results of therapy. The planning and organization of the health care system and the allocation of resources within that system are based upon these disease concepts and perceptions.

Only physicians are allowed by society to make medical diagnoses, even though considerable imprecision exists in that process. An individual physician using the best professional judgment available may diagnose one disease in a particular patient, but this assessment may not be shared by other doctors. Attempts to link *illness* (the individual's perception of loss of functional capacity) with *disease* (the professional's definition of a pathologic process) are even more complicated. Illness may occur in the absence of real disease, and disease may be present in the absence of perceived illness. The law says (and so do the health plans) that only a physician can tell the difference, a clear statement of the authoritative position.

The dominance of the medical profession sometimes spills over its clinical boundaries, however, into arenas of moral and political action for which medical judgment is only partially relevant and often incompletely equipped (Starr, 1982). As expert medical scientists trained in the scientific method, physicians sometimes allow the strong ego that enables them to deal daily with disease, birth, and death to run away into fields of emotional interests that are not scientific at all. It is a matter of history, then, that this authoritative profession has been able to turn its authority into social privilege, economic power, and political influence. In the distribution of rewards, the medical profession is the highest paid in our society, excepting, of course, basketball players, rock-and-roll singers, and drug dealers.

Things Were Not Always This Good

In eighteenth-century England, while ranking above the lowlier surgeons and apothecaries, physicians stood only at the margins of the gentry class, struggling for the patronage of the wealthy in the hope of acquiring enough wealth to buy an estate and a title. In nineteenth- and early-twentieth-century France, doctors were mostly impecunious, and the successful among them, conscious that medicine was an inadequate claim to status, pursued an ideal of general cultivation rather than mere professional accomplishment. There were very good reasons for this state of acceptance. Only a rudimentary technology was available for the treatment of disease. The scientific base of medicine was very narrow, and the number of effective medical treatments was very limited. Indeed, a great deal of energy and effort could be expended on treatment, but whether a patient recovered from an illness usually depended more on the patient and the disease rather than the treatment (Torrens, 1993).

Physicians during this period were poorly trained and practiced alone. They usually obtained their skills by serving apprenticeships with physicians already in practice and then taking short courses at unsophisticated medical colleges. What physicians had to offer was usually contained in their black bags, which they took with them wherever they went. They spent a good deal of time in patients' homes and almost no time at all in hospitals. In general, their practice was little different from that of their predecessors for centuries before them.

As time went on, physicians began to have more effective tools with which to work, and the range of their capabilities expanded rapidly. They still continued to spend the majority of their time in patients' homes, but now they also began to look to the hospital for the care of their more severely ill patients. A small but gradually increasing number of physicians began to specialize in a particular area of medicine; however, by 1940, more than 80 percent were still in general practice (Torrens, 1993).

In the rest of the world, not all societies with scientifically advanced medical institutions have a powerful medical profession such as exists in this country. Even in a Western society quite similar to that of the United States, Great Britain, most general practitioners are only moderately well paid, and they work within a national health service whose budget and overall policies they do not control. Hardly anywhere have doctors been as successful as physicians in the United States in resisting national health insurance and maintaining a predominately private and voluntary financing system. The growth of science, while critically important in the development of professionalism as in the rest of the world, does not assure physicians elsewhere the broad cultural authority, economic power, or political influence physicians have achieved in this country (Starr, 1982).

Doctors in the United States were not always the powerful and authoritative professionals that people see around today. A century ago they had less influence, income, and prestige. "In all of our American colleges," a professional journal commented bitterly in 1869, "medicine has ever been and is now, the most despised of all the professions which liberally-minded men are expected to enter" (Starr, 1982). In the nineteenth century, the medical profession was generally weak, divided, insecure in its status and its income, unable to control entry into practice or to raise the standards of medical education. The profession itself had little unity and was unable to assert any collective authority over its own members, who held diverse and incompatible views. In the twentieth century, however, not only did physicians become a powerful, prestigious, and wealthy profession, but physicians succeeded in shaping the basic organization and financial structure of American medicine (Starr, 1982).

Individual Physicians Become a Profession

The forces that transformed medicine into its present position as an authoritative profession involved both its internal development and broader changes in social and economic life in this country. Internally, as a result of changes in social structure, as well as scientific advances, the profession gained in cohesiveness toward the end of the nineteenth century and became more effective in asserting its claims. With the growth of hospitals and specialization, doctors became more dependent on each other for referrals and access to facilities. Consequently, they were forced to adjust their views to those of their peers instead of advertising themselves as members of competing medical sects. Greater cohesiveness, in turn, strengthened professional authority. Professional authority also benefitted from the development of diagnostic technology, which strengthened the powers of the physician in the physical examination of the patient and reduced reliance on the patient's report of symptoms and superficial appearance (Starr, 1982).

The dependence of patients on the professional authority of physicians increased with such developments as the increased importance of hospitals in the treatment of disease. As more technology developed, it tended to be concentrated in hospitals, with the result that patients and physicians began to go more to hospitals for the technology to be found there. Earlier, there had been no reason for private patients to go to a hospital, because they could usually get the same type of care in their homes. Then, with the continued progress of medical science, hospitals began to offer services and skills that were not available anywhere else. The voluntary shift of seriously ill patients from their homes to general hospitals increased the dependent nature of the sick. At home, patients may quite easily choose to ignore the doctor's instructions, and many do. This is much more difficult in a hospital. For the seriously ill, clinical personnel in the hospital, with a duty that is subordinate to the physician, have, in effect, replaced the family as the doctor's vicarious agent. They not only administer treatment in the doctor's absence but also maintain surveillance, keep records, and reinforce the message that the doctor's instructions must be followed (Starr, 1982).

Other institutional changes have also made people dependent on medical authority regardless of whether they are receptive or hostile to doctors. As the various certifying and gatekeeping functions of doctors have grown, so has the dependence of people seeking benefits that require certification. Laws prohibiting laymen from obtaining certain classes of drugs without a doctor's prescription increase dependence on physicians. In the twentieth century, health insurance has become an important mechanism for ensuring even greater dependence on the profession. When insurance payments are made only for treatment given by physicians, the beneficiaries become dependent on the doctors for performing services that can be reimbursed.

In their combined effect, the mechanisms of legitimation (such as standardized education and licensing) and the mechanisms of dependency (such as hospitalization, gatekeeping, and insurance) have given a definite structure to the relations of doctors and patients that transcends personalities and attitudes. It also regulated the professional and personal relations of physicians to each other. The doctor whose personal authority in the nineteenth century rested on his imposing character and relations with patients was in a fundamentally different situation from the doctor in the twentieth century, whose authority depends on holding the necessary credentials and institutional affiliations. While lay people have become more dependent on medical professionals, those professionals have become more dependent on each other (Starr, 1982). Nowhere is that relationship more apparent and intertwined than in the medical staff of the modern American community hospital.

PROFESSIONALISM CONTRADICTING THE MARKET

The emergence of a market for health care services was originally inseparable from the emergence of professional authority and autonomy. In the isolated communities of early American society, the sick were usually cared for as part of the obligations of kinship and mutual assistance. But as larger towns and cities grew, treatment increasingly shifted from the family and lay community to paid practitioners, druggists, hospitals, and other commercial and professional sources selling their services competitively on the market. The transition from the household to the market as the dominant institution in the care of the sick—that is, the conversion of health care to a commodity—has been one of the underlying movements as medicine transformed itself from slavery to specialties.

Through most of the nineteenth century, the market in medical care continued to be competitive. Entry into practice was then relatively easy for untrained practitioners as well as for medical school graduates. As a result, competition between and among doctors was intense, and the economic position of physicians was often insecure. The history of medical practice in the United States has been one of succeeding waves of alternatives for care that threatened independent solo practice. In the physicians' view, the competitive market has always represented a threat, not only to their incomes, but also to their status, authority, and autonomy because it drew no sharp boundary between the more educated and less educated. The market thus blurred the lines between commerce and professionalism and threatened to turn them into mere employees, considered only a few steps above the origins as slaves (Starr, 1982).

The contradiction between professionalism and the rule of the market is longstanding and unavoidable. Medicine and other learned professions have historically distinguished themselves from business and trade by claiming to be above the market and different from pure commercialism. In justifying the public's trust, the professions have moved toward setting higher standards for themselves than the minimal rules governing the marketplace. Professionals have maintained that they can be judged under those standards only by themselves and each other, not by lay people. On the one hand, the ideal of the market presumes the "sovereignty" of consumers' choices. On the other hand, the ideal of a profession calls for the "sovereignty" of its members' independent, authoritative judgment. A professional who yields too much to the demands of clients or patients violates an essential article of the professional code. Everett Hughes once defined quacks as "practitioners who continue to please their customers but not their colleagues." This shift from clients to colleagues in the orientation of work, which professionalism demands, represents a clear departure from the normal rule of the market (Starr, 1982).

Starr noted these feelings and attitudes in the context of late-nineteenth-century physicians, but his words apply with pinpoint focus to the current uneasiness and reservations about the growth of managed care in a competitive marketplace in the final decade of the twentieth century. A hundred years later, the more things change, the more they stay the same.

The medical profession was not helpless in the face of these outside forces, however. By augmenting demand and controlling supply, greater professional authority helped physicians secure higher returns for their work. The market power of medicine originated in part from increasing protection from the state. It also arose from the increasing dependence of patients on physicians. In the ideal market, no buyer depends on any seller, but patients are often dependent on their personal physicians, and they have become more so as the disparity in knowledge between them has grown. The sick cannot easily disengage themselves from relations with their doctors, nor even know when it might be in their interests to do so. Consequently, once they have begun treatment, they cannot exercise that unfettered choice of sellers that characterizes free markets (Starr, 1982).

One reason that the medical profession could develop market power of this kind was that it sold its services primarily to individual patients rather than organizations. Such organizations, had they been stronger and more numerous, could have exercised greater discrimination years ago in evaluation of clinical performance and might have lobbied against cartel restrictions of the physician supply. The medical profession, of course, insisted that salaried arrangements violated the integrity of the private doctor-patient relationship, and in the early decades of the twentieth century, doctors were able to use their growing market power to escape the threat of bureaucratic control and preserve their own individual and collective autonomy (Starr, 1982). Now, in the late twentieth century, the rise of health plans and payers that do evaluate clinical performance and do restrict physician supply by using closed panel medical groups are threatening that very autonomy by the application of market forces of supply and demand. Perhaps, the doctors' worst fears of 100 years are finally coming true.

PHYSICIANS' ROLES IN RECONSTITUTING THE HOSPITAL

Few institutions have undergone as radical a metamorphosis as have hospitals in their modern history. In developing from places of dreaded impurity and exiled human wreckage into awesome citadels of science and bureaucratic order, they acquired a new moral identity, as well as new purposes and paying patients of higher status. The hospital is perhaps distinctive in having first been built primarily for the poor and only later entered in significant numbers and an entirely different state of mind by the more respectable classes. As its functions were transformed, it emerged, in a sense, from the underlife of society to become a regular part of accepted experience, still as an occasion for anxiety but not horror.

People now think of hospitals as the most visible embodiment of medical care in its technically most sophisticated form, but before the past hundred years, hospitals and medical practice had relatively little to do with other. From their earliest origins in preindustrial societies, hospitals had been primarily religious and charitable institutions for tending the sick, rather than medical institutions for their cure (as described in Chapter 1). Before the Civil War, an American doctor might contentedly spend an entire career in practice without ever setting foot on a hospital ward. The hospital did not intrude on the worries of the typical practitioner, nor the practitioner on the routines of the hospital (Starr, 1982). Neither was interested in changing that relationship.

But within the next 40 years, hospitals moved from the periphery to the center of medical education and medical practice. From refuges mainly for the homeless poor and insane, they evolved into doctors' workshops for all types and classes of patients. From charities dependent on voluntary gifts, they developed into market institutions financed increasingly out of payments from patients. The same forces that promoted the rise of hospitals also brought about changes in their internal organization. Authority over the conduct of the institution passed from the trustees to the physicians and administration. The sick began to enter hospitals, not for an entire siege of illness, but only during its acute phase to have some work performed on them. The posture of the hospital became more active and purposeful. It was no longer a well of sorrow and charity but a workplace for the production of health, and the producers of that health were the physicians who practiced there.

War Changes Hospitals and Medical Practice

Although the 1900–1940 period was one of rapid growth in scientific technology, it was nothing compared to what happened with the advent of World War II. With the start of the war, this country mounted a massive effort to organize the best available talents for the care of the wounded and for the solution of the health care problems generated by the war. For the first time, relatively large efforts in medical and scientific research were begun under the direction of the federal government, and the results were impressive. The development of antibiotics accelerated rapidly, new surgical techniques for the treatment of trauma and burns were discovered, and new approaches to the transportation of the sick and wounded were developed. This remarkable dedication to organized investigation has continued and expanded to this day, with many incredible accomplishments to show for the effort, as well as the promise of more breakthroughs on the immediate horizon. It is entirely possible that the space program in the 1960s contributed as much (or more) to medical science and technology as it did to exploration.

After World War II, hospitals were no longer the same. Previously, they had been places for the care of patients, with great emphasis being placed on the caring function. Now they became extensions of the research laboratories, places where medical science was practiced and where curing was the order of the day. New procedures, new equipment, and new techniques all flourished to such a degree that the hospitals were now captured by their technology and the physicians required to use it. The technology itself and the specialized physicians that were attracted by it became the motivating force for hospitals, and most major decisions would from then on be based on that technology (Roemer & Friedman, 1971).

The effects of this technological advance altered in many ways the relationship of doctors to hospitals and to one another and shaped the development of the nation's hospital system as a whole. With the explosive growth of scientific knowledge after World War II, it was impossible for one physician to know everything, and so the trend toward specialization in a particular subarea of medicine had a strong impetus. Once the hospital became an integral and necessary part of medical practice, control over access to its facilities became a strategic basis of power within the medical community. The tight grip that a narrow elite group of physicians held over hospitals no longer seemed tolerable to other physicians, who responded by forming their own institutions or pressing for access to established ones. Under financial pressures and the threat of increased competition, the older hospitals gradually opened their doors to larger numbers of practitioners, creating a wider network of interconnected behavior that stratified and linked the profession in new and unexpected ways. What was new and different about the interconnected behavior was that it allowed for the full development and refinement of the Joint Commission on the Accreditation of Healthcare Organizations model of a hospital medical staff, which we will explore in great depth.

Before the war, approximately 80 percent of physicians had been general practitioners and 20 percent, specialists. In the years after the war, these percentages reversed. In their training and practice, physicians focused increasingly on the scientific aspects of diagnosis and treatment and, as a result, spent more time in hospitals and less time in patients' homes. House calls became a thing of the past; only a favorite memory about the American yesteryear. The hospital became the emotional center of the physician's life, since it was here that the most challenging and most interesting aspects of training or treatment occurred (Torrens, 1993).

The access that private practitioners gained to hospitals, without becoming their employees, became one of the distinctive features of medical care in the United States. In Europe and most other areas of the world, when patients enter a hospital, their doctors typically relinquish responsibility to the hospital staff, who form a separate and distinct group in the profession. But in this country, private doctors follow their patients into the hospital, where they continue to attend them. Both internally and as a system, American hospitals have had a relatively loose structure because of the autonomy of the physicians and of most hospitals from the government. As the social growth and development of the United States continued, hospitals changed along with them. As the hospital advanced its functions from caretaking to active treatment, it shifted its ideals from benevolence to professionalism and accorded its physicians greater power (Torrens, 1993).

PROFESSIONAL NURSING AFFECTS HOSPITAL PRACTICE

The rise of professional nursing also helped produce a deep change in the character of hospitals as well as an increase in their number. However, professional nursing did not emerge from medical discoveries or from a program of hospital reform initiated by physicians. Instead, outsiders saw the need first. Before the 1870s, trained nurses were virtually unknown in the United States. Hospital nursing was a menial occupation, taken up by women of the lower classes, some of whom were conscripted from penitentiaries or almshouses (Starr, 1982). Generally these untrained nurses were members of religious groups who volunteered to work in the few hospitals that existed or they were poor, desperate, discarded women who frequented these institutions anyway and were pressed into service. Their work was nonscientific in the extreme and consisted simply of assisting patients with their usual bodily functions in any way possible (Hobson, 1914).

The movement for reform originated, not with doctors, but among upper-class women who had taken on the role of guardians of a new hygienic order. After monitoring the conduct of hospitals of that day, society women in New York proposed starting a nurses' training school, which would attract the wholesome daughters of the middle class. Some doctors approved of this proposal, but others opposed it on the grounds that educated nurses would not do as they were told—a remarkable comment on the status anxieties of physicians of that day and what threatened them (Starr, 1982). But the women reformers did not depend on the physicians' approval and went over their heads to men from the same social class who had greater power and authority.

Eventually, of course, doctors come to not only accept but to rely greatly on trained nurses, who proved essential in carrying out the complex work that hospitals were taking on. The nurses training schools of that era also provided a source of cheap labor to the hospital in the form of unpaid student nurses, who became the mainstays of the hospital's labor force (Ashley, 1976). That tradition of low pay—or no pay—has haunted the nursing profession until this day. However, in more recent times nurses have used the National Labor Relations Act to engage in collective bargaining, work actions and, ultimately, strikes. These efforts bore fruit in the form of higher wages, improved grievance procedures, and a greater voice in matters of professional concern to hospital nurses.

The trends in health care delivery and the growth of medical science and technology after World War II also greatly affected professional nursing as well as doctors and hospitals. Their training became increasingly more scientific, more specialized, and more lengthy. The desire to be recognized for competence and skill led to the growth of professional nursing organizations and to formal accreditation on the basis of scientific training and ability (Torrens, 1993). It also led away from the diploma schools based in hospitals toward college- and university-based training programs and the development of advanced degree programs and nursing research.

ADVANCES IN SURGERY CHANGE HOSPITAL PRACTICE

Nursing had an undeniable effect on hospitals and the doctors who practiced there. But advances in surgery had an even greater effect by changing the nature of the doctors who practiced in hospitals and what they did there. Surgery enjoyed a spectacular rise in prestige and accomplishment in the late 1800s. Before anesthesia, surgery was brutal work. Physical strength and speed were at a premium, so important was it to get in and out of the body as fast as possible. After Morton's demonstration of ether in 1846, anesthesia came quickly into use, and slower and more careful operations became possible. But the range and volume of surgery remained extremely limited. Infections took a heavy toll in all "capital operations," as major surgery was so justly called. The mortality rate for amputations was about 40 percent. Very rarely did the surgeon penetrate the major body cavities, and then only in desperation, when every other hope had been exhausted. Surgery had a small repertoire and it stood far behind medicine in the therapeutic arsenal (Cartwright, 1967).

Lister's pioneering work on antisepsis was not generally used until nearly 20 years later, soon after which his carbolic acid spray technique was superseded by aseptic techniques. With control over infection, surgeons could begin to explore the abdomen, chest, and skull, but before they could be widely used, a variety of new techniques had to be developed and mastered by the profession. Growth in the volume of surgical work during the 1890s and early 1900s provided the basis for expansion and profit in hospital care. Starr (1982) noted that it was 1883 when the number of surgical patients exceeded medical patients for the first time. But first, certain impediments to the use of hospitals had to be removed. Before 1900, the hospital had no special advantages over the home, and the infections that periodically swept through hospital wards made physicians cautious about sending patients there. Even after the danger of cross infection had been reduced, the lingering image of the hospital as a house of death and its status as a charity interfered with its growth. Patients objected to losing the privacy and control they might have had at home; and physicians were afraid that referring patients to hospitals would mean losing the fee.

It took time to establish new understandings about professional fees and controls over patients. So in the meantime, ether and antisepsis were adapted to the home, and "kitchen surgery" continued. But performing surgery in the home became steadily more inconvenient for both the surgeon and the family as procedures became more difficult and doctors spent so much time traveling to the patient's home. To accommodate desires for privacy not available in the hospital, many surgeons first moved their operations to private "medical boarding houses," which provided hotel services and nursing. In the suburbs and small towns, doctors built small hospitals under their own ownership. Surgery had now made hospital care profitable and permitted them to open institutions without upper-class sponsorship and control, as well as legitimation. In time, most surgery moved into the growing community hospitals (Crocker, 1899).

Acute Care Replaces Long-Term, with Higher Costs

With greater pressure for admission, hospitals and physicians began to limit care to the most acute periods of illness, rather than the full course of treatment and recuperation. The growing emphasis on surgery and the relief of acute illness brought about a redefinition of purpose in some of the older charity hospitals. Active surgical and medical treatment supplanted religious and moralistic objectives and became the overriding mission. As hospitals became more generally accepted, the social origins of their patients changed, so that the occupational distribution of their adult patients became more nearly like that of the population. In the next period hospitals went from treating the poor for the sake of charity to treating the rich for the sake of revenue and, only belatedly, sometimes, gave thought to the people in between (Starr, 1982).

As hospitals came to use more of their beds for surgery and the treatment of acute illness, they had less room for recuperating patients, who were discharged earlier, sometimes to newly built nursing homes. As a result, the boundary between staff and patients became more differentiated, more fixed, and certainly more permanent. In the almshouses, patients took care of each other. They were all equal. Now, as general hospitals became more strictly devoted to acute illness, such functions were taken over completely by employees of the hospital. This meant higher costs, since attendants had to be employed to do the work previously done free by patients. As the functions and standards of hospitals changed, construction and operating costs both necessarily increased. Because of these higher costs of acute care, requiring more and better employees, higher operating costs per patient soared beyond the capacity of charity to meet them.

Private hospitals tried to turn to the government for aid, but none was forthcoming. They tried also to turn to the public for more voluntary contributions, and organize fundraising drives, but this source, too, proved insufficient. The old charity hospitals had been managed on an almost informal basis. Now they had become large institutions and there was a demand for more careful accounting, more specialized labor, and better coordination of the various auxiliary hotel, restaurant, and laboratory services that a hospital maintained (Starr, 1982).

The principal answer to the hospitals' financial difficulties proved to be greater payments by patients. New conditions brought on the increase in costs, but they also enlarged the potential for income. Many people were now coming to hospitals who could afford to pay, and since the real value of hospital care had increased, charges would not drive them away, a phenomenon that still exists. The hospitals were also encouraged to allow the imposition of doctor's fees, by physicians who objected to the free services being given to patients at the charity hospitals who could afford to pay a doctor at home but could avoid all charges by going to the hospital. Physicians who treated these cases in the hospital were prevented from collecting fees but could have charged for care provided in the home.

Changes in organization and financing gradually altered the distribution of power and authority in hospitals. The trustees' original sphere of total control diminished, while the physicians' sphere expanded. The shift was most apparent in control over admissions. Originally, at voluntary hospitals, the trustees as well as the doctors took part in deciding who of the deserving poor to accept, but as hospitals become more strictly medical institutions, the trustees' role in admitting declined. Hospitals dropped the provision that trustees might admit patients (Starr, 1982).

The devolution of decision-making power to physicians reflected the more general change in the structure of most social organizations in the late nineteenth century. There was growing importance of a salaried management in corporations, of administrators and professors in universities, of salaried editors and professional reporters on newspapers, and of civil servants in government. In hospitals, the trustees could no longer enter into the details of management. The more common pattern was for the executive of the hospital to resolve all ordinary questions and turn to the board only at intervals on major matters of policy. Unlike corporations, however, hospitals saw authority devolve more on outside professionals who were not employees, the medical staff, rather than on its own salaried management. This peculiarity of organization arose because of the special role that outside doctors came to play in the prosperity of the institution. They had replaced the trustees as the chief source of income. When hospitals relied on donations, the trustees were vital. But when hospitals came to rely on receipts from patients, the doctors who brought in the patients inevitably became more important to the organization's success.

DOCTORS PRACTICING IN HOSPITALS

The growing importance of hospitals to medical practice posed a severe problem for most members of the profession at one time. While the few physicians who held hospital appointments were gaining a more decisive role, most practitioners were cut off from access to hospital practice. Perhaps as few as 2 percent of American physicians held hospital privileges in the 1870s. This narrow monopoly may not have been of much consequence, since the few hospitals then in existence were used almost entirely by the poor. By 1910, a survey in the Bronx and Manhattan showed only about 10 percent held hospital positions, even though hospitals had grown enormously in number and importance (Starr, 1982).

While patterns of organization varied, the medical staff of late-nineteenth-century charity hospitals was typically arranged in four groups:

- A consulting staff, composed of older and distinguished physicians who had no regular duties
- A visiting or attending staff, made up of the active physicians, who supervised treatment
- A resident or house staff of young doctors in training, who carried out the details of treatment
- A dispensary staff, who saw outpatients

Of these groups, the visiting physicians were the most important. They generally served for rotating periods of three or four months per year, a system that reduced the burden on each physician, while allowing a much larger number to derive whatever advantage there might be from the name of being connected with the institution (Davis & Rorem, 1932).

Charity hospitals paid none of these doctors for their work. The house physicians gave their services for a year or 18 months in exchange for room, board, and experience. The dispensary staff gave theirs in the hope of obtaining appointments as visiting physicians and to make themselves known to patients, who might then come to their private offices. The visiting staff provided its labor in return for access to surgical facilities, opportunities to specialize, prestige, the use of capital that the community invested in hospitals, and regular contacts with colleagues, which might open the way to referrals, consultations, and professional recognition. Thus, hospital appointments became more valuable to individual solo physicians as hospitals became indispensable for surgical practice and advanced specialization.

But while their value increased, hospital appointments remained concentrated in the hands of a small professional elite. Among general practitioners, resentment of hospitals was widespread. Hospital managers were accused of arbitrary treatment to take advantage of the doctors' desire for hospital affiliation. Because of their superior equipment and personnel concentrated in one location, and because of their superior ability to reduce the threat of infections, the hospitals and their appointed physicians were killing private surgical work that had previously taken place in homes or offices. At that point in time, even well-to-do patients might enter private hospitals, perhaps paying nothing, because hospital rules permitted no private fees to be taken since physicians were considered to be donating their time and skills to charity. This widely resented rule forbidding physicians to take fees from private patients, which had been established at the older voluntary hospitals began to die out, but only gradually. The first step in this process of breaking down the old charitable tradition permitted physicians to charge patients in private rooms but still barred fees in public wards. Hospitals also began to allow physicians not on the staff to treat paying patients in unused private rooms (Starr, 1982).

Private practitioners protested against "patient stealing" by hospital staff doctors who made no charge for their services, while physicians who had formerly been in charge lost both patients and the fees that would have been theirs had the patients been treated at home. The private physicians who were not appointed to the staff wanted hospital authorities to abide by the medical profession's code of ethics, as well as guard their proprietary interests. They also wanted adherence by the hospital staff to the professional vow of silence and noninterference, so that patients would not hear disparaging remarks about their private doctor's ability. Another reason was that the hospital staff might revise the diagnosis and treatment plan. By sending patients to hospitals, private doctors could risk, not only losing their fees, but being discredited to their patients with another image of their competence (Starr, 1982).

SHAPING THE HOSPITAL MEDICAL STAFF

Physicians started asking why they did not control more of the hospital setting. One way to gain control was to be involved with a proprietary institution. Small private hospitals were built by some surgeons for their own cases, while others were joint ventures among several practitioners. To supply enough patients to make the hospitals profitable, competing doctors often had to combine their efforts. The creation of doctor-controlled hospitals was easiest in small towns throughout the country and in the rising cities of the West, where there had never been the large, charitable, trustee-dominated institutions. In the early years of the twentieth century, more proprietary than charitable hospitals were being built. They were opened mainly by physicians who had no hospital privileges elsewhere or who had positions but felt the hospitals were not providing adequate accommodations for their private patients. The increased competition from these new enterprises catering to paying patients from the middle and upper classes forced the older voluntary hospitals to find new ways to adjust because the loss of clients and revenue might become a painful reality. The threat to take patients elsewhere has an ancient history, often for very good reasons.

Soon there was a movement to open up hospitals to doctors not formerly on their staffs. It was proven that the open door to a hospital is a benefit, not only to the rank and file of doctors, but to the hospital: "It pays in dollars and cents" (*National Hospital Record,* 1907). Not everyone was convinced. Some critics saw opened medical staffs as undisciplined and wasteful, as well as potentially damaging to patients. General practitioners naturally saw closed staffing as a way to maintain privilege rather than quality, since they were usually excluded. One of the reasons expounded for allowing new physicians to join open hospital medical staffs was that hospitals served to educate doctors and that extending privileges to all members of the profession would enable them to keep up with new advances. The value of hospital-based continuing medical education (CME) has deep roots in history.

Open Staffs Bring More Patients

In the end, the decision proved to be based on financial considerations. Voluntary hospitals had multiplied in great numbers and many had fallen seriously into debt. Hospitals would fail without support from local physicians, because the income from private patients depended largely on the medical staff. If the staff could be expanded to ensure the presence of large and profitable practices, then a sufficient amount of money could be realized to defray the entire running expenses of the institution, supplying the care, not only for the private patients, but also for the charity cases (Starr, 1982).

With that hope in mind, hospital boards expanded the number of positions for doctors who could serve as "feeders" to fill their beds. The proportion of hospital-affiliated physicians rose to more than 50 percent of the profession. Almost no hospitals, except for research institutions, were totally closed, since they all generally had a courtesy staff with the privilege of attending patients in private rooms. On the other hand, no hospitals were totally open either, since even hospitals with large courtesy staffs limited their access to charity wards. The number of affiliated physicians continued to rise, to 66 percent in 1930 and more than 80 percent by 1940 (Rosner, 1977).

Even if more doctors gained entry to a hospital in their community, they did not necessarily gain equal access on the same footing as other physicians or to hospitals of equivalent status and quality. Black physicians and most of the foreign-born were almost completely unrepresented on many hospital staffs. These kinds of inequities persisted. When doctors from lower-status ethnic backgrounds obtained positions, they might do so at the lower levels of the system. Sometimes, hospital medical staff appointments depended largely on nontechnical considerations, such as personality and social background (Starr, 1982).

Doctors and Hospitals Needed Each Other

The continued dependence of practitioners on hospitals throughout their careers made them dependent on what Hall identified as the "inner fraternity" of the profession. "The freelance practitioner," he wrote, "has gradually been supplanted by one whose career depends on his relationship with a network of institutions" (Hall, 1946). Access to favored positions in that network came through "sponsorship" by a community's established physicians, who could advance or exclude aspirants at various stages of their careers by influencing professional school admissions, dispensing hospital appointments, referring patients, and designating protégés and successors. Because the hospital was essential to a successful practice, its various grades could be used as delicately calibrated rewards to signal the progress of a career. Although opening up hospitals to more doctors weakened the elite's traditional monopoly over hospital medical staff appointments, it brought greater control over the individual members of the profession. Glaser wrote that "this use of hospitalization privileges makes America one of the few countries in the world with any controls over the quality of private practice" (Glaser, 1963).

It is unclear whether this power over the quality of private practice in the hospital, if not in the office or on home calls, did raise its level, but there can be no doubt that it was used to exclude doctors unacceptable to the organized profession. By the 1920s membership in the local medical society had become an informal prerequisite for membership on the medical staff of most local community hospitals. In 1934 the AMA tried to institutionalize its control over hospital appointments by requiring that all hospitals accredited for internship training to appoint no one to their staff except members of the local medical society. Since black doctors were excluded from most of these societies, they could be excluded from hospital positions. So could anyone else, such as HMO doctors, who threatened to rock the economic boat of private practice, fee-for-service medicine. The private practitioners, who had first seen hospitals as a threat to their position, had succeeded in turning them into an instrument of professional power (Starr, 1982).

General hospitals had become a necessary adjunct of medical practice. Physicians who were excluded from the staff of existing general hospitals formed new ones. Doctors in small towns opened hospitals to prevent their big-city colleagues/competitors from drawing away their patients. The hospital medical staff had been formed and recognized as essential to the success and financial viability of both hospitals and doctors. Hospital administrations and boards wanted doctors to be members of their medical staff and practice in their hospital. Doctors wanted and needed to practice in hospitals and were both willing and eager to join the medical staff, such as it was. The hospital medical staff had now achieved reality and status. The next step would be to take its position as an equal member of the three-part organizational structure of the modern American community hospital.

What remained, now, was to develop a mechanism for developing consistency and comparability across and among these groups of doctors in hospitals. That mechanism could have been developed by some level of government, but it did not happen that way. It could have been developed by an alliance of hospital boards trying to corral and control these increasingly possessive and aggressive doctors, but it did not happen that way, either. There never was a chance that hospital administrators could act in concert to bring about such major change that would add consistency and professional control to emerging medical staffs, as they were known at the time.

Instead, the movement toward the modern hospital medical staff, the Joint Commission on the Accreditation of Healthcare Organizations model of a medical staff, was brought about by the doctors themselves, acting to exert greater control over each other regarding credentials and practice. They did it voluntarily, to themselves and to each other. No one forced them to do it.

SUMMARY

Physicians have not always occupied the same positions of honor and comfort as they enjoy today. From humble beginnings, modern medical practice has evolved into an elaborate system of specialized knowledge, technical procedures, and rules of behavior. The role and authority of individual doctors accumulated into a powerful profession with social privilege, economic power, and political influence.

While those earlier physicians were standing at the margins of the gentry class, they were usually poorly trained and practiced alone. Their skills gained from apprenticeships were usually contained in their black bags while treating patients in their homes with almost no time at all spent in hospitals. The profession was weak, divided, insecure in its status and income and unable to control entry into practice, raise standards of medical education, or assert collective authority over its members. Social changes, scientific advances, growth of hospitals, and specialization caused doctors to become more dependent on each other for referrals and access to facilities.

More technology was concentrated in hospitals, "kitchen surgery" declined, treatment shifted from the household to the hospital, and medical care became a market commodity. The radical metamorphosis of hospitals from places of impurity and human wreckage into citadels of science and bureaucracy required a transition from caring for the poor to curing the middle and upper classes, thus earning patient revenues. Hospitals needed doctors to bring patients, especially those who could pay, and fill beds, while doctors needed hospitals for their sources of personnel and equipment. The hospital medical staff was shaped, but a mechanism to exert greater control over its members was still needed.

REFERENCES

Ashley, J. A. (1976). *Hospitals, Paternalism, and the Role of the Nurse.* New York: Teachers College Press.

Cartwright, F. F. (1967). *The Development of Modern Surgery.* London: Arthur Barker.

Crocker, S. E. (1899). The invalid in home and hospital. *National Hospital Record, 2,* 7–9.

Davis, M. M., & Rorem, C. R. (1932). *The Crisis in Hospital Finance.* Chicago: University of Chicago Press.

Gerster, A. G. (1906). System of American hospital economy. *National Hospital Record, 9,* 17–19.

Glaser, W. (1963). American and foreign hospitals: some sociological comparisons. In Friedson, E. (Ed.), *The Hospital in Modern Society.* New York: Free Press.

Hall, O. (1946). The informal organization of the medical profession. *Canadian Journal of Economics and Political Science, 12,* 30–44.

Hobson, E. C. (1914). *Recollections of a Happy Life.* New York: privately printed.

May, L. A. (1993). The physiologic and psychological bases of health, disease, and care-seeking. In Williams, S. J., & Torrens, P. R. (Eds.), *Introduction to Health Services (4th ed.).* Albany: Delmar Publishers.

National Hospital Record, 10(March). (1907). Hospitals and general practitioners.

Nutting, M. A., & Dock, L. L. (1907). *A History of Nursing.* New York: Putnam.

Roemer, M. I., & Friedman, J. W. (1971). *Doctors in Hospitals.* Baltimore: Johns Hopkins Press.

Rosner, D. (1977). Bedside business. Unpublished manuscript, Harvard University. Cited in Lewinski-Corwin, E. H., (1924) *Hospital Situation in Greater New York.* New York: Putnam.

Starr, P. (1982). *The Social Transformation of American Medicine.* New York: Basic Books. Copyright © 1982 by Paul Starr. Reprinted by permission of Basic Books, a division of Harper Collins Publishers, Inc.

Torrens, P. R. (1993). Historical evolution and overview of health services in the United States. In Williams, S. J., & Torrens, P. R. (Eds.). *Introduction to Health Services (4th ed.).* Albany: Delmar Publishers.

CHAPTER

The Modern Hospital Medical Staff

The regulatory structure chosen by the medical profession to control quality was voluntary accreditation that became the Joint Commission on the Accreditation of Healthcare Organizations. However, that does not mean that there are not many other regulatory forces affecting both hospitals and doctors. Hospitals are a highly regulated industry, with external controls over

- institutional quality standards, which include licensure and certification as well as accreditation;
- construction and expansion of facilities and services by certificate of need programs, as well as local zoning requirements;

- costs or rates, federal and state payment programs, rate regulation programs, and private sector influences by insurers and health plans;
- utilization, by federal and state monitors, as well as the private payer use controls.

REGULATION OF HOSPITALS AND DOCTORS

The regulatory structure for controlling quality includes state licensure, federal certification, and the voluntary accreditation. Licensure is a state function, generally carried out by the department of health, whereby minimum standards are established and enforced regarding the equipment, personnel, physical plant, and safety features an institution must have to operate (Haglund & Dowling, 1993). Licensing agencies are empowered to set standards, conduct inspections, issue licenses, close down facilities that cannot comply with the agency's standards, and provide consultation services. In some states, the agency is underfunded and understaffed, so that standards are not en-forced stringently. Lack of enforcement does not mean that standards are not valuable for monitoring and protecting the quality of patient care; it just means that there will be a tendency to focus more on fire, safety, and physical plant standards rather than on standards for medical services.

There are also external regulatory or legal restrictions on physicians that derive mostly from federal or state legislation, including

- federal antitrust statutes, which prohibit combinations and conspiracies in restraint of trade, such as: price fixing, monopolies, boycotts, tying arrangements, and horizontal division of markets;
- state corporate practice of medicine laws, which prohibits ownership or management of clinical aspects of physician practice by persons or organizations other than physicians;
- Internal Revenue Code for not-for-profit organizations, which prohibits the receipt of benefits by insiders or of more than incidental benefits by other private parties;
- Medicare-Medicaid fraud and abuse regulations, which prohibit payment or receipt of remuneration of any kind for the referral of Medicare and Medicaid patients;
- state fee-splitting laws, which prohibit rebates or kickbacks to physicians in return for referrals (Snook, 1992).

Physicians' professional conduct is monitored closely, following the creation of the National Practitioner Data Bank in 1990 to prevent physicians, as well as other health care professionals, from hiding acts of malpractice and professional misbehavior by moving to other states and practicing under another license. Sources of data for the bank include mandatory reporting by hospitals, malpractice insurers, and state licensing boards. Hospitals must inquire from the data bank during the credentialing process.

Having now mentioned some of the external regulatory forces affecting hospitals and doctors, the focus turns to the voluntary accreditation mechanism to control quality of care, which was created by the doctors themselves, with help later by the hospital industry. In medicine, quality is not the same as quantity, cost, cost efficiency, utilization of health care, or medical care. Quality is not consistent across the board; it may vary from time to time in hospitals and among physicians. Defining quality of care can be an elusive target, but a traditional view by physicians is that quality of care must depend on the credentials of the provider. There is a deep-seated, long-standing belief that physicians who are more highly trained are usually better than those who are less well trained. There is another truism that has been accepted in recent years following the publication of a number of research studies: the doctor who performs a higher number of procedures is less likely to make mistakes or have bad outcomes than the doctor who performs fewer.

Many doctors believe that the real test of quality of care is the outcome—how did it turn out? When the physicians and the medical team treated the patient, did the patient recover and did the patient have good results? In their peer review discussions, physicians also define quality with respect to the technical aspects of care, including the quality of the diagnostic and therapeutic aspects of care. Patients may have a different view of quality, equating it with relief of symptoms, functional improvement, empathy from practitioners, and the satisfaction of psychological and physical needs, including the comfort of the hospital stay (Snook, 1992).

Some experts say that quality is a function of the medical service given patients at a specific point in time by a specific doctor to a specific patient. Peer review consists of attempting to evaluate after the fact whether there was a scientific approach to the establishment of a diagnosis and institution of appropriate therapy and management, designed to satisfy the overall needs of the patient. Patient care services should increase the probability of desired patient outcomes, reduce the probability of undesired outcomes, and be readily available, efficiently rendered, and properly documented. The quality improvement process in hospitals should be ongoing; it should measure and evaluate the professional services rendered to patients in the hospital by the doctors. It should be measured by prevailing and accepted standards of care, and its end product should be the improvement of care. The duty of the voluntary accreditation process is to verify that systems are in place in the hospital that will change the behavior of health team members, improve the overall quality of patient care, and, particularly, document that such processes have actually taken place.

THE JOINT COMMISSION MODEL

The professionally sponsored, voluntary accreditation process that has been alluded to frequently, is the Joint Commission on the Accreditation of Healthcare Organizations, which in 1987 renamed itself from its original title: The Joint Commission on the Accreditation of Hospitals. To everyone in the field, it is simply known as the "Joint Commission," and that is the way it will often be referred to here. JCAHO is a private, nonprofit organization dedicated to promoting quality health care through a voluntary accreditation process of hospital surveys (Gassiot & Starr, 1987). It is sponsored by national associations and governed by a board of 28 commissioners, composed of representatives of the major national health care professions and the hospital industry as well as six public members and one member of the nursing profession (Kent, 1995). The organizational members include:

- American College of Physicians (three representatives)
- American College of Surgeons (three representatives)
- American Dental Association (one representatives)
- American Hospital Association (seven representatives)
- American Medical Association (seven representatives)

JCAHO can trace its roots to a program called the Hospital Standardization Program that was established by the American College of Surgeons in 1918 (Snook, 1992). The program was established to enable surgeons to understand and appreciate the uniform medical records format that would enable them to evaluate members who wished to apply for fellowship status in the American College of Surgeons. ACS then joined with the other national organizations to form the Joint Commission, which began the survey program and the granting of accreditation on January 1, 1952. Although JCAHO was launched as an educational organization, it gained its present power—and took on the overtones of regulation that earn it hostility—when Medicare was passed in 1966.

When Congress created Medicare, lawmakers amended the Social Security Act to give JCAHO (then, as now, the most experienced accrediting body in the nation) "deeming authority." Under the law, the Health Care Financing Agency (HCFA) deems that JCAHO-accredited facilities meet Medicare standards of certification, subject to validation surveys by HCFA. The provider hospital (or other facility) is then eligible for Medicare reimbursement. In theory, hospitals do not need to turn to the Joint Commission for accreditation, but an overwhelming majority do. Their other options for accreditation are state agencies, most of which accept Joint Commission accreditation for licensure purposes (Kent, 1995). It has become customary for most private insurers and managed care organizations to make JCAHO accreditation a condition of reimbursement.

The original action by the American College of Surgeons was the product of a professional attempt to tighten the medical organizations of hospitals. Doctors' access to hospitals was expanding at that time, and a desire to assure minimum standards led the American College of Surgeons to adopt a requirement that hospitals wishing to receive its approval under the Standardization Program must organize their physicians into a "definite medical staff." The staff could be open or closed, with as many active, associate, or courtesy members as desired, so long as they were restricted to competent and reputable physicians, engaged in no fee-splitting, abided by formal bylaws, and held monthly meetings and reviews of clinical experiences. In 1919 the AMA's Council of Medical Education set minimum standards for hospital internships, the next year changing its name to the Council on Medical Education and Hospitals (Snook, 1992). Though compliance with these normative bodies was voluntary, and still is, they pushed the emerging hospitals and medical staffs to more formally structured, more hierarchial organizations.

More structure and more formal organization of hospitals not only continued but increased the dependence of practitioners on hospitals throughout their careers. Opening up more hospitals to more doctors weakened the traditional monopoly of an elite number of hospital-based specialists and brought greater control and homogeneity to the profession in its never-ending movement toward the organization and structure of a medical staff now recognized and called the Joint Commission model.

The Joint Commission model of a hospital medical staff is currently in use in most hospitals in the United States, whether public, private, or military. Haglund and Dowling (1993) noted that 75 percent of the nation's community hospitals and more than 95 percent of those with more than 200 beds are accredited by the Joint Commission. Kent (1995) stated that the JCAHO currently accredits—or certifies as meeting certain standards of quality—more than 11,000 health care organizations in the United States, including about 5,300 hospitals and 6,000 home care, ambulatory care, long-term care, and mental health care providers.

Standards expressed in successive versions of the *Accreditation Manual for Hospitals,* published by the Joint Commission have outlined the design, role, function, and behavior of hospital medical staffs through the years. The model that is in place now and is accepted by hospital medical staffs as the one and only "right way" has replaced models of earlier decades and is specified succinctly in the *Comprehensive Accreditation Manual for Hospitals* Medical Staff Standard MS 1 (JCAHO, 1996, p. 484):

> There is a single organized, self-governing medical staff that has overall responsibility for the quality of the professional services provided by individuals with clinical privileges, as well as the responsibility of accounting therefor to the governing body.

The manual defines clinical privileges as

> authorization granted by the governing body to a practioner to provide specific patient care services in the hospital within defined limits, based on an individual practitioner's license, education, training, experience, competence, health status, and judgment.

Further, as stated in Medical Staff Standard MS 1.1.3:

> All medical staff members and all others with delineated clinical privileges are subject to medical staff and departmental bylaws, rules and regulations, and policies and are subject to review as part of the organization's performance-improvement activities.

The original purpose of hospital medical staffs in the Joint Commission model was to assure patient safety in a time when it was less certain who the applicants were and how well trained they had been. While not losing that focus, over time the currently stated purpose has evolved and is the hallmark of present-day surveys: to review and evaluate the quality of patient care provided by private practitioners. The medical profession set out in 1919 to find a mechanism for monitoring and evaluating the quality of care delivered by its own members, and it has done that. Actually, it is the hospital that is accredited by the Joint Commission, but the medical staff is carefully reviewed, and the result of that review can threaten the hospital's accreditation. Perhaps that reality has given rise to a belief that in the name of a successful accreditation, hospital administration can make doctors do something they might not otherwise want to do, that somehow present-day members of the staff might not feel as strongly about review as did the American College of Surgeons when it began the whole process.

Sometimes, it seems almost ludicrous to hear hospital leaders and doctors rail against the Joint Commission as if it is some band of foreign invaders, when in fact it is their national membership organizations that own and run JCAHO. Hospitals and doctors pay dues to those national lobbying groups in order to receive necessary and desirable services, usually for better reimbursements. The seeming refusal to recognize and acknowledge ownership and responsibility for JCAHO by the profession and the industry calls to mind the ultimate aphorism by Walt Kelly, which has been so widely quoted in his famous line from *Pogo:* "we have met the enemy and it is us." The Joint Commission is not an enemy, of course, but it is a handy scapegoat to beat on and blame for requiring standards and conditions that hospitals and doctors should be doing on their own without being forced. For the past 30 years, the Joint Commission has had a virtual monopoly over hospital accreditation, but there are clouds on the horizon that may change the situation in the years to come, as the health care delivery system consolidates and purchasers seek more accurate, detailed, and timely quality and cost information.

Early 1995 saw a JCAHO response to criticisms by the hospital industry and the medical profession about the accreditation process. The stated problems included poor customer service, high cost, and marketing of publications and seminars: charges that were acknowledged by JCAHO as being valid, particularly that of inadequate customer response.

Some health experts believe that providers' unhappiness is a sign that the Joint Commission is doing its job more effectively than in the past (*Medicine and Health,* 1995). It could have been a coincidence, but the outcry came at the same time that JCAHO began publicly releasing individual hospital quality reports. The character and focus of the Joint Commission have come from the interests of its sponsoring organizations. The fact that the interests of those organizations also may serve well the interests and well-being of hospital patients is to the everlasting credit of all concerned. Voluntary policing, even if it seems forced, is one of the most admirable strengths of the professions in the United States.

What would happen if the major provider associations withdrew their support from the Joint Commission? Would the organization collapse? Nearly all observers, according to Christina Kent (1995), say that scenario is not likely to happen, because the main alternative to JCAHO is the federal government, and both hospitals and doctors have long maintained that they would rather be accredited by a private body than by a government regulator. It really becomes a question of "whom do you trust least?" But this struggle for control is not over, and the backstage battle will continue so long as there is power and money at stake.

Benefits of JCAHO Accreditation

In carrying out its mission to enhance the quality of care and services rendered in organized health care settings, JCAHO develops and continually refines standards, performs accreditation surveys to measure a facility's compliance with the standards, and offers assistance in improving the quality of care through educational workshops and seminars, informative publications, and a speaker's bureau. When a hospital or other surveyed facility demonstrates substantial compliance with the standards, the Joint Commission awards a certificate of accreditation, which hangs on the wall of the hospital somewhere near the front entrance.

The standards of the Joint Commission are focused on the quality of patient care and the safety of the environment in which care is provided. Every effort is made by the staff and surveyors to reflect the state of the art in health care and to provide reasonable guidelines. New standards are adopted only after extensive field review and only after national consensus is achieved. As a result of the application of this national program that grants accreditation in a similar manner all across the country, there are several benefits gained:

• Providing a motivational force for continued self-improvement and representing to the public a recognizable commitment to excellent quality care

- Designating "Deemed Status," which qualifies a hospital to receive Medicare and Medicaid reimbursement without undergoing routine federal or state certification inspection
- Expediting reimbursement from insurance companies and other payer organizations and agencies
- Fulfilling all or major portions of state licensure requirements

The hospital that has become accredited says to its community, patients, and staff that it wants to meet high standards and that it has taken the time and effort to have the recognized national accrediting body, the Joint Commission, come in to measure it against a set standard. Accreditation says to a hospital's medical staff, employees, and patients that the environment is of high quality and that the doctors and personnel are qualified to provide high-quality care. And, the process of accreditation says to the community that the board, administration, and medical staff together are a responsible institution that takes its obligation for patient care seriously and has asked an independent, objective group to come in and review it (Snook, 1992).

The Survey Process

A facility seeking Joint Commission accreditation asks to be surveyed. The Joint Commission sends the hospital a detailed questionnaire that cites the standards for a hospital. After the hospital staff completes the questionnaire and returns it, a survey team is assigned by JCAHO and a date is selected for a site visit to the hospital.

The questionnaire, and thus the standards, are concerned with three major areas: services, organization and structure, and the physical plant. There is a major emphasis placed on the scope and quality of services the hospital renders to the patient. The survey team reviews the medical staff organization and systems, the nursing procedures, the dietary procedures, the pharmacy, the laboratory department, the x-ray or imaging department, and the emergency services department. The point of these reviews is to determine whether the services provided are adequate for patients.

Surveys also study the principles of organization and administration: whether there is an effective hospital bylaws structure; whether there are written and updated policies and procedures. The surveyors determine whether the hospital requires its departments to meet on a regular basis and to render written reports. Appropriately, there is close attention paid to the physical plant and the overall environment in the hospital. This includes life-safety code problems, adequate sprinkler systems, large and uncluttered corridors, proper safety exits, and the like.

A more recent focus of Joint Commission surveyors has been to spend a great deal of time and effort on quality assurance reviews in patient care areas. The surveyors review patient medical records to determine whether the care given was appropriate for that specific case and whether the documentation supports the actions taken.

In turn, JCAHO sends out presurvey materials designed to aid a facility in its preparation for survey. The length in days of each individual survey depends on the size and complexity of the facility being surveyed. The survey team, usually a doctor, a nurse, and a hospital administrator, arrives at the institution, observes its operation, interviews key staff members and physicians, spends time reviewing pertinent documents, and holds educational training sessions. Each member of the survey team has specific areas to investigate and study. During the survey, which is actually an inspection of the hospital, the surveyors write down in detail any deficiencies they observe and then make certain recommendations. Before they leave the hospital, they give their lists with recommendations to the hospital administrator. The chief of the medical staff should be a full participant during the entire survey, but it is particularly important for the chief to be present and involved at the end of the process.

Summation conferences and full exit briefings are held upon the completion of the review. The survey team goes over with the administration, medical staff leaders, and appropriate board officers exactly what they found that needs improvement and what they recommend on the basis of their experience in conducting surveys all over the country. This should be an open and candid discussion about how the hospital can improve itself. There have been complaints in the past that at these important exit conferences, surveyors held back on their opinions and descriptions of problems found. Then, when the final report came out, things that were said to be in good shape at the exit conference showed up as violations.

The team's findings and recommendations are then sent to the central office of the Joint Commission for analysis and review before an accreditation decision is rendered, based on the findings of the survey. About 85 percent of the hospitals surveyed receive accreditation, some with modifiers (Snook, 1992). That decision is made to the hospital administration in confidence, and it is the choice of the hospital to publicize the notice or to just put the plaque with the certificate of accreditation on the wall and forgo any public announcement. Accreditation may be awarded for a maximum three-year period. There can be other provisional or contingent awards, including focused resurveys on stated items in question, usually conducted at specified intervals. If the hospital has received the three-year accreditation, then in the year before the next visit it must complete a detailed questionnaire identifying what it has done about the deficiencies noted in the previous survey.

Joint Commission accreditation surveys, sometimes frustrating, always time-consuming and expensive—paid by the hospital and not the doctors—are also frequently helpful and educational. The survey serves the useful purpose of forcing internal self-discipline on health care institutions, causing self-examinations of policies and procedures when it would be much less bother and more comfortable not to pay attention to such details. Some of the other reasons why accreditation matters include

- possible loss of reimbursement from nearly all payers
- possible increase in fees for professional liability insurance
- loss of eligibility to maintain an accredited residency program
- significant loss of prestige and public image
- challenges from the medical staff, nurses, medical groups, and payers concerning the hospital's dedication to patient care quality
- difficulty in establishing contracts to provide service to HMO or other managed care programs
- difficulty in recruiting young physicians who must work in fully accredited institutions before becoming eligible to take board examinations (Gill, 1993)

Throughout its history, the JCAHO has filled a major gap in the evaluation of hospitals in this country. Continuing the unique historical pattern of combined public-private approaches, the Joint Commission is a unique organization that legislates and regulates in a world where government and bureaucracy seem to control so much. The Joint Commission has been responsive to the hospitals and to the federal government through Medicare. It has provided an inconspicuous but very real service to patients and communities. It has elevated and maintained high professional standards while acting as an advisory group to hospitals. It has been influential in urging them to improve their life-safety measures, their quality improvement programs, and their overall organizations—all of that without being forced by government intervention. However, it must be noted that there has always been some amount of sentiment that hospital compliance with standards and regulation is a proper function of government and that there should be public surveillance rather than the voluntary, cooperative, private agency approach represented by the JCAHO.

MEDICAL STAFF ORGANIZATION AND STRUCTURE

The governing board delegates responsibility for the provision of high-quality patient care to the medical staff, which is formally organized to carry out this responsibility and is accountable for it to the board (Haglund & Dowling, 1993). As has already been noted, the medical staffs of community hospitals in the United States are composed mostly of private practitioners who are not employees of the hospital. This approach stands in direct contrast to the hospital medical staffs of most other advanced countries, which are composed of salaried physicians who are hospital based. The relationship between the hospital and the medical staff is mutually dependent, in fact, and is mutually supportive, in theory. Sometimes, of course, it is downright stressful. The hospital is dependent on the medical staff to admit and care for patients and monitor the quality of care. In one sense, the customers of the hospital are the doctors, since it is they who admit the patients, decide how long they will stay, and order hospital services to be performed by the employee staff. On the other hand, physicians—particularly specialists—are dependent on hospitals because, in order to practice modern medicine, they must have access to the diagnostic and therapeutic services available nowhere else.

Thus, a quid pro quo relationship exists. Physicians agree to abide by hospital policies and medical staff rules and to devote time to the medical staff's quality monitoring program. In return, they receive the privilege of using the community's accumulated assets to care for their private patients. At one time, they also contributed their efforts to care for patients who could not pay. As the number of public patients on Medicaid grew, and there was an increase in the number of no-pay patients, now some doctors not only will not care for those unable to pay but will not care for those not able to pay enough.

In carrying out its delegated responsibility for ensuring the quality of care, the medical staff governs itself, establishes qualifications for appointment to the staff and for clinical privileges, establishes standards of care and rules and regulations to guide the provision of care, and supervises the professional performance of its members. These duties are accomplished within the written provisions of the medical staff bylaws, which set forth the form, functions, and responsibilities of the medical staff. The bylaws must be approved by both the medical staff and the governing board (Gassiot & Starr, 1987).

The elected leader of the medical staff organization, who functions in an administrative as well as political role is the chief of staff, sometimes now called the president of the medical staff. The chief or president is responsible for

- acting as a liaison among the governing board, the administration, and the medical staff (increasingly, the chief performs liaison duties with the hospital employees and the larger outside community);
- chairing the executive committee of the medical staff and serving as an ex officio member of all committees and usually of the governing board (most chiefs now sit as a part of or at least as a regular invitee of the management council or whatever the name is of the group chaired by the CEO or administrator);
- establishing medical staff committees, ad hoc work groups, or special purpose investigative groups, and appointing members of all those bodies;
- enforcing governing board policies, as well as sponsoring reviews of those policies and revisions when the hospital would be better served by revisions of those policies;
- enforcing medical staff bylaws, rules, and regulations, even at great personal risk when that enforcement is not politically popular with some members of the staff;

- maintaining standards of medical care within the hospital, which can be a difficult process given that there are so many strong egos and personalities involved;
- providing for continuing medical education for the physicians and encouraging participation and involvement by the technical staff when that presence will help improve the quality of patient care.

Later chapters will delve much more deeply into the many roles of chiefs. That person also serves in a sense as one of the hospital's administrative and governance structure. The chief of staff is consulted by the board for advice on medical matters, as well for assurance that the medical staff collectively are carrying out their responsibilities in such a dedicated manner that the hospital is not in a position of needing to worry about risk management. Supervision, administration, management: by whatever name, the role of chief is guaranteed to be a time-consuming job, particularly because, in most modern American community hospitals, the chief also attempts to maintain the semblance of a busy private practice.

Most of the organizational responsibilities of the medical staff are carried out by some sort of committee structure. The executive committee is the key administrative and policymaking body of the medical staff. It governs the activities of the medical staff, and all other committees are advisory to it. Executive committees are usually composed of the chief(s) of staff, the chiefs or chairs of the various clinical departments, and members at large elected by the active medical staff. In some hospitals, a joint conference committee can function as a formal liaison link between the governing board and medical staff and includes members from both groups as well as the administrator. In some hospitals, a joint conference committee is a standing group that meets regularly. In others, a joint conference committee can be called to convene as needed, on the call of either the administration or the chief. The purpose of this party of the three parts is to provide a forum for discussing medical matters or problems of mutual concern to all.

Most hospitals have a credentials committee, or subcommittee, which reviews departmental recommendations as to the qualifications of applicants to the medical staff for initial appointment. Credentials committees do some of their best work in reviewing reappointment applications, since the members of the credentials committee are probably fairly senior in their service and know an appropriate application when they see one. Their gatekeeper function is irreplaceably valuable when it works correctly. Similarly, nothing can be quite so damaging as their dereliction of duty when the credentials committee acts to rubber stamp all the "familiar faces" without real review. Credentials committees make recommendations regarding initial appointments and privileges and reappointments and privileges. Credentials committees do not single-handedly make decisions; their recommendations are forwarded to the Executive Committee for consideration. That body's recommendations are transmitted to the hospital governing board, which has final decision-making power. There are sometimes some misunderstandings about who actually makes these decisions. It is not the clinical department, although that group has a large responsibility for making good recommendations, since they are truly the peers who should know the technical capabilities of the applicant. It is not the credentials committee, it is not even the executive committee. Only the board may make these decisions.

A second type of medical staff committee oversees specific functional areas, or departments; examples include emergency, pharmacy, special care, and disaster committees. A third type of committee is the evaluative or quality improvement committee, which might have been formerly called quality assurance. Its job is to monitor the patient care provided by individual physicians and to monitor their behavior as well. Monitor does not mean see that it is happening, say that it is happening, and adjourn the meeting. It means documenting departures from standards of care and recommending corrective action. The names of quality improvement committees differ from hospital to hospital, but some common ones are medical audit, utilization review, resource consumption, and (sometimes) tissue committees for surgery. In addition, there is a continuing medical education (CME) committee that plans and carries out education programs for the medical staff and hospital technical employees (Snook, 1992).

The structure of the medical staff and the behavior of that structure affect quality of care and other aspects of the hospital climate, culture, and performance. The degree of structure of the medical staff and the way that structure carries out its mission influences the costliness, quality, and scope of hospital services. What matters most are clearly specified policies, rules, and regulations; thorough documentation of medical staff activities; a core of full-time, hospital-based physicians (e.g., radiologists, pathologists, anesthesiologists, emergency department physicians), and, above all, a willingness to disturb the status quo. This type of organizational pattern offers the private physicians who use the hospital the benefits of full-time hospital-based physicians who provide leadership, administrative support and supervision, and forward movement in developing standards of care and educational programs. The medical staff works well when the core of full-time physicians stimulate the other doctors to take their quality monitoring responsibilities more seriously. What does not work well is when those full-time physicians who have an exclusive contract for their specialty act together as a partnership to not monitor their colleagues and to not lead the other attending physicians in a productive manner. Protectionism never has worked well in national politics and it does not work well in the medical staff either.

At best, the mix of hospital-based and private physicians tend to provide an environment that is conducive for change and quality improvement. When the medical staff as a group and the chief, the department chairs and other leading physicians as individuals participate in hospital decision making, then there is a powerful tool available for strengthening the overall quality of care, which is the reason the organized medical staff exists in the first place.

PATIENT SAFETY TO REVIEWING EACH OTHER

Through its history, the JCAHO has filled a major gap in the evaluation of doctors and hospitals in this country. Continuing the uniquely American historical pattern of combined private-public approaches, the Joint Commission itself is a unique organization that legislates and regulates in a world where government and bureaucracy seem to control so much. The Joint Commission truly rules with the consent of the governed. It has been responsive to doctors and hospitals, as well as the government through Medicare. It has provided an inconspicuous but very real service to patients and communities. It has elevated and maintained high professional standards while acting as an advocate group to hospitals and their medical staffs. Joint Commission surveyors have been influential in urging hospitals to improve their life-safety measures, their quality improvement programs, and their overall organizations. All of this has been done without being forced by government intervention. It must be noted that there has always been some undercurrent of sentiment that hospital and physician compliance with standards and regulations is a proper function of government and that one or more federal agencies should be doing the surveying and accrediting. That sentiment obviously believes that there should be public surveillance rather than the voluntary, cooperative, private agency approach represented by the JCAHO.

Thus, it can be seen that the traditional structure of JCAHO model hospitals is the familiar mix of a governing board with legal authority and responsibility, an administration carrying out board policy and economic strategic plans, and a medical staff divided into subgroups in some manner. To most practicing physicians on hospital medical staffs, an organizational chart would apparently be viewed like an industrial or military hierarchy, such as the one shown in Figure 3-1.

It does not actually work that way, of course, but it seems self-evident to private physicians who do not really care much about what the hospital does so long as the services, personnel, and equipment they want are immediately available when they want it. When all of those things are not on instant recall 24 hours a day, seven days a week, there can be much resulting friction and hostility, such as happened during the fee-for-service era when doctors had more leverage. Hospital administration was cast as the enemy of doctors, expressed in volumes of rhetoric in doctors' lounges. Hospital administrators and their staffs were cast as scapegoats, readily identifiable and available targets for every sin imaginable, including both sins of omission and commission.

Of course, tensions are never only one way, and there has always been reaction and resentment among administrators about the constant stream of abuse, demands, and

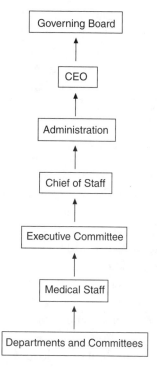

FIGURE 3–1 Hospital–medical staff relationship: apparent view.

table pounding by the medical staff as a whole, and some doctors in particular. The difference usually is that doctors can complain in loud voices and be as obnoxious as they want, while administrators are frequently unable to do much more than swallow the guff, grin and bear it all the way to the bank. Hospital administration in recent years has become a reasonably well-paid profession with very short tenure in office and no job security to speak of. But do not forget that there are solid nuclei in every medical staff of good guys, who like the hospital and enjoy practicing there. They are sympathetic to administration and behave as decent and civil human beings. Sometimes, though, the problem is that they do not stand up in medical staff meetings and say those supportive things they are thinking. They do not offer open gestures of support even though that is the way they really feel. In private they are warm and compassionate, in public they are silent.

Through all of the arm-wrestling contests between hospital administrators and medical staffs, the boards of directors or trustees have tried to continue to function in their governance role, with attention to financial success, philanthropy, and desire to perform in a service role. They delegate management to one group and quality of care to another, trusting to the good works of both that the hospital will serve the community and prosper at the same time. In general, they have done a very good job of it, as the roles of boards have evolved through recent waves of changes. However, entry into the managed care era will change the structure and function of hospitals boards of trustees or directors forever. They will find themselves searching the unknown even more as they try to find the just right balance, between caring, which is their mission, and stewardship, which is their survival (Seay & Vladeck, 1987).

SUMMARY

The regulatory structure chosen by the medical profession to control its members and the quality of their care was voluntary accreditation—the Joint Commission on the Accreditation of Healthcare Organizations. There are other regulatory pressures on doctors and hospitals by state and federal agencies, legislation, and the effects of precedent court cases. But what the doctors created, with help from the hospital industry, focuses on hospitals and their medical staffs to evaluate and ensure high quality care. Medical staffs are reviewed in surveys, but it is the hospital that is accredited, using JCAHO standards that are continually refined.

The survey process is highly organized and complicated, with differing perspectives on how to prepare for the team visit. Whether to stay in a continuing state of near readiness is one way some hospitals and medical staffs do it, while last minute panic and stress is another popular approach.

Responsibility for high-quality patient care is delegated by governing boards to the medical staff, which is organized to carry out these duties. In most community hospitals in the United States, private practitioner physicians are not employees of the hospital, but they agree to abide by the hospital policies and medical staff rules in return for the privilege of being allowed to practice in the hospital. Over time, the Joint Commission model of a hospital medical staff has produced a typical organizational structure.

REFERENCES

Gassiot, C. O., & Starr, P. J. (Eds.). *Principles of Medical Staff Services Science.* Education Council, National Association of Medical Staff Services. Privately printed.

Gill, S. C. (1993). [Presentation material for medical staff leadership training workshops]. Sharp Healthcare, San Diego, CA, and Physician Management Resources, Westmont, IL.

Haglund, C. L., & Dowling, W. L. (1993). The hospital. In Williams, S. J., & Torrens, P. R. (Eds.), *Introduction to Health Services, (4th Ed.).* Albany: Delmar Publishers.

Joint Commission on the Accreditation of Healthcare Organizations (JCAHO). (1995). *The Complete Guide to the 1996 Hospital Survey Process.* Oakbrook, IL.

Joint Commission on the Accreditation of Healthcare Organizations (JCAHO). (1995). *1996 Comprehensive Accreditation Manual for Hospitals.* Oakbrook, IL.

Kent, C. (1995) "Fix it or forget it": The JCAHO in crisis. In *Perspectives, January 23, 1995.* Washington, D.C.: Faulkner & Gray.

Medicine & Health, 49(3, January 16). (1995).

Seay, D., & Vladeck, B. (1987). *In Sickness and Health.* New York: Hospital Fund of New York.

Snook, D. I. Jr. (1992). *Hospitals: What They Are and How They Work (2nd ed.).* Gaithersburg, MD: Aspen Publishers.

CHAPTER

Medical Staff Roles
and Responsibilities

Since 1992, the Joint Commission has considered its *Accreditation Manual for Hospitals* to be a work in progress, in a transition from requirements for structures and processes as an end in themselves to one that relates performance of essential processes to patient outcomes. The number of actual standards to be used in surveys has been reduced during that time by more than two-thirds. The nature of the change process is so dynamic that accounts and descriptions put forth in this text could very well be changed or replaced by the time you read about them. In the 1995 version of the manual, the following principles were expressed (JCAHO, 1994):

- Standards should emphasize actual performance, not just the capacity to perform
- Standards should address what counts: the care provided to the patient and the management of the organization

- Standards should focus on important activities or functions that significantly influence, directly or indirectly, eventual patient outcomes
- Standards should set forth performance expectations in a quality improvement context. (The objective is not to punish competent practitioners and staff but rather to improve the internal systems and work environment that help them and their organizations realize their primary goal. That goal is excellent care that improves over time.)
- Hospitals should be doing the right things and doing them well

Another feature of this 1995 volume is that all previous accreditation documents have been combined into a single guide. The standards revision process has added a new emphasis on performance that requires multidisciplinary teamwork involving many hospital departments and services. Thus, the new standards envision the hospital as an integrated system rather than as a collection of discrete, independent units. Less attention is now placed on how to achieve the objectives of a given standard, which are replaced by a set of consistent performance expectations that could be achieved in more than one creative approach. The new survey process has moved away from evaluation of specific departments and services. Instead, it focuses on assessing performance of important functions across the organization.

These changes are obvious in the standards affecting the medical staff. In the past, required medical staff functions were carried out in splendid isolation from the rest of the hospital with little or no reference to the other components. Experienced medical staffs, wise in the ways of surveyors, paid attention to the specifics of such recognizable details as:

- departmental review of patient care provided by individuals with clinical privileges
- review of surgical and other invasive case procedures
- drug usage evaluation
- medical record review
- blood usage review
- pharmacy and therapeutics review
- other review functions, possibly including infection control, disaster plans, hospital safety, and utilization

Those medical staff services personnel and the physician leadership who are fixated on these relics of the past need some powerful relearning so that their hospitals will not suffer from any worse cultural shock. The new standards are very specific about the language that must be in the bylaws and whether those provisions are carried out without fail by the medical staff. Also, there is a strong emphasis on whether departments actually perform their jobs as described in bylaws, rules, and policies.

WHAT THE MEDICAL STAFF PRACTICES

In general, it is appropriate to state that, contrary to appearances and instinctive perception, there is a major difference between individual doctors and their medical practices and the organized medical staff as an organization. Most lay persons and, perhaps, most incoming board members are not aware of this difference and the existence of a precise and complex structure. The difference is that the organized medical staff does not practice medicine. Individual members of the staff may or may not practice medicine, but the medical staff as an organization does not. As an organized body described in the JCAHO *Accreditation Manual,* recognized in federal and state law, regulation, and code and by precedent court cases, the medical staff practices credentialing, privileging, reappointment, and peer review. There may also be payer-required utilization review.

Individual physicians, in solo or group practice, who compete professionally for patients and recognition of their medical practice, who pay malpractice insurance against the increasing likelihood of lawsuit, who are highly trained medical experts in the use of the scientific method, are required by the JCAHO model to wear another hat that nobody warned them about in medical school, and probably not in residency either. This hat is that they would somehow join together and put aside their individual differences to become a JCAHO model of a hospital medical staff. Thus, the medical staff as an organization functions as an unincorporated association for self-governance, as expressly referred to by the California Supreme Court (Willett, 1984).

The medical *staff* does not practice medicine. The *organized* medical staff in the Joint Commission model does not collectively or organizationally practice medicine. What it does do is to have overall responsibility for the quality of the professional services provided by individuals with clinical privileges, as well as the accountability of accounting therefor to the governing body. The definition of clinical privileges is the authorization granted by the governing body to a practitioner to provide specific patient care services in the hospital within defined limits, based on a practitioner's license, education, training, experience, competence, health status, and judgment (JCAHO, 1994).

This other hat, about which doctors were not taught in school, is not visible in residency, and is certainly not an integral part of office practice or physician personal life. Physicians as a group are delegated by hospital boards of directors to perform professional duties. The medical *staff* practices:

• credentialing: who is the person that wants to be on the medical staff?
• privileges: what can that person do?

- peer review: how well does that medical staff member perform?
- reappointment: should the member be recredentialed and granted the same or other privileges again?

Through the years there have been various trends in conducting these activities and various names have been attached, particularly in the peer review/quality of care arena. Medical audit, quality assurance, quality assessment, quality improvement—all have the same general meaning and intent: colleagues must look at and evaluate the care given or ordered by each staff member in relation to prevailing standards. Over time those standards change, usually growing higher, but one thing never changes: the obligation of hospital medical staffs to look and listen about care and behavior, to be willing to ask questions, to confront colleagues or peers, when necessary, and in those rare instances, take firm and bold remedial steps against one or more of their peers/colleagues/friends. And, all of this is to be done in the name of patient safety and improved quality.

Hospital medical staffs over time take on unique characteristics that reflect their members, hospitals, communities, and professional specialty organizations. Staffs use different names and words to describe their structures and different names for processes and committees, but they are all performing the self-governance responsibilities described in JCAHO standards, federal and state law, and precedent court cases. The Joint Commission model of a medical staff is thus an unincorporated association for self-governance. It is possible to be incorporated, of course, but that refinement is not required or contemplated by JCAHO standards and is not usual among hospital medical staffs. Further movement in the direction of integrated health care delivery systems or networks may show the advantages to becoming an incorporated body or group practice with a business relationship that is very different from this Joint Commission model, but more of that will be discussed in Chapter 27.

MEDICAL STAFF SELF-GOVERNANCE

There was a time in California, and perhaps other states as well, when the words *self-governance* as proposed by state medical society leaders frightened some administrators and board members into thinking that the doctors were taking over the hospital. While that might or might not have been a good thing to do at the time, self-governance simply means that the medical staff is responsible for, and allowed to elect, its own officers and for adopting bylaws, rules, and regulations that will accomplish the delegated and assigned tasks of

- credentialing
- privileging
- reappointment
- peer review

By adopting its own bylaws, the medical staff organization becomes self-governing, but those bylaws must be approved by the governing body of the hospital to become effective. Thus, the medical staff and its bylaws are the creation of the hospital board and its bylaws and derives its authority to act from this source.

The medical staff constitutes a participatory democracy, like a New England town meeting. It is truly a one-person, one-vote approach where each doctor has a chance to be heard on each issue, even if there is much heat, little light, and no action produced. Cynics might say that the main purpose of medical staff democracy is to protect the doctors from each other. Seeking consensus within this culture of equality will try the patience of every chief of staff and CEO/administrator. In the 1980s, Joseph Boyle, M.D., stated, in a keynote speech to the Physician and the Hospital Conference in California, that medical staff democracy meant that only 7 of 10 doctors would walk out of a burning building together. In the 1990s, Joe Boyle might amend that number down to 3 of 10, and maybe even fewer than that if they are competing specialists.

The medical staff participatory democracy lives by a strict and legalistic code of rules. It is always interesting that physicians turn to attorneys for help in establishing and running their own medical practice business, while complaining all the way that lawyers are not subject to credentialing and peer review processes that even approach those in medicine. Never mind that physicians also complain that lawyers are not subject to reappointment by their peers and are certainly not responsible for utilization management of the consumption of resources. Bylaws are written by the hospital attorney or the medical staff attorney or someone; or models of bylaws written or used elsewhere are adopted. Then these bylaws are accepted by the eligible voters on the general medical staff, usually following executive committee action. After that, approval is sought from the appropriate governing body of the hospital. The major emphasis of the bylaws must be to coordinate all of the efforts of the members of the medical staff in the fulfillment of institutional goals. Medical staff rules and regulations are appended to the bylaws and contain provisions that specifically relate to the delivery of patient care.

It is a measure of the respect for medical staff self-governance and its success that approval of bylaws may not be "unreasonably withheld" by the board. Unreasonably withheld means arbitrary and without a notice, discussion, and hearing process intended to allow for resolution of issues. Sometimes resolution cannot occur, and the courts have become involved. Sometimes the issues have been real enough to seek outside resolution. Sometimes there are simply stiff-necked people on both sides who want to show the other who is boss no matter what the cost. When hospitals needed doctors to bring patients, when doctors controlled medicine and could always take their patients somewhere else, when boards and administrators wanted to act in a hierarchial manner such as shown in the organizational chart in Chapter 3, then lawsuits resulted. What also resulted were feelings of animosity, dislike, distrust and damage to working relationships, which happens to be the exact opposite of the climate needed in the 1990s to succeed in a managed care world.

Medical staff bylaws are rules that must be followed. Examples are numerous of those chiefs and executive committees that just could not, would not, or did not bother with the details until finally a quality or discipline problem became a judicial review and the medical staff was unable to sustain its case that was correct in its intent but doomed to failure by lax, careless, sloppy attention to the details of due process or by intentional failure to observe the bylaws.

One more word about bylaws: They must be constantly in a state of change and revision to meet new issues and circumstances. As the world changes, as the law changes, as medicine changes, so must bylaws. It is annoying for physicians to go to required general staff meetings, to be asked to vote on language changes they have not studied and could care less about. So they complain about wasting time with bylaws changes. But this task needs to be done. Whose job is it to stay abreast of changes needed in bylaws? Maybe the medical staff coordinator is a bylaws fan. Hopefully, the chair of the bylaws committee will fulfill that task, which is usually thankless. Some bylaws chairs see their job, unfortunately, as opposing change and freezing the bylaws in a state of grace at some earlier time in history.

The commonsense definition of the purposes of a medical staff can be simply said but not so simply carried out. The staff exists to establish mechanisms for reviewing and controlling the quality of care rendered by medical staff members and to provide a structure whereby there is physician input into decision making within the institution (Gassiot & Starr, 1987). The typical structure for accomplishing this purpose includes officers, departments, and committees.

Officers

While there are local variations, the usual officers of the hospital medical staff in the Joint Commission model are the chief of staff (sometimes now called president), the chief-elect (or vice chief or vice president), and secretary-treasurer. The chief or president is elected or selected to act as the presiding officer and is accountable to the board for all activities of the medical staff. The bylaws specify the method of selection, tenure, and qualifications of all officers.

Departments

Most hospitals with more than 30 to 40 medical staff members are departmentalized, or organized into some manner of subgroups. The most common of these is the pattern of medical specialties found in most medical schools and colleges or universities where like interest groups cluster together for mutual benefit and protection. Large hospitals with hundreds of staff members may have 10 or more clinical departments made up of specialties such as internal medicine, surgery, anesthesia, pediatrics, obstetrics/gynecology, family practice, pathology, radiology, psychiatry, and, more recently, emergency medicine. Each of these could be further subdivided by formation of services or subsections within departments. But each medical staff member must be appointed to one department, even though holding privileges in another department. Usually, the application process is a request to join the particular specialty department.

When departmentalized, each department elects or selects a chair as presiding officer, as specified in the bylaws. Jurisdiction includes being responsible for all professional and administrative activities within the department and continuing surveillance of the professional performance of all members of the department. The chair is also personally responsible for the implementation of a program to monitor and evaluate the quality and appropriateness of patient care provided by members of the department.

The Joint Commission requires departments to assess and improve the quality of care and services provided in the department and to perform continuing surveillance of the professional performance of all individual members. Without trying to name all of the duties of the chair of a department in this chapter, they include being responsible for all clinically related as well as administratively related activities. Recommending criteria for clinical privileges and recommending which clinical privileges each member should have are other responsibilities of the chair. When the medical staff is departmentalized, the general medical staff must meet as a whole at least annually but usually meets quarterly in most hospitals.

In small hospitals with fewer than 30 to 40 staff members, the medical staff is usually nondepartmentalized and acts as a committee of the whole to perform the required functions. In that case, the nondepartmentalized staff is still required to have designated mechanisms to perform their functions. Being small does not mean that there is no need to pay attention or that good self-governance is related only to size.

In addition to departments, medical staff committees are the working units of the medical staff. While JCAHO only requires only one committee—the executive committee—there are usually numerous others. As a rule, in the traditional workings of the Joint Commission model, there are usually committees to carry out the required functions, such as credentials review, surgical case review, pharmacy and therapeutics, and so on, as specified in the list earlier in this chapter. Committees are usually stated in the bylaws as standing, while others are appointed by the chief or department chairs, including special or mission-specific ad hoc groups.

The Executive Committee

This is the only medical staff committee required by Joint Committee standards, although there must be two other hospital committees (infection control and safety).

The executive committee is the focal point for changes in the medical staff, whether they be organizational, functional, or attitudinal. The executive committee is the one element of the medical staff that exercises the greatest influence on the medical staff as a whole. The executive committee is the overseer of the functions performed by the medical staff. It should be the watchdog of the bylaws and the guardian of due process when there is no one else to do that job. When the executive committee is dysfunctional, there may be no one at all to do the job.

The executive committee is usually composed of the officers and department chairs, as well as, sometimes, at-large members. Representatives from administration and nursing are sometimes members, although more frequently they are invited guests who make reports and leave during the peer review session. The committee receives and acts on reports and recommendations of departments and other committees. It is the body that holds the medical staff accountable to the board of directors for the quality of care rendered in the hospital and also serve as the vehicle for medical staff input into hospital planning and decision making (Gassiot & Starr, 1987).

When the executive committee works well, it offers quality leadership in dealing with the issues and problems that inevitably confront the organized medical staff in these turbulent times. When it functions badly, it is a body of politicians who act to prevent progress from being made and try simply to protect their turf. Like all legislative bodies, executive committees change with each election, going from bad to good or, unfortunately, the other way at times.

MEDICAL STAFF MEETINGS

The vehicle for carrying out the responsibilities of self-governance are the medical staff meetings. No matter how many there are, there are probably too many. But meetings, and the accurate documentation thereof, are the means most often employed to demonstrate compliance with medical staff monitoring mechanisms required by the Joint Commission. The key issue is whether the meetings are efficient and effective in accomplishing their purpose or whether they are social events that are not really intended to do the work.

Time spent in arranging proper scheduling and adequate facilities, along with a well-planned agenda, are the only way to facilitate the successful accomplishment of objectives. Working with the chief and/or the committee chairs, the medical staff office should plan on a long range basis and schedule the meetings a (medical staff) year at a time. Day, week, hour: all of these variables should be worked out in advance. Once scheduled, then it is the chair's obligation to be there, as well as all of the members who agree to serve on that committee. Nothing is so devastating as a missing chair, especially when that meeting was scheduled exactly when that person wanted it. The fault probably lies in the fact that the practice office was never notified by the doctor that a regular standing committee meeting would take place every month on that date and that their "doctor" was the chair and a patient could not be put into that time slot. Practice office life and hospital staff life are frequently at odds with each other. Only the doctor is the common link. The medical staff office may not know the practice office people, and the practice office staff will almost certainly not know anything about the hospital and about medical staff procedure.

Medical staff services offices have learned, to their chagrin, that mailed notices are not entirely dependable as communications vehicles, and the smart coordinators always follow up with a phone call to the person who can influence the doctor's schedule. A coordinator can put out notices and posters in all the conspicuous places and expect them to be no more than 50 percent effective. That is true not only of doctors. Lots of other people just do not read signs and posters. Also true will be the effect that someone will show up for a canceled meeting. That message did not get through either, and the physician came to the committee meeting out of sheer habit. Some doctors keep coming to the same committee meetings long after they are not even on the committee any more.

Agendas are the blueprint for the meetings, defining directions for action and serving as guidelines for the direction in which matters under discussion should go. *Should go,* that is, not *will go.* An agenda prepared in advance of the meeting is crucial as a helpful tool in the decision-making process. And, a badly prepared, or even unprepared, agenda is a blueprint to inadequate or unwise decisions, or at least a lot of time wasted in flailing around. The agenda should carry forward unfinished business or other matters deferred from previous meetings. After key members of the committee have been consulted in advance about items they want included, the medical staff services coordinator sits down with the chief or chair for two reasons. One is to go over the draft for final choices, and the other is to make sure the chair has seen the agenda and discussed it, so that at the meeting the chair can't say, "I've never seen this before."

Medical staffs should have a standard format for all committee meetings, so that there is uniformity of appearance and things can be found easily. This is also as a way of keeping the committee's attention on the real business to be done, not the personal or pet items someone wants to use to take over the meeting as a way of preventing the work. The National Association of Medical Staff Services (NAMSS) training manuals have perfectly laid out examples for all of these details. Lack of available training materials is not the problem, when there is a problem. Chairperson behavior and member behavior are the problems, not the format or layout. Another helpful resource is an excellent consultant or facilitator who offers training on running successful meetings.

Minutes deserve some attention in this discussion. They can be the most effective tool available for use by the leadership and members for maintaining a progressive, functioning organization performing self-governance. The minutes are the primary source of documentation for many accreditation requirements. The minutes are also legal documents that show a meeting was held and furnish a record of all actions taken. There are extremes in the art of minute taking, ranging from the completely documented level to the soul of brevity type that mean nothing except to those who actually heard the conversation. Neither is appropriate.

A skillful notetaker is a blessing for any committee. Listening to, interpreting, and recording information are skills that must be acquired. An excellent medical staff services professional develops an almost intuitive recognition of what is pertinent and what is superfluous. It is the intent of the majority present that is most relevant to the record, although the record may not reflect the actual language used by a particular doctor (Gassiot & Starr, 1987). It is more than just taking notes, and the coordinators are more than just "secretaries." If a committee has been blessed by the work of a good medical staff coordinator, members will have saved themselves literally hours of wasted time and made better decisions because everyone could read and understand the minutes. Remember, almost no physician attends every meeting, and some do not attend much at all. The minutes are the only constant.

Minutes show results, recommendations made, actions taken, items tabled or postponed, and appropriate reasons for each. They record the highlights, the progress achieved, and the summary of any substantive discussion. Assignments made must appear in the minutes, as well as the specific reporting responsibilities. Unfortunately, sometimes, minutes show the amount of time spent on an insignificant item rather than the degree of importance of the item, which should have more attention focused on it. Finally, the minutes become binding documents and cannot be changed arbitrarily. Minutes are the official record on which judicial review trials are conducted, and they must be accurate. Any "corrected" material remains in the minutes, and corrections are added, with a notation. Frequently one doctor goes on a verbal rampage, and then asks to have those remarks stricken after seeing them in print. Or, the angry doctor blames the medical staff services coordinator by denying having said those things at all.

It is at that point where the chief of staff and the department chairs must stand firm. If the chief is unable to prevent or interrupt the misbehavior, then do not compound the matter by trying to ease it out of the minutes as though nothing ever happened. Only the Congressional Record can be edited later with the insertion of new or different material to create virtual reality. The medical staff leader must then sign the minutes. Some chairs are notoriously difficult about dropping by the medical staff office to sign minutes, which are not official and cannot be included in the executive committee packet until legally signed.

Parliamentary procedure is included in every set of model medical staff bylaws and is ignored most of the time, usually because the leaders or the members do not want to be bound by the rules. Observing good procedure seems to some physicians as a trick, and anyone who knows something about parliamentary procedure seems like a charlatan. Some chiefs adamantly refuse to follow good procedure, because it would ruin their down-home image, and they must live with those people when their term is over. Without procedure, there are endless meetings and much time-wasting. Any doctor can put on a filibuster that is personally important but may or may not have anything to do with the agenda of the meeting. Running a tight ship may offend a few, but the chief or chair will be loved by many. Even the use of such devices as an egg timer will help end the executive committee meetings before midnight. Give each agenda item a time limit, and when the minutes run out, the timer goes off. The committee must then vote whether to give that subject any more time, in five minute increments. Although the abrupt end to some dialogues may leave some physicians' egos slightly bruised, everyone will get home at least an hour earlier (Koska, 1992).

SUMMARY

As JCAHO accreditation standards have been revised over recent years, the hospital and the medical staff are now viewed as an integrated system rather than a collection of discrete, independent units. Newer standards emphasize whether medical staff officers and departments actually carry out the provisions of the bylaws, rules and policies. There is a major difference between individual doctors and their medical practices and the organized medical staff in the hospital. The medical staff performs self-governance, as described in the JCAHO manual with overall responsibility for quality of services provided by individuals with clinical privileges, as well as being accountable to the governing body. Self-governance is the other hat that doctors wear—a hat not taught in medical school or residency and that is not a part of office practice.

Self-governance includes credentialing, privileges, reappointment, and peer review. There may be different local names, but the meaning is the same: a participatory democracy with a strict and legalistic set of rules, the bylaws, to protect the doctors from themselves and each other. Bylaws are in a constant state of revision, to reflect changing times, and changing missions of the hospital, but increasing attention is being focused on the officers, departments, and working units of the medical staff.

REFERENCES

Gassiot, C. O., & Starr, P. J. (Eds.). (1987). *Principles of Medical Staff Services Science.* Education Council, National Association of Medical Staff Services. Privately printed.

Joint Commission on Accreditation of Healthcare Organizations (JCAHO). (1994). *1995 Comprehensive Accreditation Manual for Hospitals.* Oakbrook Terrace, IL.

Koska, M. T. (1992). Making mandatory medical staff meetings more physician-friendly. *Hospitals, Oct. 5,* 38.

Willett, D. E. (1984). *What Physicians Should Know about "The Legal Status of the Medical Staff."* San Francisco: California Medical Association.

CHAPTER

Credentialing

The hospital governing board, through delegated duties to the medical staff, has the obligation to the community to assure that only appropriately educated, trained, and currently competent practitioners are granted medical staff membership (Gassiot & Starr, 1987). The right to exercise clinical privileges is also based on a detailed review of the applicant's education and experience. Clinical privileges should not be granted unless there is adequate evidence that the physician is qualified. While this is the rule, there have been, nevertheless, examples that doctors have been granted privileges just because they asked for them, with the question of adequate evidence never being a part of the process. Joint Commission standards on quality assurance reflect this primary responsibility to see that patient care provided in the hospital is on a level commensurate with the recognized standard of practice.

Medical licensure has often been used as a source for measuring the competence of a practitioner, but the license itself cannot serve as a reliable resource for judging competence. Licensure board requirements are too broad, and the large volume of licensure requests make it difficult for boards to act swiftly. There is little or no feedback to individual hospitals about action taken on a practitioner's license, other than a query to the National Practioner Data Bank. There is also a great length of time involved in having any type of action initiated to curtail the license of negligent physicians. Licensure must be verified by the medical staff services office as a part of the credentialing process but cannot be relied on solely for the determination to grant approval. There must be a careful, objective process for reviewing each application to protect the public, as well as to protect the rights of the applicant. There must be ample documentation of the reasons for both acceptance and denial of membership and privileges. The hospital and the organized medical staff can then demonstrate that the credentialing process is applied to all applicants, fairly and evenhandedly.

THE APPLICATION PROCESS

Each medical staff should design an application form that meets its needs, although there are numerous examples that can be used as models. The medical staff coordinator can find many models in publications by NAMSS or the state association or by asking for assistance from colleagues at neighboring hospitals. Whatever the form, there should be provisions for the applicant to account for all of the time since graduation from medical school up to the time of the application to the hospital. Gaps in the yearly chronology are immediate reasons to ask for further information before proceeding with the processing. Other examples of necessary information include pertinent questions about malpractice claims history, disciplinary actions taken by other hospitals, licensure boards, health plans, medical groups, and so on, as well as voluntary relinquishment of license, medical staff membership, and/or privileges.

Each applicant to the medical staff fills out a standard form supplied by the medical staff services office requesting information about the candidate and requiring a number of mandatory pledges to be made by the candidate. One pledge is to obey the bylaws as written at the time of candidacy. If the bylaws are up to date, that pledge should also contain language that obligates the signing physician to also comply with bylaw changes as those may occur later with the approval of the general medical staff and board of directors. Other necessary pledges by the physician applicant that must be a part of the application form, no matter what its format, are to provide continuous care, to prohibit fee splitting, a statement authorizing a release of information by all other sources that will assist with the credentialing process, and an assurance to preserve confidentiality about medical staff matters.

From time to time, a doctor balks at some of the provisions in the application or some of the pledges contained within. One frequent example of this situation may confront the medical staff that considers emergency room backup to be a condition of membership. It is simply not possible to have people serving as members of the organized medical staff opting in or out of those portions of the bylaws that seem most convenient or favorable. Everyone observes everything in the bylaws all the time. The most difficult part of this process is finding and keeping physician members of the staff who will pay attention to the constant updating of the bylaws that is necessary to keep them current and effective.

There is another pledge that is vitally important to the conduct of medical staff business: the business of self-governance. Applications contain a pledge to disclose or allow verification of information about past history, past practice, derogatory information, quality improvement findings, judicial review outcomes, and privileges denied or withdrawn. That means information in files or records can be transmitted from one medical body to another with the proper confidential safeguards. It does not mean releasing that information to the press or the general public, but it might mean releasing quality-related sanctions to the state licensing board or the National Practitioner Data Bank.

The real world problem in credentialing and peer review that occurs frequently is when a physician has gotten in trouble at one hospital, goes to another, and fails to report that problem. When asked by the second hospital, the first hospital also fails to report vital information related to safety and quality from some misguided sense of protecting the physician's reputation. The code of silence in these instances works against self-governance and prevents integrity in the credentialing/privileging process. Furthermore, the physician has already given signed permission allowing disclosure by signing his or her application. Falsification of information or failure to disclose is sufficient reason for immediate termination of candidacy or membership on the staff. Any chief of staff or department chair who believes a staff candidate or member has some sort of right to conceal matters of patient safety or lack of compliance with the basic responsibilities of membership is misplaced in a leadership position.

A flowchart of the credentialing process, allowing for local variations, would generally follow the pattern shown in Figure 5–1, which shows upward movement from the submission of an application, continuing on through the medical staff process, and culminating in consideration by the governing board of the hospital. The key point of this process and the flowchart are that there is a well-defined pathway. There is nothing whimsical or capricious about the way it is done. The process does not change, no matter whether the applicant is a friend of the chief, the administrator, or the board chair. Data are gathered, verified, and presented for review and evaluation the same way every time.

The flowchart of the credentialing process shown in Figure 5–1 may vary locally by different names or by fewer or more boxes, but the principle remains the same. A new applicant who wishes to join a Joint Commission hospital medical staff submits an application, which is verified in writing by professional medical staff services personnel. The applicant may also pay a fee for handling and processing the application. Although

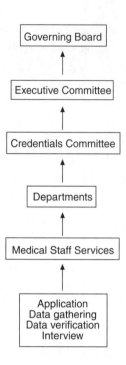

FIGURE 5–1   Credentialing.

doctors may want to verify by phone the acceptability of a candidate's credentials, that should be good staff work handled with timely and careful attention.

Good staff work is important, and so is good medical leadership support for those staff who do the good staff work. One of the crisis points in medical staff process occurs during the completion of the application, where the staff is unable to send an application forward to the committee because it is incomplete. Incomplete means that reference letters have not arrived or that recommendation letters from residency program directors or case summaries (if required) have not been presented. The application cannot go forward for consideration so long as it is incomplete, no matter who it is that wants to hurry it along. But the absence of these required materials—required by medical staff rules—may not always prevent bullying and harassment of the staff by doctors in a hurry. At that point, some protection is needed by the leadership. The in-a-hurry applicant should be told to spend the same amount of effort in securing the missing letters that is being spent maligning the staff, who are only doing their job as required.

MEMBERS OF THE MEDICAL STAFF

Who are these applicants to a Joint Commission model medical staff? State law is the determinant, and there may be differences, but in California those eligible to apply are:

- physician: Medical doctor (M.D.), doctor of osteopathy (D.O.)
- dentist: General (D.D.S.), oral surgeon
- podiatrist: Doctor of podiatric medicine (D.P.M.)
- clinical psychologist: Ph.D. trained and eligible to perform psychometric testing or cotreat where appropriate in a mental health center

To what positions may practitioners be appointed if they wish to become members of the hospital medical staff? With allowance for local variations, the following categories are usually the various levels of appointment specified in medical staff bylaws (Haglund & Dowling, 1993).

Active Medical Staff

These members are physicians who have full hospital privileges and provide most of the medical care in the hospital. They are responsible for the administrative management duties of the organized medical staff. They can vote, hold office, and serve on committees.

Associate Medical Staff

This group may consist of members who are being considered for advancement to the active medical staff. The period to be served in the associate medical staff is defined in the bylaws. At the end of this period, usually two years, the associate member is considered for advancement through the mechanism established in the bylaws, which is usually by recommendation of the appropriate department. If an associate is not advanced at the specified time, then it will probably be necessary to point out why advancement has not occurred and what steps will be necessary to achieve that target. Associate medical staff can usually be members of committees, can sometimes hold office at the department level, but cannot usually vote or hold office in the general medical staff.

Courtesy Medical Staff

These members are physicians and dentists who are eligible for active membership on the staff but who admit patients to the hospital only occasionally, usually because they are on the active staff of another hospital. They are not involved in any administrative functions, cannot vote, and cannot hold office.

Consulting Medical Staff

This group includes physicians, dentists, and podiatrists who are recognized for their professional expertise and who are willing to act as consultants to the hospital's medical staff, although they practice primarily in other hospitals. It has been customary to grant consulting privileges when the physician provides a specialized skill not otherwise available in the hospital. In those instances, some bylaws may allow for consulting staff to admit, prescribe, and discharge, although that is not commonly done by consultants. Consulting staff do not vote or hold office.

Honorary Staff

This special group consists of physicians and dentists who are recognized for their noteworthy contributions and/or outstanding service to the hospital or to the medical staff. Honorary status is sometimes attained at a certain age as specified in the bylaws, but it is usually granted at time of retirement on the recommendation of the department or nominating committee. Some medical staffs have specific criteria for the honorary staff, while others simply call it the retired staff.

Provisional Status

This category of membership is a condition for initial appointments to the staff, except for the categories of honorary and consulting. The status may continue as long as it is done according to bylaws provisions. It is possible for a member of the staff to be in one or another category while still having some provisional privileges.

House Staff

This title refers to interns and residents who function under the supervision of attending or faculty physicians but are employees of the hospital. Several court cases have taken place to establish whether house staff are students or employees, and the latter status has resulted from that litigation. Because of some of the rigors of such service, unionization of house staff has occurred in many locations. But, in any case, house staff are not members of the organized medical staff of the typical community hospital and do not take part in the self-governance activities.

After the Application Submission

In the credentialing process as shown in Figure 5–1 an application is submitted, the fee (if any) is paid, and a privilege form is completed. Written verification includes letters or documents showing

- medical training
- internship

- residency
- fellowship
- board certification
- status of board qualification
- other memberships
- ECFMG certificate
- practice in other hospitals
- valid state licenses
- proof of insurance
- valid Drug Enforcement Application (DEA) permit to prescribe controlled substances
- professional references (usually three in number)
- abstracts of previous hospital cases (when required)

For many years, the term *board eligible* was used in the context of progress toward board certification, but the term lost its useful meaning and has been discarded. Instead, the medical staff should insist upon a statement about the applicant's precise position in the board certification process (Gassiot & Starr, 1987).

In other states, there is some legal statement on the eligibility question that either specifies as to which categories of professions may be received, or there is a permissive law or regulation that leaves the discretion to the hospital board.

The medical staff office must query the National Practitioner Data Bank to find out if there are entries in the applicant's file, but it is not necessary to wait for an answer before moving on with the process. When the listed materials are in hand and the data bank query has been made and paid for, the application is now complete and can be moved from the staff work category to begin consideration by peers and colleagues.

DEPARTMENTAL AND COMMITTEE REVIEW

The process continues on past a completed application form to some sort of specialty departmental scrutiny through a chain of actions leading to granting of membership and recommended privileges by the board. The process of review by specialty supervisory committees can vary widely depending upon the attitude of the peers in the group and the leadership ability of the chair. Supervisory committees can ask for more information, more references, more cases, more explanation by the candidate, and an interview with direct questioning. Forming a complete application can take weeks or months, but so can departmental review, with or without good reason. If there are legitimate questions about the applicant's background, past practice, or qualifications, then a reasonable investigation based on the interest of quality care is obligatory. When a committee stalls the consideration of an economic or competitive rival because there are too many of that specialty here now, then members are treading on the brink of restraint of trade for reasons not at all connected to quality.

Applicants have rights, too, particularly the right to due process in a reasonable manner within a reasonable amount of time. It happens too often that a departmental supervisory committee allows its agenda to drag on too long, leaving not enough time to consider the applicant's credentials package. There is no medical staff self-governance principle or tradition that should tolerate this cavalier treatment of a good faith applicant. If there is suspicion that the application is not in good faith, then by all means identify the issues and investigate those with whatever action is necessary. But do not ignore the packet. Medical staff coordinators are usually good about pointing out those tasks that remain undone, and can advise on what action is needed. A smart chairperson soon learns that the coordinator is the best friend the committee will ever have.

EXECUTIVE COMMITTEE AND BOARD ACTION

Some medical staffs use a credentials committee as the body that recommends appointments to the board, but it is more likely that the executive committee has that duty. The role and responsibility of credentials committees can vary from place to place, but perhaps the most effective arrangement is that of the credentials committee serving to oversee the activity of the departments, sending back applications that are unclear or without appropriate recommendations. Then the executive committee can receive a clean set of recommended candidates with the assurance that someone has ensured accuracy and completeness. The executive committee can also seek more information from either the credentials committee or departmental supervisory committee and can send back an application in question so that more preparation can be done.

Once in a while an executive committee takes an action that is solely within its power: denial of an application for documented reasons related to quality of care. No other reason to deny is supportable in the due process of judicial review that will likely follow denial. Personal reasons, restraint of trade, or professional jealousies are easily exposed when a decision of the executive committee is challenged. Only quality of care will win as a supportable reason for restricting or denying privileges. The board needs to be assured that the credentialing system leads to executive committee recommendations that have been carefully reviewed and that something better than an old buddy system is in place. The arguments against allowing a credentials committee to make decisions that bypass the executive committee are that accountability is thus undermined and that too much responsibility is placed on an appointed group that can lead to kingmaking and turf guarding. In any case, neither credentials or executive committees take final actions: only the board actually appoints members of the staff and grant privileges. Only the board actually makes the decision to restrict or deny membership on the medical staff and privileges. Doctors make innumerable decisions each day in diagnosing and treating patients, in managing their own offices or clinics as small business, and in their personal lives. So it comes naturally to want to make final decisions about credentialing and peer review issues. But these individual doctors acting in groups as committees can only make recommendations to the board for the ultimate decision in the Joint Commission model.

Experienced boards of directors or trustees frequently say that the most difficult decision they make is to approve the credentialing recommendations from the medical staff. Financial decisions they know something about, facing those every day in business or private lives. But can they trust the medical staff to be careful and accurate? Who are these unknown people being allowed to perform heart or brain surgery or do other procedures on patients? Only rarely do boards have some opportunity to actually see or hear new medical staff members. It is difficult enough for other doctors to know about new members of the staff. How many times has it happened that new appointees names are read at the general staff meeting and when asked to stand and be recognized, none are present? The board is proceeding on trust, assuming that the chief of staff, often their only link to the medical staff, can be trusted in recommending new staff members.

Boards can also ask for more information, can send back a recommendation to the executive committee for further work, or ask questions about a candidate. No board should be forced to be in the position of actually reviewing application packets because the medical staff has not provided sufficient information or the assurance of a competent and trustworthy credentialing system.

Boards can also refuse to approve a candidate recommended by the medical staff, which invites major turmoil since the board has not had access to all the information built up during the medical staff credentialing process. Often, a board denial is not for quality of care reasons and is based on something less objective and documented. The next step will be meeting each other in court, where the board is likely to lose unless there are good and sufficient reasons for having denied the application.

Whatever the outcome by board action, approval of membership and privileges or denial, must be conveyed to the physician applicant in writing, specifying (if applicable) the date of the appointment and the date of its expiration, which forms the basis for the Joint Commission two-year reappointment cycle.

ECONOMIC CREDENTIALING

An artifact of the movement toward managed care is the growing use of and concern about *economic credentialing,* defined as any use of monetary rather than traditional medical standards in making decisions about whether to appoint or reappoint a physician to the hospital medical staff. Economic credentialing has not been allowed in the Joint Commission model as traditionally used, since most hospital medical staff bylaws specify that any physician may join the staff if training and experience are adequate and acceptable.

But it can be a different story for medical groups and managed care integrated networks. The rules governing minimum professional requirements for hospital medical staff acceptance can be changed to add criteria regarding economic efficiency of practice. Some organizations are demanding more in terms of their doctors' levels of learning, skills, and experience than the traditional Joint Commission expectations for acceptance to a hospital medical staff.

They demand evidence that the physician practices in a cost-effective manner. If the record shows that the doctors have not added to bottom-line profits or the risk pool, they may very well be denied privileges. Of course, it should go without saying that it is necessary as a prerequisite that there must be an information system in regular use that is capable of producing data on a severity-adjusted basis and that is immediately available at points of service.

The courts have not yet developed broadly applicable rules defining when hospitals and health plans can weigh bottom-line considerations when deciding who can obtain practice privileges. However, one legal principle that the courts have tended to uphold is that those groups—hospitals or provider networks—might violate the law if they applied economic credentialing criteria in a way that made it impossible for doctors to practice (Kent, 1994).

The issue on the one hand is that a provider group under pressure from local employers to hold down costs or struggling not to lose money treating patients for a flat-fee schedule may be anxious to eliminate from the panel a physician who routinely orders too many tests or procedures. Saving money may also be good medicine. Every procedure eliminated not only reduces the chances of iatrogenic injury but also reduces the stress that interferes with recovery. So even when the motivation is economic, eliminating unnecessary services can also improve outcomes.

On the other hand, many physician groups maintain that medical competence in the tradition of the Joint Commission model is the only way to judge a practitioner. While some doctors see economic credentialing as a threat to their incomes and practice style, it is not just that pocketbook pinch that motivates their resistance and backlash. For some doctors who bring lawsuits against economic credentialing, there is an attitude of feeling cheated that they prepared themselves to be judged by the set of standards contained in the Joint Commission model, as they had been taught in medical school and residency, and suddenly, they are being measured by new and unrelated criteria.

One of the more frequent ways that economic credentialing disputes get into the courts is exclusive contracting for hospital-based services, thereby snuffing out the practices of current providers who had been granted privileges in an open department that is characteristic of the Joint Commission model. The issue here is thus one of privileges already granted that are being taken away or terminated because of the move to an exclusive contract and whether there is a property right attached to staff membership and privileges.

A growing number of lawsuits have claimed that the process by which physicians' previously held hospital privileges were terminated was unfair. The physicians filing the suits say that the same due process protections that apply in the medical staff bylaws to doctors charged with medical incompetence or unethical behavior should apply to doctors whose privileges have been terminated by boards, on the recommendation of administrators, for economic reasons. In other words, they are asking that the protections contained in the Joint Commission model should be extended to economic credentialing arguments.

In a recent move that may add fuel to the controversy, the Joint Commission seems to be agreeing with this viewpoint. The 1996 standards will apply the medical staff hearing process to all hospital appointment and privileging decisions regardless of whether they are based on quality of care, behavior, or business-related issues (*Medical Staff Briefing,* 1995). The 1995 standards said only that medical staffs must have a mechanism in place for addressing adverse decisions for applicants and that those mechanisms must include a fair hearing and appeal process.

To date, in an effort to keep the medical staff from becoming involved in hospital decisions about business-related issues such as exclusive contracting, some bylaws have specified that decisions not directly related to quality of care or professional behavior affecting appointment or privileges will not trigger the medical staff hearing process. If there are new standards that are more specific and that say that when hospital boards use criteria in making appointment and privileging decisions that go against the traditional posture by involving issues not related to quality, and if the standards then require imposition of the entire process of hearings and even judicial reviews, then the doctors will suddenly gain enormously more influence over hospital and system business deals than they have had before.

The immediate fallout of this change will be the need to revise bylaws to recognize the new standards. There will also be more hearings and department meetings, and the committees or the executive committee could be asked to second guess hospital or system business ventures. This is not to say that the medical staff has not already been second guessing those same ventures in private, but now there may be the opportunity to decide things the medical staff knows little about, such as breach of contract and antitrust violations. Some physicians would argue that hospital business decisions have always been directly linked with quality of care.

In those cases of quality of care medical misconduct, the accused doctors are given the opportunity to argue their side of the issue as described in Chapter 7. They have the opportunity to persuade their specialty colleagues in the department, on the executive committee and possibly even a judicial review committee that they do, indeed, measure up to medical staff standards. In the Joint Commission peer review process, accused doctors are presumed innocent and the medical staff must prove there is a quality infraction. In an economic credentialing case where there is a partnership agreement, there is less presumption of innocence, no necessity to prove the case, and no chance for defense, in the words of those who oppose the actions taken.

The hospitals or health care networks that are taking economic credentialing actions argue, in response, that failure to abide by system or network standards that have been set by physicians within the organization represents an inability or unwillingness to practice in a manner that will benefit all parties concerned, including patients. That line of reasoning goes on to say that the health plan or provider organization is a business arrangement that was made clear to all participating physicians; there must be present the ability to make a business decision regarding an overutilizer physician. This argument has long since left behind the Joint Commission model, which is incapable of offering a solution.

A number of specialty medical societies oppose the provisions of exclusive group contracts that deny other doctors the chance to practice that specialty in the hospital, particularly when privileges formerly held have been taken away. Some state medical associations are seeking relief from legislatures through the vehicle of "any willing provider" laws. California hospital and physician groups hammered out an agreement in 1992 so that terminating or granting medical staff privileges cannot be made merely on economic criteria not related to clinical qualifications, professional responsibilities, or quality of care. Both groups acknowledge that there may be times when it is wise to give an outside group an exclusive contract to provide services, but stipulate the step should be taken only after weighing the recommendations of the medical staff. That agreement contemplates that the medical staff to be consulted is performing as a Joint Commission model that is being asked to give an opinion on a business decision that will help some members of the staff and hurt others.

The disputes between doctors and hospitals over who will get medical staff privileges are setting some precedents for managed care networks. The courts have tended to recognize that when an insurer or network is selecting a panel, the promise that there will only be a few members of a particular specialty can be a strong inducement for doctors to join. Exclusivity can "foster a closer cooperative relationship between the plan and its participating physicians, lower administrative costs, and clarify the differences among competing health care plans" (Horshak, 1994).

Where a functionally integrated group of doctors such as an HMO have joined together, the courts have reasoned that in such arrangements, "persons who would otherwise be competitors pool their capital and share the risk of loss as well as the opportunities for profit. In such joint ventures, the partnership is regarded as a single firm competing with other sellers in the market" (U.S. Supreme Court, 1982). A Joint Commission model does not fit into this definition at all, since members remain competitors, have not pooled their capital, do not share any risk for either profit or loss, and are not a single firm competing with other sellers in the market.

The legal issue of selectivity and exclusion is likely to narrow as provider networks increasingly merge with hospitals and inpatient facilities, forming a handful of giant integrated delivery systems in regions such as Minneapolis or San Diego. Typically, in those regions there are too many specialists to ever be included in any network, or even all the networks combined. Then the question will be whether the selectivity or exclusion reduces competition in the marketplace, thereby harming consumers or patients. The exclusion of physicians through economic credentialing by medical groups and integrated delivery systems may raise antitrust concerns if competition is harmed because those doctors are no longer able to compete effectively, as they once did. However, provider networks may have valid procompetitive reasons for exclusion of certain doctors who have shown unproductive practice patterns in the utilization review. Their competence and willingness to meet the network's cost containment goals could work against a competitive environment. It could also be that network membership restrictions through economic credentialing may turn around and become procompetitive, by forcing those nonmembers to develop incentives for forming new and different networks to compete more vigorously on the basis of both price and quality.

SUMMARY

Credentialing is the name given to the responsibility of the hospital governing board, through delegation to the medical staff, for assuring that doctors granted medical staff membership and privileges are appropriately educated, trained, and currently competent. Applicants must demonstrate education, experience, and competence appropriate to the hospital, which is in excess of state medical licensure. Application forms have grown larger, requesting standard information and requiring mandatory pledges by the candidate to obey the bylaws and authorizing release of certain informatioin.

The credentialing process flows from the staff work done to verify and assemble necesary data through committees or other review by appropriate peers to the executive committee and on to the board of trustees/directors for final approval. Boards frequently receive and act on physician applicants with no information other than trust for the recommendation of the organized medical staff.

Problems can arise when a physician applicant fails to disclose pertinent background information or when one hospital medical staff organization conceals vital information related to safety and quality. New on the horizon is economic credentialing, an artifact of the managed care era where membership in medical groups, HMOs, or, possibly, hospital medical staffs could depend on financial performance.

REFERENCES

Gassiot, C. O., & Starr, P. J. (Eds.). (1987). *Principles of Medical Staff Services Science.* Education Council, National Association of Medical Staff Services. Privately printed.

Haglund, C. L., & Dowling, W. L. (1993). The hospital. Williams, S. J., & Torrens, P. R. (Eds.). *Introduction to Health Services (4th ed.).* Albany: Delmar Publishers.

Horshak, M. (1994). Bureau of competition. Federal Trade Commission. *Perspectives—Supplement to Medicine and Health, 48 (40, Oct. 3),* 1–4.

Kent, C. (1994). Economic credentialing moves forefront. *Perspectives—Supplement to Medicine and Health, 48 (40, Oct. 3),* 1–4. (Adapted from an article by Moskowitz, D. B., 1994, *Journal of American Healthcare, Sept./Oct.)*

U.S. Supreme Court. (1982). Arizona v. Maricopa County Medical Society. Cited in Horshak, M. (1994). Bureau of competition, Federal Trade Commission. *Perspectives—Supplement to Medicine and Health 48 (40, Oct. 3),* 1–4.

CHAPTER

Reappointment

Changes that may affect a physician's performance, or the hospital where practice occurs, may take place at any time. For that reason, periodic reappraisal and reappointment is a good principle to follow. This reappraisal of the doctor's qualifications and practice patterns serves several purposes. It allows for a planned process of data gathering from various quality improvement activities that should present a profile of each medical staff member's performance, and the review of that performance by peers.

The reappointment process also presents the opportunity to make needed changes in clinical privileges allowed. A physician may have completed further training or have sufficient experience to apply for additional or different privileges. Or, there may be evidence that some privileges granted previously should now be changed or, perhaps, taken away. Such changes may be requested at any time during the year, but reappointment presents a perfect opportunity for updates and renewing the profile of what it is that the doctor does in the hospital and how well is it being done.

REASONS FOR REAPPOINTMENT

There may have been changes in the health status of the physician that would change the ability to continue in the practice of privileges previously granted. A staff member may have become involved in liability suits, and these need to be disclosed to determine whether the hospital needs to be protected. Reappointment also presents the opportunity to review the overall pattern of the physician's citizenship as a member of the medical staff and ask these important questions about performance of professional responsibilities (Gassiot & Starr, 1987). Did the doctor

- attend the required meetings?
- participate appropriately in committee work?
- comply with medical staff and hospital bylaws, rules, and regulations?
- complete medical records in a timely manner?
- display disruptive behavior in the hospital or service areas?
- become subject to disciplinary action or sanctions?

Joint Commission standards require each medical staff member to be reappointed to the staff at no more than a two-year interval. Standards specify that the reappraisal include information concerning current licensure, health status, professional performance, judgment, and clinical/technical skills, as indicated by the results of peer review, quality improvement activities, and any other reasonable indicators of continuing qualification. All of these parameters must be included in clear language in the bylaws.

Reappointment could be done more frequently than at the two-year intervals required by the Joint Commission, but this usually does not seem practical in view of the work load. Reappointment means completing a new application that repeats some of the initial application, adding anything that has changed in the two-year interval. For many large hospitals with sizable medical staff memberships, reappointment is rather like painting the Golden Gate Bridge: start at one end, paint to the other end, paint back to the beginning, and by then it is time to start all over again. There are several alternative ways: by one-half the membership each year, all at one time, monthly, by birth date, anniversary date of joining the staff, or some other alternative. But whatever procedure is chosen, reappointment represents a major expenditure of medical staff services resources and attention, sometimes to the point of affecting the rest of the ongoing work load.

INDICATORS AND MEASURING TOOLS

The clinical indicators used in the reappointment process might include the following (Gassiot & Starr, 1987). Did the doctor

- display appropriate professional competence and clinical judgment in the treatment of patients?
- behave in a manner showing proper ethics and conduct?

- exhibit appropriate physical and mental capabilities?
- cooperate with hospital personnel?
- show an ability to practice medicine in a cost-effective manner?
- make appropriate use of the hospital's facilities for patients?
- demonstrate productive relationships with other doctors and practitioners on the staff?
- exhibit an appropriate and professional attitude toward patients, the hospital, and the public?
- maintain a regular pattern of documented continuing medical education efforts appropriate to practice?

In some hospitals, there can be major differences between the reappointment application and the initial credentialing as a result of the care being taken in the two processes. Getting on the staff in the first place may be much more difficult than staying on the staff once a doctor is there. Reappointment done badly is a rubber stamp activity that displays the worst features of the old buddies club. There is a failure to use all of the multiple sources at hand to review performance, instances of quality improvement and behavior, and contribution to medical practice, the staff, the hospital, and the community. A physician profile needs to be prepared for each reappointment candidate that includes patient contact information and satisfaction studies, peer review findings, opinions and observations by colleagues and the department chair, as well as other sources, such as severity-adjusted data systems. This presentation is not intended to be a how-to manual, but the principal decision points are shown in Figure 6–1.

Teaching materials are available from NAMSS or the state affiliates of that organization, as well as periodic training sessions and the precertification study course.

THE REAPPOINTMENT PROCESS

As Figure 6–1 shows, the flow of reappointment information and review follows the same essential pathway and the same essential checkpoints of the credentialing flowchart as it makes its way to the board for approval. Once again, medical staff committees only recommend and the board approves. Reappointment usually means continuing mountains of work for the staff, but decisions may or may not come more easily to the board. On the one hand, it may not seem so chancy since the board granted approval previously and some board members may have met some of the physicians. On the other hand, it is still not likely that members of the board can objectively assess physician performance and feel their only choice is to accept the report of the executive committee as vouched for by the chief of staff.

If there is a weakness with the reappointment process, it lies in the paucity of profile material sought and supplied. Mechanisms for quality improvement should contain

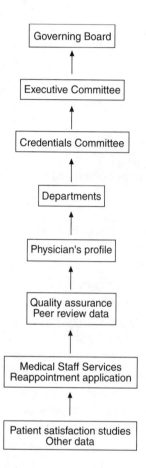

FIGURE 6–1 Reappointment.

screening criteria that can objectively identify examples of patient care requiring further review. Mechanisms for aggregating data, in the form of tracking and trending reports, serve as an ongoing measure of hospital and medical staff performance in specified areas. Mortality rates, complication rates, hospital-acquired infections, and appropriateness of procedures, drugs, and transfusions are but a few of the data elements needed for a composite picture of physician performance in the hospital practice. With the aid of the medical staff, a board could establish generic performance standards that will objectively measure and ensure continuing and improving quality (Lang and Hopkins, 1988).

By the time of a medical staff member's first reappointment, there can already be reasons for suspicion or question about practice, but not many fail to pass this reappointment hurdle. Since it is easier (but not easy) to deny membership or privileges in the first place than it is to fail reappointment, that makes credentialing the most important step in medical staff self-governance.

In the medical staff, there are credentialing, reappointment, and peer review, and the greatest of these is credentialing. That is why boards wonder about the safety of the medical staff credentialing process. Are they making a mistake and accepting a bad doctor who will bring strife, grief, and lawsuits to everyone just because the medical staff was lazy or careless about credentialing?

NATIONAL PRACTITIONER DATA BANK

Much legislation is passed by federal and state governments to remedy a loophole or solve a real-life problem. So it was when it became widely understood that interstate truckers carried multiple driver's licenses and could always use another if trouble occurred in some state. A few well-publicized examples of physicians moving from place to place to evade or escape practice problems resulted in creation by Congress of the National Practitioner Data Bank. Perhaps, the most remarkable of these examples was the cardiovascular surgeon at a major hospital who was discovered to be not a surgeon, not even a doctor, but a medical equipment salesman. That he had a very good mortality rate and low rates of infections was not a sufficient defense against the need to establish a database available to those hospital medical staffs or medical groups that perform credentialing and legitimately needed to know about the past history of those applying for membership and privileges.

A few basic points about the Data Bank should suffice for purposes of this book. A fee must be paid for each query, a query is mandatory for each credentialing and reappointment, and medical staff services professionals know very well how to do these tasks.

Doctors worry about what kind of information is entered into the computer files of the Data Bank and to whom it is accessible. Three main areas of reports are required, under penalty of fines:

- disciplinary actions taken by medical staffs or groups for reasons of quality of care
- credentials or privileges denied or taken away for reasons of quality of care
- malpractice actions where a payment has been made by an insurer

Not required to be reported are actions taken for administrative reasons such as voluntary withdrawals of applications, incomplete applications that pass a deadline for completion, or medical records suspensions. The Data Bank will be many years in the accumulation of information that can equal the expectations of its sponsors, but there is one particular item that deserves mention. Insurance companies are required to enter in the Data Bank any settlements or payments made on behalf of a physician to settle a case that would never appear anywhere else in the public record. A vigilant medical staff services office that discovers such an entry must then bring that finding to the department or the credentials committee, so that the applicant can be asked to explain how the whole event happened. Giving a false response or failing to cooperate with such a reasonable investigation is, of course, immediate grounds for termination or denial of reappointment.

Another item of information that is important for a medical staff reappointment process to know about is the physical condition of the applicant and the corresponding ability to carry out the privileges being requested. Even the act of asking that question could be considered an invasion of the privacy of the applicant under the provisions of the Americans with Disabilities Act, but there is a patient safety issue to consider also.

REAPPOINTMENT: A COMPETENT PROCESS

The real issue connected with reappointment is that it can become an automatic process, wherein a physician can routinely be regranted the same privileges over decades, without real in depth consideration of current clinical competence. Does the physician still perform all of the same privileges 40 years after first credentialing? Have the technical demands of the specialty changed without the doctor keeping up with those changes? Does the physician regularly attend the annual meetings of the specialty society and read the appropriate journals? Does the physician do all of those things but does not perform the procedure frequently enough to ensure familiarity and competence? Does anybody know? Does anybody care? Do the specialty colleagues know very well that the doctor is no longer as capable as before but do not have it in them to break the heart of an old friend by taking away those long-held privileges? If those things are happening in the reappointment process, then the members deserve the accusations that doctors protect their incompetent colleagues in a conspiracy of silence.

SUMMARY

Joint Commission standards require the medical staff to reappoint each member no later than two years from the last appointment. Reasons for this rule include further training, changes in health status, involvement in liability suits, and a review of the member's "citizenship" performance related to medical staff requirements. Tools and indicators are available to assist with the assessment process, which flows through the medical staff services employees (responsible for assembling a new application and relevant exhibits), thorough committees and the executive committee, and on to the governing board. Once again, the board should worry about whether reappointment is a competent process that does not protect incompetence.

Concern about the possibility of not knowing about the past performance history of physician applicants led the Congress to create the National Practitioner Data Bank. Hospital medical staffs are required to query this information source before reappointment can be completed.

REFERENCES

Gassiot, C. O., & Starr, P. J. (Eds.). (1987). *Principles of Medical Staff Services Science.* Education Council, National Association of Medical Staff Services. Privately printed.

Lang, D. A., & Hopkins, J. L. (1988). Trustees responsibility for professional standards. *QRC Advisor,* 4(7), 4–7.

CHAPTER

Peer Review

The term *peer review* is used for the sake of consistency and simplicity. Through the years, physicians have always been conscious of the need to be aware of the practices of colleagues and peers. The procedures for accomplishing this highly professional obligation have changed names many times. It is common for the jargon of the era—medical audit, quality assurance, quality assessment, PSRO, PRO, quality maintenance, quality improvement, clinical outcomes, or whatever follows next—to accept the fact that patients deserve to be comfortable in the knowledge that the watchdog role and function is being carried out. Even though carried out in privacy, with confidentiality safeguards such as Evidence Code 1157 in California, there must still be scrupulous attention to detail.

IDENTIFYING PERFORMANCE PROBLEMS

As hospitals invest in screening systems for the evaluation of patient care, medical staffs are now confronted with much more information, previously unavailable, about physician performance. As a consequence of current and retrospective review of all clinical services, the number and seriousness of cases for physician review has risen. Each month now, the Joint Commission medical staff is presented with a range of problems, from minor policy deviations to major clinical performance failures. In addition to individual cases, modern data processing allows for trend development: by physician, by service, hospitalwide, across integrated systems, and by diagnosis. Inferences, if not judgments, about effectiveness and efficiency of care are now within reach of the medical staff. This information flow creates an unparalleled opportunity to monitor care and strive for its continuing improvement (Lang, 1991).

Recognizing that questionable medical practice is taking place is one thing. Not recognizing questionable practice because of unwillingness to make the effort is not acceptable. Worst of all is the attitude by the members of the medical staff that all doctors are doing a good job or that it is some sort of ego attack or insult to study a physicians' cases: an insult that either threatens the doctor's complete freedom to practice medicine "my way" or dares to question the doctor's judgment. As Daniel Lang (1991) said, "at the core, the doctor believes he or she is without peers."

WHY CONFIDENTIALITY FOR PEER REVIEW?

The purpose of confidentiality shields is to protect the minutes, reports, and findings of a properly conducted medical staff peer review process from discovery by a plaintiff's attorney. The purpose of confidentiality in medical staff peer review is not to protect incompetent physicians or to conceal the fact that the medical staff is not doing its duty of due care in an effective manner. Confidentiality is also intended to encourage candor in the peer review process, to protect records and proceedings, and to prohibit compulsion of testimony in court proceedings. It is also true that confidentiality breeds suspicion that the medical staff is hiding something important to patients and is protecting its own members from deserved exposure and punishment.

Lessons from *The Verdict*

There is a Metro-Goldwin-Mayer film released in 1982 that should be required watching for participants in the medical staff peer review process. In the screenplay, a suit is brought on behalf of a plaintiff who has been rendered comatose during a delivery. The plot of *The Verdict* concerns the inexorable move in the courtroom toward the disclosure that shapes the decision by the jury. A prominent anesthesiologist, who indeed, "wrote the book," has been accused of negligence in the case. The patient vomited in her mask, which caused oxygen deprivation leading to brain damage. There seems to be no way the plaintiff's family can win the case, until her attorney locates a new and surprise witness, the nurse who had admitted the patient.

There was no mention of the hospital medical staff in the script, but there are several events that should have happened. The assistant chairman of the anesthesiology department tells the plaintiffs attorney that "the doctors killed her. They gave her the wrong anesthetic." The defendant physician, the world-famous expert was, of course, the department chair. When it came time to testify, the assistant or vice chair was nowhere to be found. He had gone on a sudden vacation to a remote island in the Caribbean. Sometimes doctors refuse to testify against each other, even when they know what actually happened. That conspiracy of silence is suspected by the public.

As the story unwinds and the tension builds, as the forces against the plaintiff's lawyer seem more overwhelming all the time, the admitting nurse describes how she filled out and signed the form stating that the patient had eaten a meal only one hour before anesthesia was induced. Prior testimony had established that at least eight hours would be required and that anything less would constitute negligence. Now working in a child care center in another city, the nurse is a sympathetic figure as she describes how the anesthesiologist had told her that he had been through five difficult deliveries that day and just did not take time to look at the admitting form that showed one hour since a meal. After the incident had happened, he went to the nurse and forced her to change her signed form to show nine hours since a meal, under the threat of having her fired. She kept a copy of the original sheet and had left nursing as a sad and disillusioned person.

Her testimony showed two lessons for the medical staff. The first is that there was actually negligence, since the doctor had failed in his duty to consider the matter of food present in the body. That failure to observe the standard of care is something the medical staff could have and should have detected and dealt with during peer review. The other issue was the criminal behavior of altering the admitting form by force of dismissal.

For those who like endings of movies that are justified, the jury recommended a settlement greatly in excess of the plaintiff's request. That was particularly rewarding for its dramatic effect, since for most of the script, there seemed to be no chance of winning the case at all. The anesthesiologist was guilty of both negligence in his care of the patient and in an unprofessional cover-up. Both of those actions are violations of the bylaws and of the spirit and intent of peer review. Could it really happen that way? Not in those hospitals where the medical staff is paying attention to all patient care, even that delivered by big shots.

These two points of view about confidentiality—it provides an atmosphere wherein candid discussion and fact-finding can take place, or it is the means by which wrongdoing can be concealed—are ofttimes irreconcilable. There is no practical way for the medical staff to defend itself or explain to the board, the patients, and the public that appropriate review procedures are taking place and that substandard care is being detected and corrected. Obviously, the best protection for the medical staff is that there is a process and that it does have integrity. All physicians on the staff will be reviewed, either by a chart falling out against criteria or else by random review. No doctor is so good or so famous or has been around so long so as to be immune from review. To err is human: to mistake symptoms or test results or miss a diagnosis is possible. To refuse to spend adequate time, to ignore appropriate staff work, to get carried away by ego, taking the position that certain doctors do not need or deserve to be reviewed: those are the real enemies of the medical staff peer review process that has integrity. And those are the lessons of *The Verdict*.

SOURCES OF REVIEW INFORMATION

There are many sources for problem identification that can lead to review of clinical performance by an appropriate peer group, including:

- committee-established screening criteria
- patient or family complaints
- reported incidents by nurses or staff
- claims or suits
- patient satisfaction surveys
- concerns expressed by other physicians

Each of these sources leads to the same process, which requires staff work to organize and present data. There are chart reviews and abstractions of important facts and issues that can be separated from the larger mass. The medical record is the key document in the peer review process, as well as in a malpractice lawsuit. Office records and hospital charts are the documents that reflect patient care and communication. The Cooperative of American Physicians advises its members to make each entry in the chart as if it were to be reviewed by a jury, because it might be. There should be no jesting, no sarcastic remarks, no finger pointing, and no insulting entries about the patient. Of course, there should be no alteration of a medical record, an act that is sure to destroy the defense of a case (Smith, 1988).

THE REVIEW PROCESS

In the review process, written reports are gathered; verbal reports are documented in writing or not considered; there are expert witness testimony and, perhaps, even case profiles of past performances by the physician in question. But the key event in the sequence occurs after the data has been collected and assembled. A physician peer member of the committee must first look at the data presentation and make one of three recommendations:

- More information is needed to complete the file and no further action can be taken until that staff work is completed

- No patient care issue appears and the case should be filed with no further attention
- An issue does appear, the data seems to be present and appropriate, and the case should next go to the agenda of the peer review committee

Anyone connected with the peer review process has heard immeasurable complaints that nurses should not review doctors or that some nurse in particular in out to "get" someone. That may all be true: nurses should not alone review doctors and a particular nurse may indeed be out to "get" a doctor, just as some doctors are out to "get" some nurses or other doctors. Remember this slogan about peer reviews: "staff screens; peers review."

Staff, whether nurses or not, collect and present data according to criteria and guidelines developed by the committee. But only a peer physician decides whether the case should be reviewed by the committee. Only a peer has the authority and opportunity to place the case on the agenda. Unfortunately, merely by being placed on an agenda constitutes a mortal insult to some physicians who will act out that reaction by a show of temper directed at the chair or, more likely, against the peer review or medical staff services clerical personnel.

NOTIFY THE PHYSICIAN

At the point where a case is to be reviewed, the offending medical staff member should be notified that complaints, claims, or incidents have been reported. Here is the opportunity for real mistrust and lack of faith in the integrity of the review process to arise. A group of peers, some of whom are strong economic competitors, are going to sit in a closed room talking *about* someone who is not present and does not yet know about the meeting. The committee is not talking *to* that person, yet. Facing an accuser in court is a basic tenet of the law, but in the medical staff, facing the accuser when that person is a nurse, employee, or other person vulnerable to retribution or retaliation by a powerful physician is not exactly the same thing. That is the reason why written statements are so important: so the review does not degenerate into a verbal shouting match that usually is won by the surgeon with the loudest voice or by the internist who admits the most patients.

Chiefs of staff and supervisory department chairs must be careful, wise, and judicious in handling these complaints and situations, which are almost always complex. But failing to notify the physician who is being discussed in the fact-finding portion of the committee work is inexcusable and inappropriate. Besides being basic fairness, early notification of the medical staff member can sometimes lead to the discovery or presentation of additional information that could lead to a quicker and simpler explanation of the circumstances and thinking process, resulting in saving everyone a lot of time and effort.

The purpose is improvement of quality and the search for good patient care, not the carrying out of a vendetta or simply a time-wasting committee meeting, such as happens all too frequently.

OUTCOMES AND ALTERNATIVES FOR ACTION

There can be several results or outcomes to a peer review process. The first outcome is, of course, to say that there was no harm, no foul, no significant or major issue involved and to return the case to the file. If there are one or more issues, the most frequent action taken is to write a letter from the committee expressing its views on the case and requesting the physician to pay attention to some particular way to remedy the problem. Usually committees ask for a written response that explains the case from the viewpoint of the one or more physicians involved. It is a simple request for information without threats or condemnations.

The habits and preferences of chairs differ, but a very successful way to proceed is for the medical staff coordinator to draft a letter based on the notes and minutes of the meeting and discussions that had taken place. It is successful because it can be more timely, more objective, and more inclusive. The physician is entitled to receive some documentation of the committee's action—something other than word of mouth from friends or enemies. An even better way to add to that written communication would be some helpful suggestions by the chair or one of the senior members of the department. Those helpful hints from respected colleagues can be a powerful stimulant toward accomplishing the goal of peer review. The goal should be to improve quality and not to harass or punish other members of the staff, except in those rare instances when further action is necessary.

A more formal result of the review process is to place the physician on an intensified review of some sort, whether retrospective chart review of all cases, or all cases of a similar nature. This level of committee action is essentially staff work with summary reports being brought to the designated committee reviewer who can then report at the next meeting. Any intensified review should be a standing item on the agenda of the committee as long as that special scrutiny is in progress. It should be in progress for a specified period of time or a specified number of cases. Left wide open without specifying an end point can, and will, drag it on for a long time, leaving the physician in question dangling without any clear idea of what the committee is looking for or what it wants done in the way patients are being treated. Besides, the process of justice needs to move at a deliberate speed. Staff members are entitled to due process. As well, the medical staff services and peer review staff need to know that they are not continuing to collect data and schedule agenda items in a useless pursuit.

Another useful outcome of case review is to direct the physician to attend appropriate continuing medical education (CME) programs intended to assist with the quality improvement process desired by the committee. There should be a certificate or program director's statement or some evidence that the physician actually attended the course. There should also be some description of the course content so as to determine that it was the appropriate learning material that will satisfy the remedial purpose. Signing in and leaving is not CME and it is not acceptable. Does that mean that the committee does not trust the physician? Maybe or maybe not, but documentation of education is always appropriate when dealing with safety issues, quality of care, and self-governance, and it assures the board of directors that a process is in place that has integrity.

These remedies suggested are all involved in actual patient cases—the acts of diagnosis, admission, treatment, prescribing, and discharge—those functions over which a departmental supervisory peer review committee has jurisdiction. With no limitation or required change of practice, there is no requirement to report to any other body, such as a licensing agency or the National Practitioner Data Bank. However, the next most formal level of review could affect practice: concurrent review. When the committee determines that an issue is sufficiently important to impose this requirement, each patient admitted to the hospital by the physician in question will be reviewed each day by a peer member of the committee or by a special monitor appointed for that purpose. Do not assign this job to a nurse or staff member. If it is important enough to do, then it is important enough that peers must shoulder the work load burden.

WHAT SHOULD BE REPORTED?

However, as long as there is only chart review, even done concurrently, there is still not enough practice restriction going on to report. That condition changes when a monitor or proctor is required by the committee to speak with the physician before any further patient care action can be taken. This further requirement may be imposed with or without the consent of the physician being reviewed. Usually, a monitor or proctor must be notified in advance of the admission, then the monitor watches and listens to the progress of the case and the thinking process involved; and no action may be taken without the permission or concurrence of the monitor. When things have progressed to this point, there must be a really serious question about the competence of the physician being reviewed, and a distinct possibility exists that membership and/or privileges may be affected.

Concurrent review at this level is an infringement on practice and has crossed the line into a probably reportable status if the monitoring extends for a month or more. This level of monitoring should be reported to the administration. If such a relationship exists that a physician of this questionable competence is being watched but that information is concealed from the people who must deal with the possible aftermath, then some major issues need to be confronted and resolved in the hospital/physician relationship. The medical staff and administration may pull and tug at each other for a number of reasons, but they must be united in their pursuit of quality improvement. However, the review would not yet have to be reported to the board, except possibly through the mechanism of a joint conference committee. At a minimum, though, the board should be made aware at the next reappointment.

Similarly restrictive, and reportable, is the required presence of a proctor during surgeries or procedures, if that requirement has been put in place during a reasonable investigation of quality issues. That does not mean that a proctor used during initial credentialing must be reported. This situation is quite different. Initial proctoring, as recommended by the California Medical Association and others, is simply a verification process leading to the decision to grant membership and privileges. Imposition of forced proctoring as a result of quality problems noticed is altogether different. Once again, duration of the restriction becomes a factor, and good medical staff services coordinators or managers will know exactly what the reporting requirements are for the licensing board having jurisdiction.

A restriction on practice, after having been applied, must be exercised promptly and effectively, if the peer review process is to have integrity. Allowing physicians to slip through the net by not notifying monitors or proctors about impending cases is a severe breakdown of the process and should be dealt with immediately by the committee chair. Or, if the committee itself is at fault, the chief of staff must take vigorous action immediately, including summary removal of the chair if that is where the fault lies. The other reason for prompt and decisive action by the committee is that the physician deserves and is entitled to due process and no unnecessary entanglements on practice.

Although department chairs are elected by their colleagues, since that is one of the benefits of medical staff democracy, the chairs have very clearly defined roles and responsibilities. The duty of maintaining the integrity of the peer review process is comparable in importance to the duty of careful examination during credentialing and reappointment for the chair. Sometimes, during the review process, it becomes apparent that one of the issues involved is a policy problem, whether the existing policy is in error, is inadequate, or has become obsolete or there is no policy at all that covers the situation. It is an obligation of the chair to remedy the policy problem by whatever means are appropriate.

ABUSIVE BEHAVIOR IS NOT ACCEPTABLE

Peer review that leads to clear, precise, and well-written policies is a worthwhile accomplishment since there will now be guidelines for quality improvement in the future that will apply to everyone. Sometimes, also, an unexpected but worthwhile outcome of peer review is a rethinking or restructuring of the administrative process. Raised consciousness about verbal abuse, sexual harassment, or other safety issues have caused hospital managers to create or rewrite policies, add counseling services, and offer lectures or presentations to the general medical staff as well as to employees. Besides, physicians are equally responsible in their offices to follow the same guidelines. Doctors cannot harass their own employees any more than they can hospital workers.

Thankfully, the world has progressed far enough that abusive doctors are no longer allowed to exhibit their bad dispositions and bad professional behavior to patients, families, nurses, or other hospital employees without being called to account for it. If you have someone in your hospital who still behaves like that, the chief of staff and chairs should demand that it be stopped immediately. Administrators, chiefs, department chairs, medical directors, and board members must not only act together in a timely proactive manner to inform present or future culprits about the consequences of their actions, but they must also respond in a timely manner to instances of abuse as soon as those occur. It is unacceptable to excuse it away. It is the chief's duty to tell the person she or he is wrong. If a staff member continues in her or his misguided way, then take prompt and appropriate remedial action.

One innovative response by a hospital CEO, with willing concurrence by the medical staff, to an incident of abusive behavior by a doctor was to ban that offending physician from the hospital buildings and grounds. He was declared a trespasser, so to speak. No official action was taken by the medical staff for reasons of quality, so there was nothing to report, but that surgeon had a month or six weeks to think about it and make a living only in the office. Whether or not most bylaws would permit this sort of infringement on practice is a real question.

Another feature of this incident was when the chief of staff, also a surgeon, met with the operating room staff to find out what happened. During the discussion, it came out that the O.R. staff did not think much of the chief's temperamental behavior, either. So he also had a learning experience that he was able to relate to others as an object lesson. To his credit, he made the situation amusing but instructive.

For too many years, medical staffs have accepted or tolerated offensive behavior by ignoring it or shrugging it off because people were hospital employees, and doctors considered the hospital their enemy or rival, so it was all right to treat nurses and technicians as subhuman.

ARE PEER REVIEWERS LIABLE?

At times, members of review committees say they are, or act as if they are reluctant to deal with instances of inappropriate or improper care because they will be taking an action against a colleague for which they could be sued. There is no question that the rejection of an application for medical staff membership and privileges, termination of membership and privileges, or reductions in privileges can adversely affect a physician's professional reputation and ability to earn money. Reasons for legal recourse against members of peer review committees based upon damage to reputation or economic injury include defamation, tortious interference with the right to practice, and restraint of trade under antitrust laws (*Hospital Law Manual,* 1995).

To help reassure medical staff members who participate in the peer review process and thus are potential defendants, a number of states have enacted statutes granting qualified immunity from liability to members of peer review committees [e.g., California Civil Code Sections 43.7, 43.8, 47(2), and 47(3)]. Also, Congress enacted the Health Care Quality Improvement Act of 1986, which includes qualified immunity from antitrust liability to encourage thorough peer review.

"Qualified" immunity means less than total immunity. Typical qualifications are that the peer review committee act without malice after making a reasonable effort to obtain the facts of the matter. Since absence of malice is a factual issue, qualified immunity is no certainty for the hospital medical staff team. Therefore, hospitals often provide insurance coverage for peer review committee members to cover both liability and defense costs, including attorneys' fees.

The peer review committee process consists of staff work to gather and present data, committee deliberation, and, if appropriate, a discussion to evaluate the data with the physician involved, leading to a recommendation for action to be taken. That recommendation must be sent to a quality improvement committee or executive committee for further discussion. Then, if it appears appropriate, and supported by data, an action is taken by the executive committee that can affect the membership and privileges of the doctor. The right to a judicial review committee hearing satisfies the due process requirement. Willett (1984) has also pointed out this prohibition against the imposition of liability on individual members of quality assurance committees.

It is also possible that a departmental committee might act more boldly, in the opposite manner from being hesitant about being sued. That is, the committee may attempt to take some sort of definitive unilateral action not within the committee's power. Experience shows that almost every instance where quality of care proceedings against a medical staff member moves eventually to court review and are won by the plaintiff, as Peter Ellsworth (personal communication, 1994) points out. The reason why the medical staff lost the case can be traced back to defective data or lack of due process.

TOWARD REMEDIAL ACTION

So here is the scenario. A departmental committee has found one or more egregious cases or a pattern of poor quality care. The physician has met with the committee, the problem could not be resolved through letters or more CME, and the case proceeds to the executive committee with a recommendation for sanction. The executive committee makes a decision that remedial action is indicated. Some executive committees have found that the use of a secret ballot is useful in arriving at such a conclusion.

For this scenario, the decision is to take remedial action, having reached that conclusion in the peer review closed session portion of the agenda. The next step is to notify the offending doctor in writing immediately: not at the chief's convenience, or some other delaying tactic, but immediately, with the exact terms of the action and all applicable dates that apply.

The next move is up to the physician. Whether or not to appeal the decision of the executive committee and any remedial action imposed that would affect membership or privileges is the prerogative of the physician in question, but that appeal must be made in the manner specified and within the time limits required by the bylaws. The physician should be very accurate and very precise; this is no time to be playing fast and loose with the bylaws.

JUDICIAL REVIEW

If there will be an appeal, then due process enters the judicial review stage. Any set of medical staff bylaws that is maintained in reasonable condition of modernization and update will have a section describing the judicial review procedure. Here follows a description of one model that will work, but is not the only acceptable way that will satisfy due process requirements.

A judicial review is a trial that follows courtroom procedure in general, although with some important differences. Counsel for the medical staff should have been involved from the moment an agenda item came to the executive committee that had the possibility of resulting in remedial action. Some medical staff leaders still cling to a notion that such matters are to be kept away from lawyers for some reason or another, but not when a physician's career and reputation or the good name of the hospital is at stake. Many medical staffs have found great support and advice from the hospital's attorney, while at times an independent counsel seems indicated. If that is to be the case, the question of who will pay the lawyer needs to be worked out well in advance of a judicial review crisis.

The executive committee plays the role of prosecutor, forced to prove by the weight of the evidence that the decision to affect privileges or membership was reasonable, appropriate, and warranted in order to protect patient safety. The physician appealing the action taken becomes the defendant, arguing that the decision to sanction, and the punishment imposed, were wrong and should be reversed and removed. If the physician is an applicant for initial medical staff membership and privileges, bylaws often provide that the applicant shall have the burden of proof (*Model Medical Staff Bylaws,* 1989).

At this point in the process, there are several caveats to follow, and several more to be observed as the drama continues to unfold. The proper role of the chief of staff has been to chair the executive committee, as well as to assure that the departmental procedure was carried out properly. The chief has another duty of supreme importance: appointing a judicial review panel of medical staff members to serve as a jury able to see and hear the data, to read minutes of previous meetings, and hear such witnesses as may be necessary to both sides.

The judicial review panel of five to seven members must be impeccable in their credentials to serve. Recognized leaders, incorruptible in their devotion to high-quality care, at least one from the same specialty as the plaintiff physician, while others should be from other specialties and departments that are related to the specialty involved or at least can understand the work of the physician on trial. Primary care physicians should always be included in judicial review panels, since they give referrals, not just receive them. Conflicts of interest must be guarded against scrupulously, such as partners or strong competitors. Fairness is the issue now, and whatever steps are necessary to ensure fairness should be taken. No person who has been a participant in previous proceedings in this case is eligible for the judicial review panel, including the department chair, review committee members, any member of the executive committee, and any of the chiefs of staff now in office. The role of the chiefs is to ensure good management of the process in order to protect the integrity of the medical staff self-governance, not to serve as some sort of personal avenging angel.

An attorney or judge (possibly retired) is used as the hearing officer, paid for by the hospital or medical staff. A court reporter produces a transcript, at hospital or medical staff expense. The plaintiff physician is entitled to a copy, if desired, but should pay for duplication expenses.

Both sides should be represented by counsel, who should be as completely familiar with medical staff law as possible and as competent as possible. This is the first opportunity for the defendant to be represented, since it is totally inappropriate for defendant's counsel to participate in any of the preceding peer review due process. There is no place for attorneys during the medical staff peer review process. They may be retained by the physician and give advice and plan strategy but they may not attend peer review sessions and listen or participate. When the entire medical staff/hospital board process is completed, then the defendant and attorney have access to the entire legal system in which to seek redress. Some bylaws even have a provision prohibiting medical staff members from moving outside the peer review/judicial review process until it has been completed and all administrative remedies have been addressed.

The medical staff attorney, acting as prosecutor, then presents the case that is intended to support the sanction taken. The defendant's attorney argues on behalf of the client, presenting evidence and witnesses, the hearing officer conducts an orderly process that does not need to observe all formal courtroom rules of evidence, while the jury of colleague physicians listens, reads exhibits, and renders a verdict. All of this should be done in a timely manner, without unseemly haste or delay.

What is the verdict? If the jury agrees with the executive committee, the action previously taken has been ratified and is presented to the board of directors for decision. If the executive committee action is not upheld, then the verdict may specify restoration to membership or restoration of privileges. The executive committee is notified in writing by the chair of the judicial review panel, and next steps must be determined. If there is no real sentiment to continue the issue, then the case is dropped, and hard feelings will undoubtedly linger for years, if not lifetimes. The idea of being put through the ordeal of a judicial review, of being talked about by other doctors, the fear that patients or the press might find out—all of those are horrible to consider, particularly when the medical staff accusers could not prove their case to the satisfaction of a panel of respected colleagues who tried their best to be objective.

If the departmental review committee still feels that a quality of care issue has been left unresolved, then new data and new monitoring or review must begin. Care, however, must be taken that rights are preserved and that retaliation does not occur by anyone. But what if the committee members are still convinced that the physician should have been punished? Now is the time to reexamine procedure to see if the committee gathered and presented data that was clear and conclusive or if there was really an attempt to "get" someone, and the preparation was done emotionally and not through the scientific method.

ROLE OF THE BOARD

If the verdict by the judicial review panel was to reject the action of the executive committee and the executive committee does not request an appellate review, then the board of directors is not yet directly involved since no issue was ever presented to them. However, the board must be made aware of the process and be satisfied that it was conducted properly. The board is not yet able to take any independent action of its own, such as removing membership or privileges, since the remedies provided for in the bylaws have not been completed. Thus, the board remains a spectator on the sideline, waiting to see the outcome.

On the other hand, if the verdict is to uphold the action of the executive committee and the physician requests an appellate review by the board of directors, then the board or appeal panel of less than the full board will hear the appeal. The role of the board at this point is very important but seems unclear to many people. The board does *not* retry the case but acts as an appeals court to assure that due process was carried out. Commonly, the grounds for appeal are that there was substantial noncompliance with the requisite procedures so as to deny a fair hearing; the decision was not supported by substantial evidence based on the hearing record; or the action taken was arbitrary, unreasonable, or capricious. The proceedings of the appeal board are based on the written record, including exhibits, of the hearing held by the judicial review panel or committee (*Model Medical Staff Bylaws,* 1989).

Assume that the board satisfies itself that due process was observed and that the bylaws were followed scrupulously to safeguard both the rights of the accused physician and the integrity of the peer review process. All of that happened exactly as it was supposed to. The physician is then notified in writing with a description of the exact sanction and any and all dates involved. The peer review process is now complete and the role of the hospital medical staff in carrying out its duty of self-governance has been carried out. Now litigation can begin, or any other action the physician wants to undertake, if there is a wish to continue the struggle at his or her own expense, as it has been all the way through. The physician can go to court, resign from the staff, or accept the penalty, but some important issues remain. If the review process was performed appropriately, with protection of rights, with an abundance of carefully documented data, without conflict of interest, in the reasonable belief that a quality of care problem was being improved, then the medical staff can believe that it did its job as well as possible. Whatever comes next will be played out as it happens. However, if those conditions are not as secure as they should be, then maybe there is reason to worry.

Rarely is there any other action taken by the board that is different from the considered wisdom of the department, the executive committee, and the judicial review panel. But if the board, for some reason, chooses to reject all of the agreed-upon findings, then there are probably some major issues going on in the hospital that are more complicated than the performance of one doctor in one or more cases. The entire set of relationships among the administration, board, and the medical staff and maybe even the survival of the hospital could be in jeopardy.

So what is the role of the administration in all of these proceedings? The answer is that the administration and board are partners with a large stake in both process and outcome. Their roles are to support the process but be careful not to interfere with it. As well, the administration and board should supply resources and information, be kept informed by the chief of staff about patient safety issues, and support nursing and other staff in their activities of providing documentation, but without direct participation or influence in the peer review process. If the hospital uses a vice president for medical affairs officer, that person can be a vital link in the necessary communication flow, can muster the resources needed, can support the chief and the medical staff mechanism as it grinds its way forward (probably too slowly), and can represent administration and the board. Under no circumstances, however, can the VPMA run the show, chair the judicial review panel, or give any other appearance of controlling the process.

Should the administrator chair or sit as a member of the judicial review panel? To most members of the medical staff that would produce instant discredit and reversal of the entire affair. The administration should participate by furnishing appropriate information and cooperation when needed but offer no interference while the process is playing itself out, lest it should give to the medical staff the appearance of some kind of purge. In some hospitals, there is such an extreme wall of confidentiality by the medical staff that administration and the board are unaware that an untoward event has even occurred and that a jury trial is in progress. People only find out when it is time to pay the legal bills, which the medical staff will certainly send to the administration. Such a hospital is quite disconnected in its relationships and its process and could not be termed in any way a partnership.

What is the role of the board during the conduct of the peer review process, the judicial review, and the executive committee's recommendation against a sanctioned physician? The board plays no active role, allowing the process to unfold without trying to overtly (or even covertly for that matter) influence the outcome. Individual board members should stay out of it. Do not try to put in a good or bad word to any of the medical staff participants. The *worst* enemy of the process is the member of the judicial review panel who titillates colleagues in the doctor's lounge by describing all of the events and evidence being discussed and who said what about whom. It is equally improper to discuss peer review matters of any kind on the floors and units of the hospital to other physicians who are or are not participants. Confidentiality means to never discuss it with anyone anywhere.

Since the board sits as an appeals body, its role is to ensure fairness and that the rights of the physician were safeguarded, particularly that the accused was represented by counsel. After all, the same board admitted that physician to the staff and granted privileges at some earlier time. Under no circumstances should a board allow itself to be drawn into a discussion of the merits of the case or to listen to the physician's defense, even if by a friend of the board members. Follow the bylaws, which were approved by the board and which bind board members as well as the medical staff to follow the due process described within.

Being a friend of board members will not stop an aggrieved physician from suing for damages after the medical staff review process is completed, and that person is entitled to the right to seek redress. At that point, tampering by individual board members or even by administration will not serve the hospital well. The best defense the board has against suit is that the medical staff process was impeccably clean, with adequate and appropriate data, with a peer review process performed without conflict of interest, in a reasonable belief that a quality of care issue was involved, and (particularly) that the punishment recommended is appropriate to fit the crime. The physician who sues after a process like that may still win, the litigious climate being what it is. This is all the more reason to follow the rules as the best and only protection.

If all those conditions prevail, then the board will have a strong defense for its sanctions against the offending physician. If, on the other hand, the department review committee exhibited personal bias or a noncompetitive attitude; if the executive committee did not demonstrate proper oversight; or if the judicial review panel was wrongly chosen or did not function in a fair, objective manner, then the board may very well lose a suit without doing anything wrong itself. Yet, it did do something wrong: it allowed a medical staff to avoid or evade its responsibilities to perform self-governance, and it did not hold the chief of staff accountable to provide good information in a timely and cooperative manner. The word *partner* is tossed about by those players in the health care delivery game, but this is one time when they better act that way.

DO MEDICAL STAFF FUNCTIONS MATTER?

A lot of time has been spent discussing common as well as some not-so-common everyday medical staff functions. Do those functions—credentialing, privileging, reappointment, peer review—actually matter? Is the whole thing a monumental waste of time as some staff members have charged? Why are these things being done at all? Why are there so may meetings? In the doctors' lounge there will be plenty of grumbling that medical staff functions *do not matter:* They are being done only because the Joint Commission requires them. JCAHO is a unwelcome intrusion into the lives and practices of physicians. The organized medical staff is too bureaucratic and time-consuming. Its functions are important only to the hospital so as to maintain JCAHO accreditation. On the contrary, these functions are important to individual physicians as well as to the delegated organized medical staff because they are intended to:

- protect patients
- protect physicians from themselves and each other
- improve quality of care

SUMMARY

The term *peer review* is used for consistency and simplicity, standing for all references to the evaluation of physician performance. The desire to better accomplish peer review was, in fact, the original reason for voluntary accreditation by structures that became the Joint Commission. Uses of screening systems, data systems, and current and retrospective review are characteristics of the unfolding technology. More worrisome to hospital administration and governing boards is the fear or suspicion that some members of the medical staff are unable or unwilling to make a real effort. Confidentiality shields have been erected by state legislation and generally protected by the courts where there is a good faith effort at peer review in reasonable belief about a quality issue.

The review process lives or dies with good staff work to assemble and array data, according to criteria and guidelines developed by medical staff committees. For the organized medical staff, the key ingredient is due process for the physician involved, as well for the hospital and the patient. Sometimes, review committees are reluctant to deal with problems for fear they may be liable individually, but state and federal immunities exist. When an egregious problem has resulted in a physician being recommended to the executive committee for sanction, there could be further due process through formal judicial review that resembles a court trial. Eventually, if action must be taken, that will occur only by action of the board on recommendation of the medical staff.

REFERENCES

Hospital Law Manual, Attorney's Volume. (1995). Section 7, Medical Staff. Gaithersburg, MD: Aspen Publishers.

Lang, D. A. (1991). *Medical Staff Peer Review: A Strategy for Motivation and Performance.* Chicago: American Hospital Publishing, Inc.

Model Medical Staff Bylaws (1989). Sacramento: California Association of Hospitals and Health Systems.

Smith, D. L. (1988). *Loss Prevention for Physicians.* Los Angeles: Cooperative of American Physicians, Inc., Mutual Protection Trust.

Willett, D. E. (1984). *What Physicians Should Know about The Legal Status of the Medical Staff.* San Francisco: California Medical Association.

CHAPTER

Chief of Staff

The American health care system is undergoing change unprecedented in both magnitude and velocity. Nowhere else is that change more apparent than in the need for a higher degree of physician leadership than the health care system has previously demanded. Doctors must realize that no matter how much they think health care has changed in the past decade, it is only the beginning. Each year the existing system dissolves more. Some organizations are trying to create a form of order out of the apparent chaos of change by leaving behind the strategies of management and patterns of medical practice that were simply reacting to regulatory and payer attempts to control quality and cost. For these organizations that seek not simply to survive but to excel, effective physician leadership will be key for both the medical staff and the hospital. This new breed of leadership can be defined as the ability to transform vision into a force that successfully mobilizes people to achieve common goals deriving from this vision (Merry, 1993).

LEADER OF THE MEDICAL STAFF

Whether called by the traditional name chief of staff or the newer form, president of the medical staff, we mean the elected leader of the Joint Commission model of a hospital medical staff. The job of the chief (or president) has grown from one of being essentially honorary to the present day tasks of being the identified spokesman and policy guide for an organization that shows all the attributes of a political party, including lack of unity and lack of respect for the leader. A formal approach for recognizing the duties of the chief is shown in the job description presented as Appendix 8–1. But there are many more subtleties and a wide variety of informal relationships that shape the basic position in addition to the formal job description. Each chief brings unique qualities to the job. Each chief invariably faces some sort of crisis that shapes the character and personality of that Chief as a leader from that point on. And, the job itself, in a particular hospital, is shaped by each chief's handling of critical issues.

There should be a formal job description for the position of chief of the medical staff, or president of the medical staff, if the hospital uses that title. If the hospital does not have a written version, then it can use the example supplied in the appendix or else write a more appropriate description of what the chief is expected to be and to do. Do not just continue to ad lib the selection and preparation of this crucial leadership position. It has always been a standard joke among doctors that failure to attend the committee meeting or annual general staff meeting makes the absent person vulnerable to being elected. The days should be gone when a chief is elected to the office on the night (or two weeks before) the term begins. The days should be gone when the new chief then stands at the microphone at the banquet where the vote was announced and in time-honored tradition says: "Well, I don't know what I'm supposed to do, but I'll try hard." Why is it that a leadership position is considered something a physician might be stuck with if he or she is not present to refuse the honor? (Merry, 1993). There should be no mystery about what a chief does in the hospital, and there should be a long enough period of training and preparation before taking office to ensure that the new chief is ready and able to pick up the continuing burden of the office.

Physicians have traditionally shied away from organizational leadership roles for a number of reasons. Organizational leadership in health care has traditionally been performed as well as perceived as a nonclinical function, something that administrators do. Doctors have traditionally seen the purpose of administrators as caretakers more than real leaders. In medicine, real leaders are outstanding clinicians—clinical virtuosos, master practitioners of both the art and science of medicine. Master clinicians have made marvelous strides in the advancement of medical practice but rarely as outstanding managers. The best physicians and the most admired teachers exhibit a flexible, patient-based approach that requires a great degree of clinical autonomy. Physicians regard themselves as independent agents in their medical practice, in the hospital or network, and in the medical staff. Autonomy is a core value.

Autonomy may produce clinical mastery, but it does not produce team players. Autonomous physicians are at the top of the clinical decision-making hierarchy. The difficulty of moving groups of them in response to someone else's vision should be apparent. Many physicians are not only averse to taking leadership roles themselves, but act even naturally rebellious toward anyone, including chiefs of staff who attempt to take them in a direction they might not value or find relevant. As Martin Merry (1993) said, they tend to be deeply suspicious of any form of leadership that might compromise their autonomy. This resistance to accepting direction or suggestion is the exact opposite of the kinds of teamwork demanded by modern organizational excellence. Physicians are likely to want to elect leaders who will not direct them but will advocate their tradition of autonomy in response to any party, particularly the administration, who might challenge this tradition. Chiefs who seek to genuinely lead their colleagues with the best motives and the best interests of the medical staff at heart are often astonished to find themselves doing so at their peril.

JOB OF THE CHIEF

In the Joint Commission model, the job of the chief of staff is to see that

- medical staff systems of credentialing, reappointment, and peer review are in place;
- systems comply with standards or regulations;
- systems comply with the bylaws;
- systems actually function well with the help of medical staff services and peer review professionals;
- results and outcomes of the systems are reported regularly to the board.

In a recent study of medical staffs in a nationwide group of hospitals, chiefs of staff in those institutions responded that their three top reasons for accepting the position were new opportunities, an obligation to their colleagues, and professional growth (Medical Leadership Forum, 1994). The chiefs who responded that the most important skills that a chief can have is to be a listener, a communicator, a decision maker who can facilitate the exchange of ideas, objective, skillful at running meetings, and able to work under stress. Those were the ideal skills. The chiefs noted that their actual skills include being a listener, a team player who is confident and a physician advocate. Their self-confessed greatest weaknesses were being too reactive, hesitant, talkative, too process oriented, and rigid.

Other study data shows that the ideal length of term to assure quality leadership would be two years, although historically, most chiefs have served one-year terms. Almost one-half of the hospitals surveyed compensate their chief, at a median level of $25,000, with a range of $10,000 to $50,000. The average chiefs of staff in this study spend 10 or fewer hours per week in the role and report that assuming the position had little impact on their practice and that their patient base remained the same. Approximately 30 percent of chiefs worked more than 10 hours per week, and the same number reported that their patient base had declined. Chiefs are active in continuing education classes aimed at management skill development, with a median of 30 hours (ranging up to 50 hours) per year devoted to this effort.

Another interesting aspect of the study responses is the chief of staff opinions about medical staff executive committees, which had an average of 18 members. Executive committees meet on a monthly basis, for 1½ hours. The chiefs ranked the effectiveness of their executive committees highest in credentialing, with much lower ratings in peer review, participation in activities, and direction regarding mission, goals, and strategies. Overall, chiefs of staff in participating hospitals indicated they were generally satisfied with the effectiveness and efficiency of the executive committee, but there were considerable degrees of ambivalence or dissatisfaction. The chiefs were asked to rate each of several traits or attributes of potential candidates for membership on the executive committee. While a long list of traits were named, the five most important were considered to be demonstrated achievement in medicine, objectivity, ability to work with other executive committee members, support of other medical staff members, experience on other hospital committees, leadership and patient advocacy. Furthermore, the chiefs thought the executive committee is too detail and process oriented and does not contribute to the hospital's larger strategic decision making. The committee falls short in its responsibility to assess its own performance and assess the performance of its individual members.

The chief of staff is personally responsible for working with administration and the board in the best interests of patient care and safety, creating a harmonious workplace environment for nurses and the employee staff, and fostering a good image for the hospital. A chief is not charged with righting all the perceived wrongs that have been previously done by the world to the medical staff in the minds of some of its individual members. The chief is a leader in person and in example to other physicians and is always aware of the enormous respect that accompanies the office.

When there are medical or quality issues that make the papers, the chief should function as the representative to speak publicly. Never should a junior member of the public relations department be put out in front of reporters or television cameras to try to talk about a medical matter. There are examples too numerous to mention about administrators who were nervous or hesitant about discussing the problem and tried to get away with a "no comment" answer. Prepare the chief well with good information and the policy position if there is one and count on his or her wisdom and judgment to respond intelligently and protectively. When the matter is medical, the chief *is* the expert. Of course, this advice succeeds best in a hospital working relationship where a feeling of partnership exists and where problems are something to be solved, not covered up, in the interests of quality improvement.

The roles and responsibilities of medical staff leaders have become so large and complex that the time has passed when chiefs of staff and department chairs served on a rotation or "turn" basis. Maybe the worst of all systems of succession are those that rotate alphabetically. A better idea now is to enact position descriptions such as the example provided. The job and its components differ, of course, depending on the location, size, and local culture situation, but the main tasks remain the same. Chiefs should serve at least two-year terms and should be compensated. That stipend should take into account the importance of the job—and job it is indeed, no longer just an honor or a gentleman's obligation to colleagues to do a share of service. The chief should be paid for the importance of the medical staff and that position to the hospital, for the number of hours spent in meetings, and for recognition of lost patient care income.

Many chiefs find that they cannot possibly maintain a full practice load, and this dose of reality needs to be made very clear before taking office. The same explanation of reality needs to be made clear to the administration if that has not yet occurred, and it certainly needs to be explained to boards, who might not have a clue what the chief does besides attend their meetings. Ask the medical staff coordinator some time about how much correspondence there is that needs to be read, drafted, approved, and signed. Ask also about how much time is involved in working out agendas for the executive committee and preparing reports to the board. It is not just an honor, it is lots of real work.

THE GOOD, THE BAD, THE CHIEF

Most of the time, it is truly an honor to be regarded well enough to be elected chief. Only a very small percentage of the medical staff ever achieves that honor, while a very high percentage never wants to be so recognized and would not take the position under any circumstances. Perhaps the old saying applies here. Attributed to Mark Twain, a man who was being tarred and feathered and ridden out of town on a rail supposedly said "If it wasn't for the honor, I'd rather be somewhere else."

It is a sad fact that chiefs cannot merely exist, much less act as a leader willing to challenge the status quo, without offending someone who might have sent a referral patient. Hard work, long hours, loss of referrals, constant abuse from doctors who refuse to change their ways or the status quo as the world changes around them: these are some of the rewards for the modern day chief of staff, along with a real sense of accomplishment, the knowledge of having solved some real and important problems, and the perception that overall patient care was improved. Some incidents are tribulations, such as when the orthopedic surgeons refuse to do E.R. backup during the Christmas–New Year week and threaten a boycott. There are also the rewards created by the association with some truly fine and outstanding people on hospital boards and in administrations, to go along with the pleasure in working with fine staff in medical staff services and the peer review analysts.

By and large, most chiefs seem to grow into the job and usually exude a sense of responsibility and service. Soon after taking office, they learn to develop the thick skin necessary to maintain sanity in this changing world of evolution and transition from doctor–centered and controlled hospital medical practice to the next world of shared control with others. But what are the new challenges facing these leaders in a changing environment? They must, of course, try to succeed in mobilizing colleagues in pursuit of medical staff goals, if there are any. There should be attention to improvement of the executive committee and concern for more efficient practice patterns in a capitation world, as well as internalization of the general principles of quality improvement by whatever faddish name. But chiefs cannot be just cheerleaders. Merry (1993) proposes the following characteristics as a definition of successful physician leaders.

Vision

Leaders must think globally, act locally, be able to grasp the big picture, understand where their organization is going, and contribute actively to the formation of an ongoing institutional vision.

Communication Skills

In acting locally while thinking globally, successful physician leaders now and in the future should genuinely hear their colleagues at the same time they are articulating organizational direction. Moving toward a shared vision, once there is, indeed, a higher degree of sharing that vision, will require high levels of ongoing and repetitious communication. Many specific tasks must be accomplished, some of them routine and repetitive, before there is any progress to be made.

Trust

Trust might be defined as the end result of commitments consistently kept. Leaders must follow through. They must do what they say they will do. No one, particularly not a suspicious and distrustful doctor, can be verbally persuaded to trust a leader whether self-proclaimed or elected. The leader must earn trust through actions. The problem is, frequently, that the physician leader is left twisting slowly in the wind by a sudden turn in direction by the administration and the board, after the physician leader has spent months persuading medical staff colleagues that something else would take place.

Self-Confidence

By definition, leaders foster change. There was a period some years back, when leaders were urged to become "change agents." The term died, but not the general idea. The medical staff is the bastion of status quo, while their good leaders are trying to take them to unknown places. Some of those places may be perceived as threatening, while others are well known to be downright hostile and dangerous. Leaders—chiefs and department chairs—cannot worry about their popularity with their colleagues. That advice is easy to give, but medical staff physician leaders cannot avoid worrying. They must some day return to their place in the ranks to associate once again with some of the unforgiving who have long memories.

Courage

In their willingness to break new ground, many leaders are inherent risk takers. With risk comes the potential for loss. The wise leader understands this and weighs specific risks carefully. One of the major risks is that the administrator or management or executive group will probably be gone by that time, taking all their promises with them, but the medical staff will still be there with enhanced distrust and more than ever resistance to change. The demonstrated willingness to face and probably actually experience loss defines the medical staff leader in these turbulent times as a person of real courage.

SUMMARY

The elected leader of a Joint Commission medical staff has been (traditionally) called chief of staff or (the newer form) president of the medical staff. The job of this official, by either name, has grown from being essentially honorary to the identified spokesman and policy guide for an organization that shows all the attributes of a political party, including lack of unity and respect for the leader.

There should be a job description for this position, such as that presented in Appendix 8–1. Preparation is necessary in these modern times of managed care, merger and acquisition, and integrated health care system building. An organized program for identification and selection of future leaders is crucial, as is a budget for training and preparation. Future leaders need skills training and should demonstrate identifiable qualities. They should be paid appropriately for their responsibilities and sacrifices. The successful growth of the Joint Commission model of a hospital medical staff through the years is due in no small measure to the fine leaders who have served their colleagues.

REFERENCES

Merry, M. D. (1993). Physician leadership for the 21st Century. *Quality Management in Health Care* 1(3), 31–41.

Williams, S., & Ewell, C. M. (1994). Medical staff leadership trends at sixty-five leading hospitals. In *Panel Survey of Hospital Medical Staffs.* La Jolla, CA: The Medical Ledership Forum of the Governance Institute.

APPENDIX 8–1
POSITION DESCRIPTION: CHIEF OF STAFF

POSITION TITLE: Chief of Staff

DEPARTMENT:

REPORTS TO: Board of Directors and Medical Executive Committee

POSITION PURPOSES: Provides medical staff leadership to assure quality of care throughout the hospital during a two-year term including:

- bylaws implementation
- JCAHO Accreditation
- verbal and written reports to the governing board
- harmonious relationships among medical staff, board, and administration.

KEY RESPONSIBILITIES: Coordinates concerns of medical staff with administration, nursing service, and other patient care services. Represents medical staff through ongoing assessment activities. Communicates quality of care issues to and among medical staff, board, and administration. Enforces bylaws, rules, and regulations, including corrective action consistent with a fair-hearing process. Appoints all members of all medical staff committees, in consultation with department chairs and other committee leadership. Calls, prepares agenda for, and presides at all general medical staff meetings. Chairs executive committee and serves as ex-officio on the board's joint conference and all other medical staff committees. Consults with CEO on regular basis to maintain quality of care and harmonious relationships.

CUSTOMERS SERVED: Board of Directors in cooperation with the CEO. Systemwide involvement with other chiefs, CEOs, and other executives.

EDUCATION
M.D./D.O. degree

LICENSURE
Management training preferred (ABMM certification, M.B.A., A.C.P.E., PIMS, etc.).

EXPERIENCE
- Active staff for at least five years
- Previous success in major medical staff responsibilities
- Excellent communication and analytical skills
- Excellent organization and management skills
- 80 or more hours a month in leadership activities
- Annual written and verbal progress report to governing board
- Holds no similar role at same time in another institution
- Participates in board and medical staff leadership planning retreat

RECOGNITION AND BENEFITS
- Stipend paid in recognition of complexity and importance of the position, and time demands
- Tuition and expenses for self and spouse in two external CME events per year
- Exemption from mandatory E.R. call, other committee assignments, and meeting attendance requirements
- Committee obligations waived for three years thereafter
- Hospital indemnification for role-related activities

OCCUPATIONAL HAZARDS
Time demands, schedule disruptions, conflict with peers, effect on practice office and referral patterns

CHAPTER

Three-Chiefs Model

A successful model used by a growing number of hospital medical staffs is that of providing for three chiefs of staff. These include, by whatever title, the chief in office, the past chief, and the chief-elect. A complete description, of this process and the duties involved needs to be written in the bylaws, of course. The chief in office, serving a two-year term, functions in the role outlined in the position description which generally includes making appointments, serving as the elected leader and spokesperson, and chairing the executive committee and general staff meetings. The chief needs to work closely with administration and represents a physician's point of view to the board.

One of the more difficult things to get used to for a new chief is to be constantly asked by managers and trustees, "What does the medical staff think about this?" The question is actually unanswerable, since the chief has neither the means nor opportunity to canvas the members individually or to seek opinions from the influentials on the staff. There was plenty of input from the dwellers of the doctors' lounge, but maybe the reverse of that opinion is closer to reality. However it is, the chief must answer *now* and must say something believable and credible if the medical staff is to be considered in the decision being studied. Chiefs also enforce bylaws, rules, and policies as well as ensure that competent systems are in place and working. Further, the chief must be able to explain those systems to the most uninformed member of the board so that they make sense. Saying that medical staff business is confidential just will not wash as an answer when the question was about a system, not a person.

THE CHIEF OF STAFF ELECT

The chief of staff elect, or chief in training, follows the role in the position description shown in Appendix 9–1. The chief elect should chair the quality improvement committee (by whatever name), which was probably called the QA committee back in the 1980s. The reason for this particular responsibility is to learn the peer review system from top to bottom to find out who the problem doctors are, as well as to find those leaders who will make good appointments when that time comes that the chief-elect becomes the chief and must make all appointments. During their two-year term, chiefs in training should attend adequate and appropriate training in preparation for assuming the duties of the chief. The bylaws must specify that the chief-elect will succeed to the office of chief automatically so that training and preparation will have a practical effect, as well as to prevent a surprise when an unknown or unprepared person is suddenly thrust into the all-important chief of staff position to satisfy the whims of a group of dissidents. There definitely needs to be the provision and possibilities for the outlet of dissatisfaction and dissension, but election of the chief of staff is not the appropriate place to spew that particular venom. If the system is not working, elect good leaders, and then help them fix the system.

Pay the-chief elect for the necessary responsibilities and time spent overseeing departmental peer review, serving on other committees as assigned by the chief, and meeting regularly with administration and the board on important issues. Furthermore, the chief-elect should have his or her office manager meet with the medical staff coordinator to arrange schedules for meeting times. Each new chief-elect should tell the office staff about the new list of duties and the new people who will be calling the office from the medical staff office, for whom there is no need to go through the normal routine. The other pervasive problem is when the medical staff coordinator has carefully and patiently gone over the meeting schedule and responsibilities, only to have the chief-elect forget to show it to the office staff person who handles the calendar. Consequently, when the medical staff office calls frantically, looking for a chief-elect who should be there chairing a meeting, the only response that the practice office can give is a limp explanation about lack of information.

THE PAST CHIEF OF STAFF

Many medical staffs do not make good use of the vast array of knowledge learned on the job and do not make good use of all that skill and experience by having specific assignments for the immediate past chief of staff. Pay the past chief also, but pay less than the chief-elect, which is less than the chief in office. Assign the past chief a set of duties, such as those in the job description provided as Appendix 9–2.

Past chiefs can serve a unique and important role by chairing special ad hoc groups appointed to solve immediate problems such as E.R. backup or some other hospital/medical staff issue that will benefit from the results-oriented guidance of a veteran who has been through all the medical staff wars and is no longer very patient with all the foolishness. If it is a dirty and unpopular job that must be done, then appoint the past chief to get it resolved. The sage advice of the past chief can be invaluable to a new chief who may not yet know all the background on long-standing enmities or feuds within the staff. Chiefs will differ in their specialties and their opinions, but what they have in common is *being* chief, in a position that cannot be delegated or performed by anyone else at the time. Past chiefs also make wonderful board members, because they bring such a wide array of perspectives and are not easily intimidated by special interest groups.

The three-chiefs model is not the only way to reduce turnover, to provide more continuity and preparedness for the most important position in the medical staff, but it is certainly one time-tested and proven method for meeting those goals. The strength of three chiefs is that it is a clean organization with a clear internal structure and well-understood relationships. There is no confusion about roles, while the structure provides ease in working with the administration and the board. The weakness of three chiefs is that it can be complex and will need executive leadership, such as that presented in Chapter 10. A successful three-chiefs model also requires a support structure and adequate staff, but then so does any medical staff leadership system. The chiefs will need weekly meetings to keep up with all the issues of a fast-moving hospital and medical staff in a rapidly changing health care environment. That means someone beside the chiefs must prepare an agenda, manage progress toward accomplishing each agenda item and report back regularly to each chief on issues as needed. The requirements of those duties will demand someone other than the medical staff coordinator who is consumed with the work load of committees and credentialing.

SUMMARY

Some medical staffs use the three-chiefs model, which has many advantages to recommend it. Using the position of the chief of staff elect, or chief in training, allows time and opportunity to learn all of the medical staff systems well in advance of the succession to chief. That is particularly important with respect to the peer review process and in determining who will make good appointees when it comes time for that responsibility. A job description, such as that provided in Appendix 9–1, is essential for the recruitment, selection, and preparation of the incoming leaders, as is an adequate pay level.

Many medical staffs do not make good use of the vast array of knowledge, skills, and experience by having specific assignments for the past chief of staff. Pay the past chief also, but pay less than the chief-elect. Assign the past chief duties, such as those in the job description provided in Appendix 9–2. Past chiefs can be particularly valuable in chairing special ad hoc problem solving groups, and they make particularly good board members.

The three-chiefs model can provide continuity and preparedness, since it is a clear and clean structure with well-understood relationships.

REFERENCES

White, C. H. (1986–1994). [Faculty workshop presentations on medical staff organization and structure]. Grossmont Hospital, La Mesa, CA; and Sharp Healthcare, San Diego, CA.

APPENDIX 9–1
POSITION DESCRIPTION: CHIEF OF STAFF ELECT

POSITION TITLE: Chief of Staff Elect

DEPARTMENT:

REPORTS TO: Chief of Staff

POSITION PURPOSES: Provides continuity in medical staff leadership with the chief of staff during a two-year term.

KEY RESPONSIBILITIES: Assists chief of staff as assigned. Member of the executive committee. Chairs the quality improvement committee. Oversees the peer review committee.

CUSTOMERS SERVED: Chief of Staff and Executive Committee

EDUCATION
M.D./D.O. degree

LICENSURE
   Management training preferred (ABMM Certification, M.B.A., A.C.P.E., IMS, etc.)

EXPERIENCE
   • Active staff for at least five years
   • Prior success in major medical staff leadership roles
   • Prior medical staff leadership education and skill development
   • No concurrent leadership office in any other hospital during the term of office
   • Stamina and willingness to serve a two-year term in office followed by a two-year term as chief of staff

RECOGNITION AND BENEFITS
   • Stipend
   • Tuition and expenses for self and spouse in two external CME events per year
   • Exemption from other committee assignments and meeting attendance requirements

• Hospital indemnification for role-related activities

OCCUPATIONAL HAZARDS

Time demands, schedule disruptions, lobbying by interest groups within the medical staff

APPENDIX 9–2
POSITION DESCRIPTION: PAST CHIEF OF STAFF

POSITION TITLE: Past Chief of Staff

REPORTS TO: Chief of Staff

POSITION PURPOSE: Provides benefit of experience, continuity and familiarity with hospital and medical staff issues and personnel.

KEY RESPONSIBILITIES: Assists chief of staff as assigned. Member of the executive committee. Chairs the risk management or utilization review committee. Chairs special ad hoc problem-solving committees. Offers senior medical leader role to the medical staff, administration, and board.

CUSTOMERS SERVED: Chiefs of Staff, Executive Committee, Board of Directors, system involvement with boards, CEOs, other chiefs.

EDUCATION
M.D./D.O. degree

LICENSURE

EXPERIENCE
• Two-year terms as chief elect and chief of staff

RECOGNITION AND BENEFITS
• Stipend
• Tuition and expenses for self and spouse in one external CME event per year
• Exemption from other committee assignments and meeting attendance requirement
• Hospital indemnification for role-related activities

OCCUPATIONAL HAZARDS
   Time demands, schedule disruptions, time away from full-time practice, conflicts with peers developed during six-year period of leadership

CHAPTER

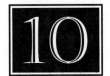

Medical Staff Executive

Consider an idea called the *association model.* Associations of all types—of doctors, of business and industry groups—all have members who have joined together for the purpose of advancing their legitimate self-interests. In this case, the members of the medical staff have joined together by choice and have agreed to abide by the rules (bylaws), which were made known to the applicants in advance. Think of the hospital medical staff as an association, just as the state and county medical societies are associations.

THE ASSOCIATION MODEL

An association has a policymaking group that is smaller than the entire membership. Think of the executive committee, for that is its function, to act on behalf of the membership.

Associations have an elected officer to represent the members and be the identifiable leader acting and speaking on behalf of the entire organization. The nation has a president, the state has a governor, and the medical staff has a chief of staff to carry out the same executive and legislative duties.

Associations have staff employees to perform the work of the organization, perform its assigned functions, and carry out policies once they have been formulated. The medical staff has its assistants in medical staff services, quality assessment, continuing medical education, the health sciences library, utilization management, perhaps a physician referral service, and others.

What the medical staff does not have that an association does have is an executive officer to implement the policies and supervise the staff. The medical staff executive represents a new generation of management whose job it is to keep the office of the chief of staff working effectively on a full-time basis (White, 1989). In the traditional Joint Commission model, the chiefs and departmental chairs come to the early morning meeting, eat the donuts and drink the coffee, then go on to their practice offices while the staff works without further leadership or supervision except for what they can accomplish through phone calls to the practice office. In contrast, in the new model, each department in the hospital has an on-site administrative manager or supervisor except the employees of the medical staff.

Executive as Manager

A medical staff executive is a full-time manager who directs the office of the chief of staff and supervises those employees that have been combined into a unified medical staff department rather than a collection of overlapping or conflicting supervisors. Those who do not believe that typical hospital supervision and authority is overlapping for the medical staff employees should ask them about it sometime and about how difficult it is to have the doctors telling them one thing to do while their hospital manager is countermanding or contradicting that instruction. An organization chart showing the medical staff executive position in its proper relationship would look like Figure 10–1.

The principal duty of the medical staff executive is to implement the policies as determined by the executive committee, the chiefs of staff, and the department supervisory committees. No chief is able to attend all of the committee meetings but an executive could be present at the important meetings for all of the important issues and key events. As a practical day-by-day reality, the executive helps to carry the burden of the chiefs and can represent them at some events to give reports and to bring back information that will be useful in making decisions. Does the executive speak for the chief or make individual statements and give personal opinions? Only if delegated that mission by the chiefs and when within a comfortable working relationship.

Effective Executive

Can a nonphysician be effective or of any value within an organization of physicians? National, state, and county medical societies have functioned that way for decades, and

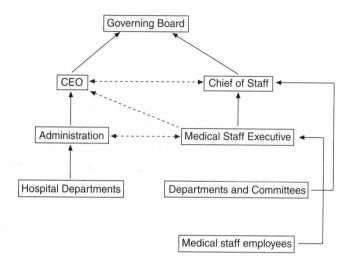

FIGURE 10–1   Hospital–medical staff relationship: Medical staff executive.

no claims have been made that having an association executive is not a good thing to do. But in the hospital medical staff is there the idea that, like a doctor's office, there should only be the doctor, a nurse, and a secretary. The doctor makes all decisions. But in a complex world of rapid change in the health care scene, a chief of staff cannot be present all day every day to make all of those hour-by-hour support recommendations for the employees. The executive manages the employees. In most hospitals, a private, independent physician or any other outsider is not allowed to supervise employees.

A good medical staff executive will have had the experience and ability to offer support and guidance on legal, regulatory, and antitrust issues by being familiar with precedent cases and what principles from those cases applies to the present issues confronting the medical staff. The executive does not act like an attorney. There should already be counsel available and the executive can be in frequent communication with that attorney for advice and to get clearance on letters and policy positions. Most of the time the best working arrangement is when the counsel is the hospital attorney. In very rare instances, a medical staff member may need to have independent counsel who is not the hospital attorney, but the doctors should be prepared to pay for that service out of their own pockets. The executive should know the bylaws cold and can apply those requirements to present situations or be able to suggest bylaw changes to fit changing circumstances.

Employment Status

The medical staff executive is a hospital employee who reports to the chief of staff as the supervisor and receives annual evaluations from the chief. The administration should provide reports and comments to the chief as a part of that process, but it does not have the ability to override the chief's opinion. This is a structure intended to facilitate communication and information sharing. It is not a vehicle for creating warfare. If that is the result, then all sides have failed to understand the possibilities and use them wisely.

The executive should sit as a member of the management group of the hospital and bring perspectives from the medical staff to persons not likely to receive that information. Personnel benefits for the executive should be the same as an associate administrator. The executive of the medical staff should also have a good office that is accessible to the doctors as they come and go through the hospital. A good office will demonstrate the attitude on the part of the administration that it respects the medical staff and is as sincerely interested in good management as are the doctors and the successive chiefs, who benefit from having a steady source of help, information, and advice.

JOB OF THE EXECUTIVE

The job of the medical staff executive is to remain loyal to the doctors even when placed in a position of being caught between power groups. The association model and the medical staff executive are ideas that will work very well in many hospitals but will absolutely not work in those places where the CEO or Administrator is king of the hill and could not tolerate the idea of the medical staff receiving top-quality support and assistance, because that would somehow endanger or threaten the administration. Where those attitudes exist, there must be some other problems that are greater than whether the medical staff is allowed or prevented good management support.

The executive needs to be the guardian of due process, reminding chiefs and departments when an application has been sitting on an agenda for too long and that the applicant has rights too. The executive can point out promptly and clearly when a committee action looks and sounds like an anticompetitive move in restraint of trade. An executive should go to chairs and point out to them how the committee is wasting time and avoiding real decisions. Likewise, the executive should advise those same committee chairs how to write an effective letter that presents clearly and understandably what the committee really wanted to do or was really trying to find out in the peer review process.

The executive should know everything that is going on in the medical staff and all its committees, with help and support from the clerical staff, who know they can ask for advice and support from their supervisor. A nonphysician executive has no temptation to enter clinical affairs and does not carry the burden of refraining from telling the other doctors how to do it. There are also no carry-over relationships with other members of the medical staff stemming from former partnerships, competitive rivalries, or former referral relationships. From either point of view, the executive can be neutral and objective, working in a very clean, clear structure that has well-defined roles.

The medical staff executive must focus on problem solving and liaison. The executive can represent the policies and positions of the medical staff and give authorized information to the board and administration, speaking on behalf of the chief when delegated that duty. Likewise, a good executive should represent the positions and public statements of the board and administration to the medical staff as their employee and advocate, able to translate what is really being meant by statements. The executive should function to deflame and demystify rather than to create dissension and disagreement. If the latter is the product, then the association model is not working correctly.

The executive should not be expected to leap tall buildings (or tall administrators) in a single bound but at the very least should be able to leap in several different directions at the same time in order to fit with the endless number of diverging-converging interests of the individual members of the medical staff with whom and for whom the executive works. The executive helps the chief and does not get in the way of the chief's performance, or function as a rival to the chief. Unfortunately, not enough hospitals have initiated the medical staff executive structure. Where such an organization or structure exists, a position description would read like the example in Appendix 10–1.

Finding and Recruiting an Executive

Once this unique person who can live up to the job description is found, who should pay the salary? This may be the critical issue in deciding whether or not to search for and employ an executive to complete the association model. Of course, the medical staff should pay it, since the person works directly for and with the doctors. Many on the medical staff will contend that unless the executive is paid by the staff, then loyalty is suspect. But the medical staff probably does not have much extra money and will refuse to vote for a dues increase that would pay the professional level salary that will be needed to attract and keep the kind of person wanted.

First, approach the board and ask that a fund be established to help support and improve the performance of medical staff self-governance. The special purpose fund is kept separate from the general administrative operating budget and is thus not at the mercy of the annual budget process. Then allow the medical staff executive to hire an excellent executive secretary so as to complete a top-notch administrative office for the medical staff. Ignore those hard-liners on the medical staff who cannot or will not see any advantage in good management or who just do not want the organized medical staff to function effectively. Let the results of good management prove to them that the executive is the right thing to do, no matter who is paying.

SUMMARY

The hospital medical staff is an association for self-governance responsible for overall quality of care in the hospital, performing professional duties of credentialing, privileging, reappointment, and peer view. Other associations, joined together for mutual self-interest, have a policy-making group and an elected official to act and speak on behalf of the members. Associations have staff employees to carry out policies and work of the organization.

The hospital medical staff, unlike an association, does not have an executive officer who works full time to direct the office of the chief of staff and supervise the employees combined into a unified medical staff department. The duty of the medical staff executive is to implement policies, help carry the burden of the chiefs, represent them, give reports, and bring back useful information. The executive does not speak for the chief, is not a rival, but does offer guidance and counsel on legal, regulatory, and antitrust issues confronting the medical staff. The executive has pay and benefits of an associate administrator, and serves on the management group, with access to administrative and board systems. This chapter presents a discussion about the job of the executive, particularly how to fund and pay for the position. Existence and success of the position demonstrates that administration and the board respect the medical staff and is sincerely interested in good management of the self-governance program. A job description is provided.

REFERENCES

White, C. H. (1989). *The Medical Staff Executive* [Faculty presentations]. Estes Park Institute, Brighton, CO.

White, C. H. (1986–1996). *The Medical Staff Executive* [Faculty and consultant presentations]. Grossmont Hospital, La Mesa, Ca; Sharp Healthcare, San Diego, CA; other state and national audiences.

APPENDIX 10–1
POSITION DESCRIPTION: MEDICAL STAFF EXECUTIVE

POSITION TITLE: Medical Staff Executive

DEPARTMENT: Medical Staff

REPORTS TO: Chief of Staff

POSITION PURPOSES: Assists the Chiefs of Staff by overseeing medical staff program functions and providing timely information regarding the status of these functions. Attends meetings of medical staff and appropriate board committees to perform coordination, documentation, and liaison functions. Conducts special studies requested by the chiefs of staff and prepares summaries and analyses of the findings. Is accountable to the chiefs of staff and ultimately through them to the hospital board of directors. Recommendation for dismissal is made with the advice and consent of the medical staff executive committee.

KEY RESPONSIBILITIES: Conducts all business affairs of the office of the chief of staff as the administrative center of the organized medical staff. Routinely attends all meetings of the medical staff. Maintains such records as are necessary to assure the medical staff administrative responsibilities regarding accreditation of the hospital are always being properly discharged. Assists the executive committee. Develops and maintains productive working relationships with the organizational structure of the hospital and its departments. Oversees the medical staff's financial affairs to assure proper budgeting documentation and procedures. Participates as a regular member of the management council, CQI council, and appropriate system activities.

Supervises and evaluates all personnel in the integrated medical staff organization responsible for completion of services necessary for medical staff activities. Supervises and evaluates the medical staff services manager and the medical staff services coordinators in the performance of medical staff committees, credentialing, and reappointment duties. Supervises and evaluates the quality resource management manager and the QRM specialists in the performance of medical staff peer review. Develops and maintains familiarity with quality resources management functions and assists the chair of the quality assessment committee. Supervises the continuing medical education coordinator and staff, the health sciences library coordinator and library assistants. Develops and maintains familiarity with continuing medical education accreditation, functions, and programs. Assists the chairs of the continuing education and library committees. Supervises the physician referral services coordinator and the physician referral services specialists in the performance of their duties. Assists the chair of the physician referral services advisory committee. Supervises the utilization review coordinator and staff in the performance of their duties. Assists the chair of the utilization review committee. Supervises the physician resource consumption program and staff. Assists the medical director as necessary.

Communicates pertinent information to the chiefs of staff, appropriate chairs, leadership, and general medical staff. Receives and routes all reports and serves as contact liaison with the individual staff members, as directed, on behalf of the chiefs of staff. Reviews all minutes to be submitted to the executive committee. Assists the chiefs of staff in preparing data for use at the executive committee meetings. Keeps the chiefs of staff informed of all committee activities and other operations of the hospital. Attends the board of directors meetings and board committee meetings, serving as assistant to the chiefs of staff. Coordinates the functions and activities of the physician leadership program as directed by the chiefs of staff.

Develops and maintains knowledge of legal, regulatory, and hospital information utilized in providing information to the chiefs of staff and medical staff members. Maintains a working knowledge of the medical staff bylaws, rules, and regulations, of Joint Commission standards, of state medical association standards, and of the state hospital licensing act. Assists the medical director for accreditation and licensing. Develops and maintains knowledge of medical staff responsibilities in the Medicare and Medicaid programs and other federal, state, and local requirements. Facilitates implementation of the medical staff bylaws, rules, and regulations, including communication with the medical staff in regard to timely completion of medical records. Assists the chair of the medical records committee, as well as the bylaws and nominating committees.

Serves as a resource to the medical staff, board of directors, the administration and the community. Enhances the public image of the hospital. Provides regular presentations on legislative, regulatory, accreditation, and peer review affairs to the executive, quality assessment and long-range planning committees. Provides legislative grand rounds annually and reports to the general medical staff at quarterly meetings. Provides periodic reports to the board of directors on legislative, regulatory, accreditation, and Medicare mortality data issues as needed. Provides reports and presentations to hospital managers, nursing staff, seniors club, auxiliary, and volunteers as needed. Maintains working relationships with colleges and universities as a faculty member or preceptor.

CUSTOMERS SERVED: Chiefs of staff, organized medical staff, individual physicians, medical staff employees, Board of Directors, administration, nurses, departments (clinical and ancillary), patients/public.

POSITION ACCOUNTABILITY: The medical staff executive is directly accountable to the chief of staff and ultimately through the chief of staff to the board of directors for performance of all assigned medical staff functions. By agreement between the hospital administration and the medical staff, the medical staff executive is accountable to the chief executive officer only for hospital-related functions, such as resource consumption studies. The medical staff executive will participate as a regular member of the management council with benefits comparable to the associate administrator.

Performance evaluations for the medical staff executive will be conducted by the chief of staff with direct input from the chief-elect, past chief, and the chief executive officer. Recommendation for dismissal is made only by the chief of staff with input from the chief executive officer and with the advice and consent of the medical executive committee. Participation by the medical staff executive in selected professional activities such as speaking or teaching is acceptable, with prior approval by the chief of staff. Any honorarium paid may be accepted.

AUTHORITIES

Policy: May recommend policy changes to the chiefs of staff, medical executive committee, and other medical staff departments and committees. Advises the chiefs of staff and assists the medical staff with necessary adherence to policies and procedures.

People: Authority to hire, evaluate, discipline, and terminate employees in accordance with established hospital policies and procedures. Makes recommendations for changes in salary range assignments and classification of employees to the chief executive officer and the director of human resources.

Materials: Full authority for budgeting and staffing. Full authority to requisition, rent, or purchase for professional services, legal assistance, and capital and noncapital equipment and supplies as called for in the budget. Full authority to approve travel for the chiefs of staff, leadership program participants, medical directors, and hospital employees under supervision.

EDUCATION

Master's degree in health care–related field, with doctorate preferred

LICENSURE

EXPERIENCE
- Lengthy experience demonstrating working productively with physicians, administrators, trustees or directors, nurses, employees/staff, and the public
- Senior-level skills in planning and development
- Knowledge of hospital organization, interrelationships of medical staff/administration/nursing is essential
- Ability to relate to physician leadership and engender confidence and trust among medical specialty groups is essential

- Skills and knowledge in quality assurance and analysis, internal hospital quality mechanisms, continuous quality improvement theory and process, performance management, outcomes evaluation, and related fields
- Effective interpersonal communication skills, particularly writing and public-speaking, and oral/teaching presentations
- Possess facilitative skills of problem solving, running effective meetings, team building and development, self-managed work groups, and conflict resolution

CHAPTER

Department Leadership

The leaders of clinical or service-line departments of the medical staff are the middle managers who make the medical staff self-governance system work, if it works (White, 1994). Sometimes, those same middle manager–chairs have also seen to it that the system does not work very well at all. Chiefs of staff are elected, and so, usually, are department chairs by a narrow mix of colleagues and peers in the same specialty. The specialty club forming the department may have a very different agenda than the leadership or the medical staff as a whole.

In a Joint Commission model, the executive committee is composed of chiefs, chairs, and, sometimes, at-large members. It is not exactly like a president and the cabinet, because in that model the president chooses the leaders that are wanted. The chief of staff must frequently work with whatever sort of leader the specialty department sends. In the medical staff, the chief who is trying to manage self-governance may be forced to take potluck with whatever chair persons present themselves at the table. Sometimes they do not present themselves at all, being absent or coming late and leaving early. Melding these various personalities with their differing agendas is often the sorest trial for a chief. Back in the provinces, the department chairs have a major job to do, as

147

shown in the position description presented as Appendix 11–1. If the hospital has not put together formal descriptions for these chair positions, then it should be strongly recommended that it be done. There are multiple examples of guidelines and suggestions by Sandra Gill, Linda Haddad, and Hugh Greeley that will help with the job of composing these requirements for department chair responsibilities and accountabilities (Gill, Haddad, & Greeley, 1995).

JOB OF THE CHAIR

Over time, the role and responsibilities of department chairs has increased greatly in scope and importance. Now, when a survey team conducts interviews, it is probable that it will spend more time with the chairpersons than with the chiefs. Department chairs are now personally responsible to review and evaluate the quality of patient care provided by those physicians who are members or have privileges within the department. JCAHO standards specify the review and evaluation of

- surgical and other invasive care procedures
- drug usage
- medical records
- blood usage
- pharmacy and therapeutics functions
- risk management
- infection control
- disaster plans
- hospital safety
- utilization of resources

In the 1994 *Accreditation Manual for Hospitals,* Medical Staff Standard MS 4.6 delineated the long list of responsibilities for the department chair, including the necessity for those duties (and any others needed locally) to be specified in the bylaws. There should be a formal training program for incoming or new chairs so that this list can be presented and discussed. Any chair, man or woman, who really does not want to follow the standards should resign immediately or be assisted in making the decision to let someone else have the honor and hard work. Being responsible for all clinically related activities of the department service is a serious burden of due care, and no one should accept the job with only the intent to protect the economic interests of the particular specialty involved. An obstructive department chair is an enemy of medical staff self-governance and should be considered that way.

Department chairs are viewed as officers of the hospital and must be included under the hospital's liability insurance coverage for all actions taken in performance of their duties that are carried out in good faith and following the bylaws. This protection is particularly valuable in the case of remedial action that must be taken during or following peer review findings that relate to quality of care.

Where to Pay Attention

Department chairs must pay particular attention to the credentialing and granting of privileges for applicants to the department, because it is the recommendation bearing their signature that makes its way through the credentials committee, the executive committee, and eventually to the board. By signature, the chair has certified that a competent credentialing or reappointment process has taken place and that the full faith and authority of the department so guarantees it. If that is not what the chair really means when signing the appropriate forms, then there is a real problem, including possibly that the wrong person is in the position as the chair of the department.

Department chairs must also be aware of the professional performance of all individuals with clinical privileges. They will be called upon to make recommendations for reappointment based on current clinical competence. Once again, the department is certifying, through the signature of the chair, that the physician in question is known to possess the competence to perform all privileges granted. Department chairs enforce clinical service, medical staff, and hospital policies, rules, and regulations. Enforce means that one of the specialty colleagues that elected the chair, and perhaps even practices with the chair, has broken the law and must be corrected or punished—a task that can be particularly onerous. Chairs also implement actions taken by the board, whether in agreement or not. Civil disobedience is not an option, although resignation is. If there is serious disagreement with a board policy or action, then relationships need to be revisited and reasons clarified.

Chairs should also report and recommend to the administration matters that affect patient care, including personnel, equipment, supplies, special regulations, standing orders, and techniques. Sandra Gill (1994) also notes that chairs work with management to help prepare the budgets, both operating and capital. Skillful chairs work behind the scenes to promote integration of the organization and coordination with other services. Perhaps no other action the chair takes will earn so much undying gratitude from the nurses and other staff as the willingness to react promptly and confront an abusive physician who is making the workplace miserable.

DEPARTMENTS: WHERE CHANGE TAKES PLACE

The smoldering issues of the actual delivery of health care are more likely to present themselves and actually occur on the units and in the specialty areas where the department doctors do their work. Those are the locations where changes in patterns of clinical practice will take place, including a combination of factors such as: (1) increased discontent with the current system, (2) the emergence of discernible and attainable options for change, (3) concrete suggestions for implementing such change, and (4) a nucleus of clinical, managerial, and political leadership to initiate and sustain the needed reforms (Shortell & Reinhardt, 1992).

Attitudes toward the delivery system of the next decade will be shaped by deeply held perceptions that come from personal experience, anecdotes, persuasions of leaders, or formally structured information from a variety of sources. Sometimes these perceptions may be an accurate reflection of the facts. At other times, however, they will rest on the most casual of empirical bases and border more on folklore and myth than reality. Unfortunately for the medical staff, the department, and the leadership, these views of the world may be deliberately manipulated through biased information supplied by particular interest groups.

There are a wide variety of approaches available for changing physician attitudes and behavior toward the delivery of clinical care at the department level. These include education, feedback, financial incentives, nonfinancial incentives, administrative restrictions, sanctions, and changing patient behavior. It seems reasonable to assume that the future points toward more complex systems for the redesign of health care delivery, such as continuous quality improvement, measurement of patient care, medical outcomes, and small-area analysis. Continued emphasis on the development and dissemination of practice guidelines will not necessarily result in their successful implementation without attention to specific behavioral changes. The most promising approach would be to reinforce such changes over time, with appropriate assessments made of their ultimate impact on patient outcomes. Then, when the changes become daily habits, there is a new basis for further guideline development and refinement (Shortell & Reinhardt, 1992).

Making an impact on the daily lives of patients and doctors at the individual level will be a result of the interaction of inhibitors and facilitators as specific components of behavioral change that influence outcomes. For example, there is widespread lack of knowledge among some specialty physicians about the specific value of clinical pathways, practice guidelines, or algorithms. This lack of understanding or recalcitrant attitude can be best dealt with by involvement of the particular physician in development of these tools. Sometimes, once an algorithm or guideline has been developed, there is disagreement with it and reluctance to follow recommended procedure. In that case, personal face-to-face interaction by those medical directors or department chairs charged with implementation is a help in facilitating cooperation.

Algorithms for Good or Evil

One of the problems with the development and use of clinical guidelines or algorithms is that slowness inherent in the process and the necessary lack of involvement by large numbers of the doctors who will be expected to carry out the practice pattern. Also, some guidelines are a radical departure from the current practice by a particular physician, in the department, or even in the community. There may be no real incentive to change because the procedure is infrequently performed. On the other hand, there may certainly be no real incentive to change because the procedure is the most commonly performed in the department.

There will need to be assistance and encouragement by the department leadership to secure the gains that are hoped for through changed behavior by the department doctors. A learning attitude forms a more receptive environment, as does an appeal to the continuous ability to learn new methods that offer to improve practice. Take care that an obscure or irrelevant procedure is never chosen as the first or test guideline developed. Instead, choose the most frequent procedure, the highest risk procedure, or, perhaps, the most costly. Choose something that the doctors will believe is worth the effort and will provide some assistance they can use but did not previously have. And, best of all, if the department has a tradition of seeking and using regularly a learning attitude and employs educational resources without being forced, then practice changes and guidelines can come as a normal progression over time.

Test of Leadership

The true test of department leadership will come when the clinical leaders support change in the department and actively work with their colleagues even when the norms of the peer group do not yet support the algorithm, guideline, or clinical pathway. In that case, the job of the chair and more enlightened colleagues will, over time, be to change the peer group pressures against developing new approaches to practice into new peer group norms that support continuous improvement. An added benefit for the department, the hospital, and certainly for patients is to change low group cohesiveness and support into strong group cohesiveness and improved morale.

If there is lack of support in the department in question toward quality improvement through the use of new practice patterns, that may be an indication that the larger culture of the medical staff and the hospital does not support such innovations, either. There may be a lack of resources supplied by the hospital to properly develop and implement guidelines and protocols. There may be poor communication, coordination, and management practices in dealing with quality measurement and improvement, particularly in handling the conflict that can result from the change process. Medical staff leadership by strong clinicians, particularly at the department level will be the key to securing adequate resources from the administration and/or the board. Even though it goes against their nature somewhat, department leadership must lead the way in demonstrating effective communication and coordination and encouraging exemplary management practices. Remember, it is not acceptable to only complain about what administration does that is bad. It is also totally necessary for the departments to loudly proclaim and complement when administration does something good, as well.

One last element of these attempts to provide value-added services is that they absolutely require effective clinical information systems that can provide accurate, relevant, and timely data that is acuity adjusted. Left alone, the hospital will buy and use information systems that serve the accountants and the finance people without any thought for also serving clinical purposes. Departments need to be able to describe what they require in order to assist their efforts in meeting external purchaser demands for higher quality at lower cost.

SUMMARY

The middle managers of the medical staff who make the self-governance system work are the leaders of departmental or service-line departments. Department chairs have a major job to do, as shown in the description provided. In the Joint Commission model, the department chair has the responsibility to review and evaluate the quality of patient care provided by the physicians who are members of or who have privileges within the department. There should be a selection and training program for these essential leaders to prepare them for the responsibility of all clinically related activities of the department service. Any chair who does not intend to follow the standards that apply should not accept the position. Neither should there be an automatic rotation or alphabetical order methods of selection.

Department chairs must pay particular attention to credentialing and granting of privileges, because the chair signs the recommendation that wends its way to the board for approval. Similarly, the chair signs the recommendations for reappointment based on current clinical competence. The department is certifying, by signature of the chair, that the physician is competent to perform all privileges granted. Chairs also are involved in budget preparation, personnel matters, equipment, supplies, special regulations, standing orders, and techniques such as clinical pathways. Departments are the place where changes in patterns of clinical practice take place.

REFERENCES

Gill, S. (1994) *To be the Best Department Chair I Can Be* [Faculty workshop presentation]. Sharp Healthcare, San Diego, CA.

Gill, S., Haddad, L., & Greeley, H. (Ongoing). [Faculty presentations and materials]. Estes Park Institute, Brighton, CO.

Shortell, S. M., & Reinhardt, U. E. (Eds.). (1992). Creating and executing health policy. In *Improving Health Policy and Management: Nine Critical Research Issues for the 1990s*. Ann Arbor: Health Administration Press, Association for Health Services Research, Foundation of the American College of Healthcare Executives.

White, C. H. (1994). *To Be the Best Department Chair I Can Be.* [Faculty workshop presentations]. Sharp Healthcare, San Diego, CA.

APPENDIX 11–1
POSITION DESCRIPTION: DEPARTMENT CHAIR

POSITION TITLE: Department Chair

DEPARTMENT:

REPORTS TO: Chief of Staff, Executive Committee

POSITION PURPOSES: Clinical department or service line primary medical administrative officer, leader, and clinical manager, including:

- Credentialing
- Reappointment
- Peer review
- Administration of quality of care
- Executive committee, board, and administrative liaison
- Collaboration with hospital managers
- Budgeting

KEY RESPONSIBILITIES: Departmental or service line quality of care among all credentialed medical staff members. Patient care evaluation and concurrent monitoring. Writes reports on quality review actions and results thereof. Makes recommendations for continuous quality improvement and other requests. Develops and implements departmental or service line programs, evaluation of patient care, ongoing monitoring of clinical practice, credentials and privileges review, medical education and utilization. Member of the executive committee, making recommendations and suggestions regarding department.

Maintains continual review of the professional performance of all practitioners with clinical privileges and of all allied health professionals with specified services in the department or service line. Transmits, as required by the bylaws, written recommendations concerning clinical privileges or specific services and corrective action in the department or service line. Appoints subcommittees as necessary and designates subcommittee chairs. Enforces hospital and medical staff bylaws, rules, regulations, and policies within the department, including initiating investigations of clinical performance and ordering consultations to be provided or sought when necessary. Implements within the department actions taken by the executive committee and by the board.

Participates in every phase of management of the department or service line through cooperation with nursing service and hospital administration in patient care, including personnel, supplies, special regulations, standing orders and techniques. Assists in preparation of the annual report, including budgetary planning pertaining to the department or service line. Performs other duties as may be requested by the chief of staff, executive committee, or the board.

CUSTOMERS SERVED: Chief of Staff with Board and administration reports as needed. Members of the department or service line as their representative and advocate. Provides leadership in initiating and maintaining systemwide communication with counterpart chairs in other system departments or service lines.

EDUCATION: M.D./D.O. Degree

LICENSURE

EXPERIENCE
- Active staff for at least five years
- May not hold officer or leadership position in any other hospital medical staff during term of office
- Prior successful service in the medical staff organization

RECOGNITION AND BENEFITS
- Tuition and expenses for self and spouse in one external CME event per year devoted to medical administrative activities
- Exemption from E.R. call, other committees
- Hospital indemnification for role-related activities

OCCUPATIONAL HAZARDS
Potential involvement in corporate negligence or antitrust, significant time demands, probable conflict with specialty peers and colleagues

CHAPTER

How Administration Relates to Physicians

The most useful and helpful way to describe how a hospital administration relates to the physicians who practice there is to explain the traditional organizational structure that is in place in most institutions, who the administrators are, and what they do. Most doctors do not really understand the breadth and depth of what administration is or does, and some do not really care. The roles are straightforward: doctors practice in hospitals, singly or in groups, and administration manages the personnel, equipment, and facilities.

ORGANIZATIONAL STRUCTURES

Traditional Bureaucratic Organization

Most hospitals in the United States tend to be traditionally organized, that is, they tend to follow the classical theory of organization. The traditional organizational structure derives from the theory of bureaucracy described by the nineteenth-century German sociologist Max Weber (Snook, 1992). Hospitals are mainly bureaucratic organizations and use bureaucratic principles. One of the principles of bureaucratic organizations that applies effectively to hospitals is the grouping of individual positions and clusters of positions into a hierarchy or pyramid. Another effective principle of hospital organization is the consistent system of rules. Hospital rules are really guidelines or official boundaries for actions within the hospital. Prominent examples of such rules include the set of personnel policies outlined in the personnel handbook or written nursing procedures for the care of patients in each nursing unit. Hospitals also generally use the principle of span of control, which in a bureaucracy says there is a limit to the number of persons a manager can effectively supervise. Another widely recognized bureaucratic principle of organization followed by hospitals is the division and specialization of labor. Specialization refers to the ways a hospital organizes to identify specific tasks and assign a job description to each person.

The most popular and traditional hospital structure is a pyramid or hierarchial form of organization used in many other places, such as the military or business. In this arrangement, individuals at the top of the pyramid have a specified range of authority, and this authority is passed down to employees at the lower levels of the pyramid in a chain-of-command fashion. In this way, hospital authority is dispensed and delegated throughout the organization. The rigidity with which this militaristic form actually takes place usually reflects the personality and management style of the administrator, more commonly now called the chief executive officer (CEO). In a traditional structure there is a difference between line and staff work. Line authority in the hospital connotes direct supervision over employees or subordinates, while staff functions in an advisory or supporting role to assist the line managers.

Individual physicians in private practice can relate to this structure according to their own personality, as well. Some religious hospitals are strongly organized with a chain-of-command structure, and that style fits some doctors as well. One of the usual characteristics of a tightly run hospital is that everything and everyone are exactly in the place they should be in. That style is not for every doctor, of course; some prefer a more maneuverable environment. Different strokes for different people, unless, of course, that hospital is the only one in town that has the equipment needed, or is the only one that offers the service performed. In that case, the doctor makes the best of it, while complaining about the bureaucracy.

Matrix Organizations

A second type of structural scheme is a matrix organization, whereby the hospital caregiving processes operate more horizontally than vertically. This arrangement is oriented more toward solving problems or managing projects, and the authority within any given project rests more with a designated project manager than with the chief executive officer or department manager. In recent years, moves toward patient care teams and self-managed work groups are a reflection of the matrix approach. They are also a reflection of a move away from the "administrator as king" attitude that has been present in some hospitals. It is difficult to be a king when the worker bees are busy running around in work groups managing themselves. Chances are that a matrix or team organization in a hospital will show a high level of morale and dedication to good patient care, and it can be recognized by watching to see who the team members are. If they include some of the brightest and most competent nurses and other professionals, then shared governance is alive and well in that hospital, and people will feel good about what they are doing. The good CEO in that situation does more by doing less.

Matrix or team management attracts some physicians who like that style and work well in it, while absolutely repulsing others who want more definition and control. Matrix or team care approaches do seem to bring out some previously or otherwise overlooked doctors who are quite good and have lots of good ideas to suggest but who somehow just never broke through the power structure in a traditional hierarchial power organization. There will be some good patient care going on in either style, but there may be a different level of employee satisfaction when tradition changes to shared governance.

Product or Service Lines

There is another organizational arrangement that needs to be identified, although more will be said about it in succeeding chapters. The product-line, or service-line, management approach divides entire hospitals or divisions within hospitals according to similar service categories. These categories are more often these days called *strategic business units,* which have budgets, staff, equipment, and facilities for the specialized use of one set of patients. They also have real profit expectations under the threat of possible termination of the service. Service-line structures look like the way of the future for many regional integrated systems as they attempt to reduce duplication and improve efficiency. From the doctors' standpoint, the service-line approach probably brings together some long-time competitors who are now being asked to consider closing some units in the hope of keeping others open.

Changing Relationships

No matter what the organizational structure, there are changing relationships between the practicing private physicians and administration. Many of the doctors are present in the hospital only part time (or nearly no time), whereas the CEO and whatever management team there is have full-time hospital responsibilities. The administration is dedicated to the long-term success and continuation of the hospital, while physicians are dedicated to the long-time success and continuation of their practices, whether they take place in that particular hospital or not. There is loyalty, a great deal of it sometimes, but there are different incentives and motives at work. As more physicians become employees or independent contractors of the hospital, and more medical staff physicians are using it full time, some of the traditional relationships are breaking down while new physicians may find it hard to establish a relationship at all.

ADMINISTRATORS/CEOS: WHAT THEY DO

At one time, the chief executive officer (CEO), probably formerly titled the hospital administrator, was likely chosen from the ranks of the nursing department (Snook, 1992). In many church-related hospitals, it was common for the CEO to be selected from the ranks of the religious order or from retired clergy. These administrators knew the hospital well, worked hard, and were dedicated to patient care, particularly in trying to follow the physicians' wishes. Another track through which some administrators rose to their positions was through the business or finance office ranks. At times, it was also common for some hospitals to place a retired businessman or maybe a physician in the administrative position.

Such upward mobility is not that common today. Most CEOs are now products of university training programs. The first university course in hospital administration started in the 1930s, and the field has continued to grow. The profession has become more complex and the demand for trained administrators has multiplied. The American College of Health Care Executives, formed in 1933, has encouraged high standards of education and ethics, and those who meet its requirements are admitted as members. A number of universities now provide formal training in hospital administration, although the curriculum might now be titled health services administration to recognize that hospitals are no longer the only source of care. The most widely accepted degrees are at the master's level, whether in business administration, public health, or public administration.

The hospital CEO of the 1930s and 1940s dealt primarily with the internal operations of the hospital, including personal daily relationships with the doctors practicing there. The administrator was concerned with matters that directly affected the patients treated in the hospital. This involved bargaining with employees, developing proper benefit packages, and determining the best methods and techniques to manage the institution. In later decades, increasingly strong labor unions, third-party payers, and governmental agencies all began to impact significantly on the hospital industry. During those years the role of the administrator became a dual one, dealing with both the inside and outside aspects of hospital management. More sophisticated and specialized management was required to operate a hospital effectively, and the CEO became more involved in activities outside the hospital. Necessarily, this attention to other affairs reduced the time an administrator could spend in day-by-day relationships with physicians, and some of them resented the resulting loss of immediate access to the CEO's office.

Today, the CEO must strike some proper balance between outside and inside activities. But the main role of the CEO is to coordinate the facilities of the hospital with its resources so as to allow the medical care mission of the institution to be most efficiently and effectively carried out. Since hospitals are also businesses, their services are capable of being measured by business yardsticks. The CEO's responsibility is to handle and manage the tangibles of money, personnel, and materials. The chief executive has been appointed by the governing board to be responsible for the performance of all functions of the institution. The board then acts in a judgmental or deliberative fashion and holds the executive accountable. Boards delegate responsibility for quality of medical care to the medical staff, and they delegate to the chief executive the administrative responsibility for all functions, including relationships with the individual physicians, the organized medical staff, the nursing staff, technical staff, and general services departments, that will be necessary to assure the quality of patient care.

Inside activities carried on by administrators include many aspects not readily apparent to the practicing physicians. Not being readily visible or apparent may sometimes mean that the doctors are not aware of these other roles and do not value them. All such activities will appear to the doctors as unnecessary bureaucracy that detracts from the real job, which is making the doctors happy. Nevertheless, the CEO must also oversee the review and establishment of hospital procedures, supervision of hospital personnel, including termination procedures when necessary. Terminations can be long and messy, are almost always expensive, and may very well end up on the front page of the newspaper. CEOs are responsible for internal relations to ensure a smoothly running hospital. CEOs are directly responsible for the fiscal and financial operation and well-being of the hospital, and that aspect is what most of the board members want to talk about most of the time.

Traditionally, it has been the CEO's job to attend to those tasks in the hospital that directly affect the patients' well-being. Examples of this include overseeing that the buildings, grounds, and facilities are in adequate order and that the personnel are qualified to fill their specific job requirements. The CEO must answer for the acts of employees under the principle of respondeat superior, with the help of the general counsel. The administrator must keep the physicians and the board informed about the hospital and its plans for the future. In these days of affiliations and mergers, the CEO will have assumed a new duty to the corporate office, its executives, and at least one more board.

CEOs schedule board meetings, arrange agendas with the approval of the board president, and attend those meetings with the obligation of communicating ideas, thoughts, and explanations and suggesting policies that will help the hospital. If the hospital is now part of a system or network, there will be the necessity to explain or inform the local hospital board about the plans or actions of the larger corporate structure. The CEO is responsible for preparation and defense of the annual budget, which must be approved by the board. Hopefully leading physicians, the medical staff leadership, and board sub-committees played a large role in the preparation of that budget so there will be acceptance and commitment before it is put on the agenda for final approval.

The administration identifies, along with the affected physicians, new services that need to be offered as well as new equipment that is needed to begin the new service or to replace technology that is no longer state of the art. Woe to any CEO who tries to perform this task alone or with only input from a close circle of management advisors. Unless the involved physicians have fully participated, there will not be a successful new service. In fact, it was probably the reverse: the doctors proposed the new service, the finance department researched it, and now the administration proposes it to the board in the budget. The finance department is also heavily involved with negotiating contracts for payment rates with health plans or insurers and preparing monthly financial statements for presentation to the board, as well as the year-end summaries. Those who have been in a situation where the finance department liked the doctors and enjoyed working with them, and vice versa, have probably seen the best that hospital medical practice has to offer.

The Inside Role

Perhaps, the most important task of the CEO or administrator is in maintaining positive relationships within and among the various hospital publics. These mean the governing body, the medical staff, employees, auxiliary and volunteers, foundation, and patients. It is an absolute given that no administrator can keep all the doctors happy or all the patients or certainly all the nurses. Nor is it wise to emulate wily politicians who keep everyone unhappy to some degree, but not to the breaking point. The official relationship between CEO and board is one of an employee and employer, but those two actually function more as partners. The administrator is the representative of the board in the daily activities of the institution and must turn the board's policies and directives into administrative action. Indeed, that partnership relation between the board and the administrator has been strengthened now that the CEO is a voting member of the board in many hospitals and systems. That pattern is quite common in other industries where the CEO is also a member of the board of directors and is an equal among equals, not just a salaried employee. Many doctors do not understand this change in the structure and relationships as they try to use an old strategy that might have been successful once: that of trying to isolate the administrator to be caught between doctors and the board. It is hard to do that now, as some physicians have discovered to their surprise and amazement. Many board members do not take kindly to that kind of treatment of their CEO, for whom they performed a national search and in whom they have invested a lot of hopes and expectations.

The CEO should act in partnership, not only with the board, but also with the individual physicians and the organized medical staff. When the movement toward managed care began, there were incessant cries that the hospital and the doctors needed to be partners. That always seemed to be a trick to the doctors, whose long-standing suspicion of the motives of the administration prevented them from yielding easily to the requests for partnership. Under the best of circumstances, the CEO or administrator will have a mutual understanding with, respect for, and trust in the individual doctors and the organized medical staff. (Although, there are some who have proven not to be trustworthy or who would not make good partners). The key responsibility and the key action are to effectively communicate with the doctors in a variety of ways. Successful CEOs are effective in keeping the doctors informed about organizational changes, board policies, and decisions that affect them and their patients. These communication vehicles need to be both inside the official medical staff structure and outside so as to reach those doctors who do not receive communications from the medical staff. Those CEOs who hide behind a bevy of impersonal secretaries and who insist on making appointments far in advance are not likely to know the mood of the physicians.

The employees must look to the CEO as their work leader, and the employee group provides many of the administrator's day-to-day challenges. Keeping them informed of the critical role their services play in the successful operation of the hospital and the provision of high-quality patient care is the administrator's job, and it is a difficult one. All employees must be continually informed, through as many vehicles as are available, about the mission and philosophy of the institution and how well those objectives are being met. In dealing with employees at all levels, it is critical that the CEO show objectivity, understanding, and fairness. Sometimes a little warmth also helps. The CEO must handle well the authority to employ, direct, discipline, and dismiss employees with these principles in mind. Another principle to keep in mind is whether a complaining doctor is enough to have a nurse fired. It has happened, and the nursing staff knows all about that kind of treatment.

CEOs have a role in patient relations, mostly through setting a tone for the employee staff to follow. In past years, administrators could stand out in the hall or down in the cafeteria, talking to patients and families, making friends for the hospital. Now, it is more likely that the CEO is sitting in a meeting with a health plan, discussing a contract that will bring more patients to the hospital—patients that the CEO will never see. But the employee staff must fulfill all legitimate patient requests for general comfort and care that will assist their treatment and recovery. The hospital staff, with the direction and encouragement of the administration, must also understand the needs of the patient's friends and relatives and the safeguarding of confidential information. Nothing will infuriate a doctor more than for the hospital staff to be rude or uncaring in dealing with patients and families.

The Outside Role

The outside activities of today's CEOs are numerous, including relating to the community, understanding governmental relationships, and participating in educational and planning activities. Sometimes, political or legislative crises are so demanding that a CEO will spend more time in the state capitol than in the hospital. One of the roles of the modern CEO/administrator is to educate the community about hospital operations and health care matters, including the plans and patient care intentions of the system or network the former freestanding hospital has joined. Various publications sent to the residents of a service or catchment area can be very helpful.

Community lectures can also help, although there are some CEOs who should not be turned loose on the public, not so much for fear of what they might say, but that they will probably not say anything. Let someone else make the speeches in that case. While it is the CEO's responsibility to present a positive image of the hospital or system, the first step in that process is to present a positive image of the CEO. That may require help from a public-speaking consultant in doing presentations effectively. There will also need to be a speech writer, who can draft scripts on very short notice, so that the CEO can make lucid and coherent statements when out in public or dealing with the media. The words *public relations* have come to possess an unpleasant image of trickery and deceit, but the concept is still valid. The hospital or the system must project a positive image and promote public understanding of the hospital programs through the media, even though the CEO is uncomfortable in dealing with those "media-type" people.

Some CEOs enjoy negotiating contracts with health plans and insurers and consider that to be one of their greatest accomplishments. Some do not and have other people to do that job. The CEO must oversee and is ultimately responsible for staying on top of governmental program changes, state and local planning bodies, and local politicians in order to keep up-to-date and to promote hospital interests. Community hospitals are part of the community and are expected to take part in community activities, even if the administration and many of the doctors think street fairs and footraces are silly and undignified.

ADMINISTRATION WORKING WITH DOCTORS

CEOs hire other people to help them with managing the hospital and its many far-flung programs and activities. Selecting and keeping a competent staff is one of the most important responsibilities for the executive officer. That staff is delegated the duties of seeing that the hospital is running smoothly and efficiently. Whether called chief operating officers or associate and assistant administrators or vice presidents, the game is the same. The management staff works with the doctors in the units and with the department managers, and they supervise the middle management ranks. It is frequently the case that relationships are strong between the administrative staff and the practicing physicians, while the CEO is unknown, unliked, or not understood.

Hospital medical staffs were first formed so that doctors could bring patients to the hospital, along with the revenue they brought with them. Until the modern era of managed care, the administration wanted most of all for doctors to fill the beds. Since a never-ending supply of doctors was needed to bring those patients to the hospital, the main task of the administration during the cost-reimbursement and fee-for-service era was to attract physicians, one way or the other. When filling beds was the objective and doctors could choose which hospital to use for a particular patient, then attracting them was the lifeblood of the hospital. Being a "doctors' workshop" was what counted. It was the CEO's job to see that the doctors had the proper tools in the right place at the right time in order for them to carry out their role in patient care in the hospital. That system worked to the advantage of the doctors who could use that leverage on each administrator for staff, equipment, office space, or other inducements.

By giving them what they said they wanted, individual physicians and the medical staff as a whole became a privileged class of specialists—sometimes humble and kind, sometimes arrogant, always demanding. Managed care will change much of that arrangement, with great turmoil, as will be shown in later chapters.

The Money

The administration provides a budget for the medical staff services personnel, peer review staff, CME, health sciences library, and staff support for utilization review. The administration controls the money, provides free meals to the doctors, serves food at committee meetings, and offers convenient parking and other amenities unique to each hospital. Rarely, if ever, during the 1970s and 1980s was a hospital administrator fired for losing money. But many, many have lost their jobs by crossing influential physicians or the medical staff as a group.

A board cannot usually stand between an angry medical staff and an unpopular administrator, even if the board chose that executive. The remedy for that situation was to provide some pretty lucrative golden handshakes for departing administrators. The average time in office for administrator/CEOs can be as low as four years, according to various study data. Just as in sports, it is easier to fire the manager than all the players (or doctors). The 1980s was the peak of the era of the hospital as a doctors' workshop, which was built and staffed to favor specialist physician practices. Managed care will change that pattern as there becomes increased emphasis on outpatient primary care.

HOW ADMINISTRATION RELATES TO MEDICAL STAFF

The administration relates closely with the chief of staff, department chairs, medical directors, and individual physicians in the best interest of patient care throughout the hospital. Administration works with the organized medical staff structure as the executive management representing the board and concerned with JCAHO accreditation, with other governmental bodies, and with local zoning or fire safety issues that affect hospital operations. The CEO/administrator should attend executive committee and general medical staff meetings and sometimes other significant groups, such as the medical staff strategic planning committee or other occasions where the present and future of the hospital represents a mutual concern.

Associate or assistant administrators, by whatever title, should be integrally involved in the clinical as well as the business aspects of the hospital as those aspects require medical staff communication, input, policymaking, advice, or other personal relationships. A hospital is a people place, in spite of the high-tech medicine going on all around. Representatives of administration present information, serve as sounding boards, carry back questions and complaints (sometimes the same thing), search for answers, convey a vision of the future, and describe the financial condition of the hospital. To many members of the medical staff, particularly those not very well informed, the hospital is an endless fountain of money that ought to be spent on behalf of the doctors, because after all, they made the money.

ADMINISTRATION IN PEER REVIEW

A continuing issue in some hospitals is whether the administrator, vice president for nursing, or comparable persons should sit with credentialing or peer review committees. The answer is: they should, if they have information to give, a perspective to offer, a board position to represent, or a safety responsibility to uphold (White, 1986). But those presences should always take place with the prior knowledge or permission of the chief of staff or department chair and never as a last minute bursting on the scene to vent some point of view that comes as a surprise to the presiding leader. Rampant emotionalism is simply not the way to conduct medical staff self-governance. At least that is not the right way, which is not to say it does not happen from time to time. Skillful or impassioned oratory will still sway the unwashed masses, particularly when not many facts are known or when facts are irrelevant to the rampant emotionalism. It is truly fun for some doctors to vent, particularly if the venting is directed at a hospital administrator who has entered into some devious plots against the medical staff, who are always right, and who agree on everything.

Administration should participate in peer review when appropriate. It is a sign of productive working relationships when administration participates comfortably and effectively and the medical staff accepts and encourages good communication. Sometimes peer review is so secret that the CEO/president/administrator *must* be barred. But sometimes it is foolish to ban the administration from the peer review deliberations when state law requires that remedial action reports to the licensing board must be signed by that same administrator. The medical staff carries on the investigation process but does not report the outcome or action taken. The hospital does. The medical staff has been delegated that function by the board, but the board is still responsible through its executive and agent, the administrator.

TRUST

If the medical staff does not trust the administrator, then there are bigger problems than one peer review hearing for a poor-quality doctor. The administrator usually should not attend judicial review, although it is not likely that the administrator wants to attend, since it would mean spending additional hours in more late-night committee meetings after a long day spent in other meetings. Judicial review is not fun. The administrator could testify, however, as a witness if there is vital information that relates to the case.

What is different now in the move toward managed care is the involvement with contracting that can bring new volumes of patients to the doctors and hospital. Doctors used to bring patients to the hospital; now the hospital brings patients to the doctors. The most important task now for some administrators is to form partnerships with physician groups so that both can participate in the managed care environment. Those are business arrangements that are natural for administration and the board, but unnatural for the organized medical staff. Business arrangements are right and proper for physicians practicing alone or in groups, but wrong for the Joint Commission model of a medical staff. This idea will be further dealt with in Chapters 20 and 21.

Some doctors have problems with differentiating employee relationships. Physician office personnel are employees of the physician (and partners), but hospital personnel are not. One of the most unlovable characteristics of the late and unlamented fee-for-service system was that hostility between doctor and hospital, whether real or perceived, was dumped on hospital employees. Nurses were dumped on, as well as technicians, dietary and maintenance workers, and medical staff services employees. Somehow, hospital employees seemed subhuman to doctors and it was acceptable to verbally abuse them, because the doctor did not like the hospital administrator. It would be a pleasure to say that the evolution to managed care has lessened the frequency and intensity of these outbursts, but to some physicians, tensions are even greater. The issue is one of safety in the workplace for employees, which is a hospital responsibility to safeguard. Too often, misbehaving physicians are left to the tender mercies of medical staff discipline systems that are more merciful to the doctor than to the employee.

However, the administrator remains the visible target for physician unrest and anger, an easy target for the doctors' lounge orators who will say many things in that backroom privacy that they would never say outside. For every administrator, there is an enormous concealed iceberg of unknown medical staff activity that could very well be threatening, particularly if the medical staff is failing to act on important issues such as quality or behavior. Despite the oratory coming from a particular small group of haters and those who enjoy agitating, the organized medical staff must go about its business every day of credentialing, reappointment, and peer review, whether it likes the administrator or not, as well as if there is no administrator in place at the moment. Medical staff self-governance knows no holidays and no relief from its constant vigilance and attention to detail.

When something goes wrong, it is not the chief of staff or the department chair who loses a job or a practice, it is the administrator. The administrator can never quite be completely comfortable with that medical staff's capacity for mischief.

SUMMARY

The roles are straightforward: administration manages the personnel, equipment, and facilities in the hospital while physicians practice medicine there, singly or in groups. The traditional hospital organization and structure is bureaucratic and hierarchial, with rules and policies in a chain of command headed by the chief executive officer. Another structural scheme is the matrix organization, which is more oriented toward solving problems or managing projects. Matrix or team management rests more with designated project managers than with the traditional chief executive officer or departmental manager. This style will attract some physicians while repulsing others. The product-line or service-line management approach is increasingly finding favor within hospitals or hospital networks. Called strategic business units, these service categories have budgets, staff, and equipment for the specialized use of one set of patients. No matter what the structure, relationships are changing with different incentives, motives, and loyalties at work.

The chief executive officer position evolved with increasing education and responsibilities, with inside relationships to handle money, personnel, and facilities, as delegated by the governing board. Perhaps the most important duties have always been to establish and maintain working relationships with the doctors who brought patients to the hospital to fill beds. The outside role of the executive officer includes relating to the community, governmental bodies, and educational or planning activities, such as the need for new or improved specialized facilities.

Communicating with the individual physicians and the organized medical staff is growing much more difficult with the advent of managed care, and the administrative leader remains the visible target for physician unreset and anger.

REFERENCES

Snook, D. I., Jr. (1992). *Hospitals: What They Are and How They Work (2nd ed.)* Gaithersburg, MD: Aspen Publishers.

White, C. H. (1986–1992). [Faculty workshop presentations]. Grossmont Hospital, La Mesa, CA.

White, C. H. (1992–1994). [Faculty workshop presentations]. Sharp Healthcare, San Diego, CA.

CHAPTER

13

Vice President for Medical Affairs

The medical staff executive structure presented in Chapter 10 is a creature in and of the medical staff itself. Far more common is the employment of a medical director, in the older terminology, or the more modern title of vice president for medical affairs. Definition of terms should now be the first order of business. What is meant by the title medical director: a clinical expert who guides and performs high quality specialized care, or a physician who is doing administrative work? Setting aside the clinical definition as a particular example that is fairly clear in its intent and use, this chapter will explore the variations of the administrative role.

DEFINITION AND ROLE

The VPMA (or medical director) is defined as a physician who has been employed full or part time by administration (Gill, ongoing). In earlier years, that person might

169

have had a lengthy career of medical practice in that same hospital, but this pattern is not necessarily true any longer. Sometimes the role is unclear or undefined. Sometimes there is no job description. Sometimes this senior doctor is used only as a problem solver with no structural relationship to the medical staff. It is even possible that the VPMA may not have privileges to practice medicine in that hospital. If that is the case, then the medical staff usually will not consider that person to be theirs, or even one of them. The VPMA will be an alien being belonging to nobody and trusted by nobody.

Other variations of the job include an assisting role to the administration through the contracting process, helping to manage joint ventures, or directing the QA process in the hospital. But the key element in the life of the VPMA is that the doctor was hired by the administration and reports there. For many chiefs of staff, that is a complication of the leadership role and can lead to misunderstanding and conflict. Sometimes, the medical staff does not accept the VPMA as another physician colleague but views that person as a traitor who is no longer one of them and is now dedicated to helping administration make life worse for the doctors.

The role can also be confusing for some board members who are not sure who speaks for the medical staff or who represents the physicians. The distinctions between the VPMA and the chief may not be clear and can often be misunderstood by board members or employees. In fact, the distinctions may not even be clear or understood by the VPMA, whose responsibilities and accountabilities were not adequately described by the administration. It is not unknown for the administration to appoint someone before figuring out what was wanted. It is not unknown for an administrator to request that the VPMA keep the doctors under control (which, at least, is a measurable objective).

Sometimes a VPMA takes part in medical staff activities and can not refrain from giving clinical opinions on cases in peer review. Some VPMAs bring a whole lifetime of histories and relationships, including referral patterns and competitive hatreds and jealousies. The baggage may be too much to allow effective performance, and that is one of the criteria that administration should take into account. An organizational chart that shows how it might look to have a medical director or VPMA is shown in Figure 13–1.

BEFORE HIRING A VPMA/MEDICAL DIRECTOR

The continual refinement of the VPMA position and its evolution, as provided by Sandra Gill, Daniel Lang, and John Lloyd in their ongoing speeches and seminars, have improved the clarity and led to much better understanding of this position. For example, the administrator contemplating creation of a VPMA or an administrative medical director position should consider these questions, among others.

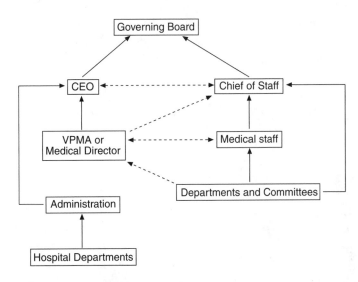

FIGURE 13–1   Hospital–medical staff relationship: VPMA.

What Problems Need to Be Solved?

These could include:

- low census
- medical staff unrest
- poor compliance with economic controls
- failing grades from JCAHO
- excessive liability losses
- low community image
- low self-image

Each of these symptoms are the product of a combination of inside management concerns and outside forces acting on the hospital and larger health care world. Low census is probably a result of the movement toward managed care and will not be solved by the VPMA acting alone. If there are signs of turmoil within the medical staff, poor attention to the elements of self-governance, and lack of pride in the hospital, then there are major issues of communication, trust, and integration toward a common culture that need to be worked on immediately. If it is the administrator's hope that a new, inexperienced VPMA will solve things quickly, there will be a considerable delay in the resolution of the issues. The VPMA cannot solve problems of this magnitude by simply giving orders, although there are probably some administrators who think that is all that is needed. Chances are that any hospital in the midst of issues such as these is also suffering from poor attention to quality of care by the doctors and poor quality of management care by administration.

What Attributes Are Valued in a VPMA or Medical Director?

These might include:

- obedience
- reliability
- popularity
- professional competence and experience
- small stipend
- communicator
- independence
- maturity
- knowing the gossip on the leading doctors

Daniel Lang has been assured that each is a valid concern by administrators seeking to employ a VPMA or medical director (Lang, 1985). If the job needs to be done, then look for competence, a better than average ability to communicate, and an unflappable nature. Objectivity is crucial, as is the benefit of some experience. No matter what the current crisis is, there will soon be another that is larger and worse. Knowing gossip on doctors will hurt much more than it helps. Those who consider this to be of utmost importance should forget the whole idea.

What Specific Tasks Will the VPMA or Medical Director Have?

These might include:

- improve the quality of care as measured objectively
- establish an acuity-based clinical measuring system
- establish a performance-based reappointment system
- deal with medical staff resistance to either or both of the clinical measuring or reappointment systems
- supervise the utilization management program
- train medical staff leadership
- pay for training and trips to national conferences

- act as facilitator for clinical groups
- learn to be a facilitator, and process the natural personality to be able to work with people rather than to simply give orders
- establish communication channels between administration and the medical staff when tasks go wrong
- establish and maintain communications channels before tasks go wrong, so that emergency behavior and bailouts are not the normal way to act
- act as a front for administration to hide behind when tensions arise
- keep the doctors in check
- represent the medical staff in administration and board matters
- refrain from direct interference in the performance of self-governance by the chief and the medical staff

There is a fertile field for VPMAs to work, along with the organized medical staff, in the area of development and use of severity-based objective data systems that can measure clinical performance. The political problems are always present, whether in a Joint Commission open staff or a closed panel, but there is no other more promising approach to reducing variations in practice. In the end, if it is necessary to reduce spending on health care, particularly in the hospital setting, reducing variations in practice will accomplish that end. Downsizing of middle management will be a short-term, one-time fix, but medical staff variation may actually increase as there are fewer hospital staff to follow physician orders and work closely in situations such as clinical pathways. Having the administration-based VPMA to be responsible for utilization review is actually a better solution than to expect the volunteer physicians to perform that act of policing each other.

A VPMA trained and experienced in the role of facilitator who can enable channels of communication and problem solving is a helpful approach that has a lot to recommend it. The problem, if there is one, will be for the VPMA to actually behave in the self-effacing and helping role that is required for good results by a facilitator who does not have a vested interest in any particular outcome of the discussions. If the VPMA attempts to use the position as one of power leverage that combines the weight of administration with the status of a physician, then trouble could result that might be worse than if the administration did it themselves. When the administration or the CEO is not good at that sort of thing and only serves to heighten tensions with the medical staff, then a VPMA can serve a useful role in standing between the two opposing forces.

The sticking point in the behavior and performance of a VPMA is in relationship to the self-governance functions of the organized medical staff. It may be possible for a VPMA to offer training in the duties of being a chief of staff and/or other staff leadership positions, but where did the VPMA learn those functions well enough to be a teacher? Hiring a VPMA does not eliminate the required functions of credentialing, reappointment, and peer review that must be performed in the Joint Commission model, and the chief of staff does not report to a VPMA. The VPMA does not have veto power over medical staff actions, although that person can be a valuable resource in planning strategy. Some medical staffs have the old reservation about the VPMA: being paid by the administration is contaminating.

Who Wants the VPMA or Medical Director?

These might be:

- the chief of staff, who has too much work
- the administrator and/or associates, who are tired of talking to or trying to work with the doctors
- nurses, who want protection from the abrasive or abusive physician whom the medical staff will not discipline
- the board, to keep the doctors in line
- everybody

The worst reason for adding a VPMA is because the other CEOs and administrators are doing it, so that must be the right way to proceed. The herd mentality is not a reason and is doomed to not work very well, if at all. There are valid reasons and there are legitimate tasks that can be performed, but there needs to be a clear understanding about the need and the job description for the position. If a CEO appoints a VPMA without discussing it with the chief of staff and the medical staff leadership, there is a guarantee of strife and conflict. The VPMA will be in an impossible position with no chance of success and will not last long, having nothing to show for the attempt but a sullied reputation.

How Much Authority Will the VPMA or Medical Director Be Allowed?

Possibilities include:

- permission needed for every action
- only the least amount of information that absolutely must be known
- disciplinary authority over medical staff doctors
- direction of the education program for the medical staff
- supervisory authority to hire, fire, and evaluate the employees of the medical staff who do medical staff services, peer review, CME, and library

- freedom to relate independently to the needs of the medical staff, board, and administration without asking for specific permission each time
- leadership of key hospital quality and other committees
- responsibility for budget preparation for clinical services as well as the medical staff organization
- responsibility for evaluating and recommending or approving the medical equipment capital budget
- responsibility for developing and supervising the residency program

It is not possible to give the VPMA appointed by administration direct disciplinary authority over doctors who practice in the hospital, because that is the legitimate function of the Joint Commission model of a hospital medical staff. Being a participant in the process can be helpful. Carrying the message that inappropriate behavior by doctors is not acceptable by either the administration and the board as well as the medical staff is also helpful. Directing the CME program can be done very well by a VPMA, unless there is already a strong CME chair and committee in place, in which case there is now a tug of war that did not need to happen. For the VPMA to direct a house staff program and negotiate residency arrangements are strong points that cannot be done well by either a volunteer chief or a lay administrator. Similarly, to be a participant in the budget process with ample information and feedback from the clinicians is an improvement over the usual process where only the finance department tries to put together a budget without seeking input.

Perhaps, the most important and useful role to be played by a VPMA is to be a member of the management team, so that there is physician input available at all times during the conduct of hospital affairs. Some fairly grievous errors could be prevented by having that perspective available. The salaried VPMA can be present in those meetings when the volunteer chief who has a practice to conduct may not have the time. The VPMA could attempt to represent the medical staff position on issues but not to usurp the prerogative and responsibility of the chief of staff and the executive committee. A VPMA does not replace the chief and does not control the self-governance functions of the medical staff.

How Will the Performance of the VPMA or Medical Director Be Evaluated?

Possible options include:

- demonstrates the ability to promote effective exchange, leading hospital and medical leadership to openly and honestly confront and resolve difficult issues

- keeps medical staff issues and squabbling out of the boardroom
- shows unswerving loyalty (but to what or to whom?)
- achieves an annual vote of confidence by the medical staff
- earns the respect and cooperative working relationships from the chiefs of staff and department chairs
- use zero-based approach (if there are no complaints, there must not be any problems)

Review and evaluation of performance is a function of the personnel process and must be done by the administration that hired the VPMA. It is not proper for the medical staff to perform that function, although an opinion and consultation with the chief is certainly in order. If the first item above has actually occurred (that is, there has been open and honest confrontation and resolution of difficult issues), then the VPMA appointment was a success and that hospital is well-equipped to move forward into the next era in the evolution of the health care delivery system. Such accomplishments are the hallmark of a talented and successful VPMA, who might indeed be a candidate for the CEO/administrator position.

How Will the VPMA or Medical Director Be Compensated?

Possibilities include:

- hourly, to compensate for time lost from practice
- as an independent professional on a par with peers
- cost shared with the medical staff organization
- allow the VPMA to supplement income as a hospital-based consultant
- incentive bonuses
- encourage the VPMA to become a surveyor or a consultant who helps other hospitals prepare for surveys, and grant the necessary time off

A salary schedule should be established within the human resources department for the VPMA and all medical director positions, based on job descriptions. Salaried positions for the VPMA will not replace the total income that might have been earned from full-time clinical practice, but it will be considerably more than the middle management schedule. There are pro and con arguments about whether the VPMA should remain in private practice. The real issue here is whether the VPMA is on all sides of every issue. It dilutes the effect of the VPMA to be first on one side then the other when issues arise. There is definite merit in having the VPMA engage in training to become a surveyor or consultant who can help prepare for surveys. That role becomes particularly important in moving from an individual hospital to an integrated system position, so that there can be survey preparation going on continually, leading toward the day of system surveys.

THE EFFECT ON RELATIONSHIPS

It should be made very clear that the doctor who works for the administration does not replace or have supremacy over the organized medical staff structure as described in the Joint Commission model. The administration cannot hire someone who will do the job of, or replace the chief of staff, just as the medical staff cannot hire a medical staff executive who will take over administration of the hospital. There is a valuable and useful role for each to perform that can make things better for everyone, whether an administrative person is added for the medical staff or a medical person for the administrative staff. Both can do well and help build better relationships and a more smoothly functioning organization, which will be necessary in the managed care era that is upon us.

But to do either of these things will require some different ways of thinking and acting by all parties. Hardening of the categories is not the exclusive property of either the administration or the doctors. It does seem obvious that there are more 55-year-old doctors who want to retreat from clinical practice than there are candidates for medical staff executive positions, but maybe the search has not been hard enough. Why not try some of the professional people who have been working in state or county medical societies or associations? That job may become an endangered species as time goes on and the societies, both medical and hospital, have less to offer their members that will justify the increased dues payments.

By reviewing the empirical evidence and by scanning the registration lists at national meetings, the number of people working in medical management is growing. Teaching hospitals moved to VPMA earlier than did some of the nonteaching institutions. Larger hospitals added the position earlier than did smaller institutions. VPMAs appear to be almost entirely white males who have left their practices in small or large part to become involved with administration and are constantly defining or redefining the role in behavioral terms of their capabilities and hospital needs. Some of the best work is being done in focusing on cost-effective care. A hospital's best advertisement in a managed care–contracting world is the presence of a single standard of care at an affordable level. Any hospital or integrated system of doctors and hospitals that is monitoring physician performance retrospectively against historical and current experience for analysis and education; that is monitoring performance concurrently for consultation and intervention; that is participating in joint resource analysis with medical staff leadership and administration; that has developed joint strategies for addressing problem areas has an enormous head start toward success.

SUMMARY

The medical staff executive structure is a creature in and of the medical staff itself, while the medical director or vice president for medical affairs is a physician employed by the administration. There can be relationship problems with the elected chief of staff and with the organized medical staff itself. Sometimes, the duties expected from the VPMA are not made as clear as in the job description provided. There can be confusion within the board if trustees are not sure who speaks for the medical staff. Continual refinement of the VPMA position has improved the clarity and provided much better understanding, as has the performance of outstanding physicians in the office.

Guidance and assistance is offered in thinking through the hiring of a VPMA, including what problems are to be solved, what attributes are wanted, what specific tasks will be given, who wants the VPMA, how much authority to give, how to evaluate performance, and how to compensate.

REFERENCES

Lang, D. A. (1985). *The Physician and the Hospital* [Faculty workshop presentations]. University of Southern California, California Hospital Association, California Medical Association.

Gill, S. (Ongoing). [Faculty presentations]. Estes Park Institute, Brighton, CO.

CHAPTER

How Boards Relate to Physicians

To community leaders that compose the majority of hospital boards, physicians can mean several things: their own family doctor, the specialist who performed surgery or another procedure, the famous practitioner who is the star of the hospital and a leader in that professional field. All of these are visible manifestations of what physicians do as practicing doctors. Board members, especially when new to the board, think generally of physicians in this practice role. Board members also look at the recommendations for individual new physicians to join the staff as independent physicians, being recommended for approval based on their own credentials. Boards also routinely approve for reappointment each two years those previous members of the staff.

Perhaps, the board understands the role of physicians as members of a group holding an exclusive contract with the hospital, although they may never have actually met any group members other than whoever negotiated the contract. More likely is it that the members of the board are acquainted with a contracted medical or service-line director who functions in a combined administrative-clinical role, since that person probably makes periodic presentations to the board asking approval of a new program or capital investment. Certainly, some committee members of the board will know the leader of a group with whom the hospital is forming or participating in a joint venture. All of these and other arrangements are practice-related arrangements.

Many new directors or trustees come to the job on the board believing that, as their fellow citizens in the community, doctors are employees of the hospital and can be made to mind or follow orders like any other employee in civilian life. Usually, in a community nonprofit hospital, those doctors are not employees but are independently licensed physicians and surgeons (the license reads that way). They may be dependent on the hospital for many things, but that does not include following orders from administration or members of the board of directors or trustees (White, 1983).

HOW BOARDS RELATE TO MEDICAL STAFF

New members bring many skills and experiences with them to the hospital board, including success with finance, bonds, land acquisition, human resources, labor relations, sales, marketing, management, law, philanthropy, and, possibly, amassing or inheriting wealth. But none of them bring any previous experience or knowledge of the medical staff and how to deal with it.

Upon learning that doctors as individuals and the medical staff as an unincorporated association for self-governance have roles, functions, rights, responsibilities, political strengths, disunity, and lack of faith in almost everything, some new trustees grow suspicious and distrustful. Boards are sometimes tempted to perform medical staff functions themselves. The duty of the board is not to personally conduct medical staff functions but to see that competent systems are in place (White, 1986).

The chief of staff is the person the board should look to for reports and assurance that competent systems are in place and that they do function effectively. Boards approve credentials, reappointments, privileges, policies, disciplinary actions, and budget requests from the medical staff. Yet the question still arises of how to ensure that the peer review process, working as it does in secrecy, is guaranteeing that bad doctors won't escape scrutiny or punishment and get the hospital in trouble. Could a conspiracy of silence be protecting its members from the consequences of their actions? Can board members be more sure that they are not personally and collectively at risk for the unknown actions of the medical staff, most of the members of which they do not know? These uncertainties can be answered by ensuring that a competent system is in place. The best guarantee that a competent system is in place comes through building trust and effective relationships among administration, the board, and the medical staff, particularly in the persons of the chiefs of staff (White & Green, 1988). A more detailed account of the reports required is presented in Chapters 15 and 16.

Why should directors or trustees not sit as members of a peer review committee to make sure the doctors are doing it right? That question has been asked or considered by practically every hospital board member who ever assumed the title. There are two very good answers to this question.

Answer 1

The presence of a trustee or director or any other outsider would inhibit the candor essential to good peer review. Head-knocking arguments; personal attacks; accusations of bad medicine, faulty decision making, poor judgment, on the one hand; or agreement, on the other hand, that nothing else could have been done to save the patient: all of these could take place during a typical peer review committee meeting. In fact, most of them usually do take place during the process that serves the same purpose as the confrontation setting in a courtroom between lawyers. Trying to arrive at the truth about the best quality of care in a profession that is still science and art combined requires candor and it *is* inhibited by outsiders.

Answer 2

Because the board will function as an appeal body if the judicial review process requires it, the member cannot have taken part in the original actions. If a director or trustee sat in on the departmental peer review meeting that originated a due process proceeding, that person is not allowed to later sit on the appeal, as a simple conflict of interest. For the same reason, chiefs of staff cannot be everywhere at the same time. They cannot be expected to sit with each peer review committee, to sit as a member of judicial review panels, and to serve as members of board and administration committees. The chief of staff should serve only as the chair of the executive committee and the general medical staff.

Law and the Board's Role

The real role of the board in the Joint Commission model is to exercise the duty of due care to patients by protecting them from incompetent doctors. Case law has clarified that hospitals and their boards are not responsible for the conduct of physicians on the staff because doctors are not their employees or agents. Hospitals are responsible as employers, of course, for the acts of an employee committed within the scope of that person's employment.

A hospital can also be vicariously liable for the negligence of "vicarious" agents. Physicians with exclusive contracts to provide services in "closed" departments, such as radiology, pathology, and emergency, are often held by the courts to be ostensible agents of the hospital. Among the reasons giving rise to the ostensible agent relationship are that the hospital selects the physician for the patient, the patient relies on the hospital's judgment in choosing the physician, and the hospital holds itself out to the public as offering these services.

If the medical staff doctor is not an employee, then what is that person? In conventional legal terminology, a person is either an employee or an independent contractor. An employer is responsible for the acts of the employees, but subject to very broad qualifications, not for those of an independent contractor. In this view, the hospital is merely a facility, or hotel, whose reason for existence is merely to provide a place or workshop where a licensed physician can practice medicine in an individual way of caring for private patients (Gassiot & Starr, 1987). However, legal theories have evolved and changed so that although a staff doctor is an independent contractor, as a physician practicing in a Joint Commission model of a hospital medical staff, that person is also a concessionaire or licensee, someone to whom the hospital governing board has granted the privilege of practicing medicine within the hospital's premises.

The hospital is the occupier of land on which it invites patients into its custody, for treatment by its independent contractors or concessionaires, the doctors. By granting staff privileges and by taking custody of patients, the hospital takes the risk of incurring liability for acts committed by the concessionaire, the medical staff physician. There is but one rule that applies here, in the words of Justice Goldberg, and that is to "use due care to see to it that those patients in custody are not harmed by the concessionaires, the independent contractors who collectively make up the medical staff" (Goldberg, 1978).

In another landmark court decision in 1965, the Darling case dramatically illustrates the changes from previous theories about responsibility and liability for the quality of patient care, and the duty of the board to assure that quality. Previously, hospitals were not considered to be responsible for the negligent treatment of patients by physicians. Hospitals were thought of as mere providers of facilities and support personnel. Physicians used the hospital facilities as independent contractors who were selected by their patients. The Darling case set the precedent that a hospital could be held corporately liable for the negligent selection or retention of physicians on the medical staff and for their actions. In the case, the physician was allowed to perform surgery he was not capable of doing, was not reviewed to bring his operative procedures up to date, was not adequately supervised, and did not request consultation, particularly after complications had developed. The hospital's defense was that only the physician could practice medicine; it was powerless to forbid or command any physician or surgeon in the practice of his or her profession. The hospital's only obligation was to use reasonable care in selecting medical doctors. The court disagreed.

There are other precedent cases dealing with negligence in reviewing credentials, negligence in conducting peer review, a physician's inability to get along with others to the detriment of patient care, and a growing number of antitrust actions. The very nature of the practice of medicine and hospital care creates new areas of potential risk that inevitably results in an increasing imposition of liability (Ludlam, 1986).

BOARDS IN SYSTEMS OR NETWORKS

An emerging issue for the hospital field concerns the structure and functions of governance within multiple hospital systems or integrated health care networks. Models for structuring governance in systems such as these have been described (Haglund & Dowling, 1993).

In the *parent holding company model,* governing bodies exist at both the system and institutional levels. In that instance, the local board continues to grant medical staff membership and privileges. Some systems have adopted a variation of the parent-holding company model in which there is a system-level governing board, but boards at the institutional level serve in only an advisory capacity. The responsibilities of the advisory boards may be generally limited to community relations and monitoring quality of care, but if members of the medical staff practice only in that institution and do not have full privileges for the system, then that advisory board is still responsible for carrying out the Joint Commission model responsibilities.

The *corporate model* occurs when only a system-level governing board exists to carry out all the governance activities of a multihospital system. Regardless of the governance model in existence, it is more likely that the corporate-level boards will retain responsibility for decisions regarding the transfer or sale of assets, formation of new companies, purchase of assets greater than a base figure, changes in hospital bylaws, and appointment of local board members (Haglund & Dowling, 1993). For other activities, the governance model affects the locus of decision-making authority. In general, the more decentralized the governance model, the more likely it is that activities such as service development, strategic planning, capital and operating budget approval, medical staff appointments, and appointment and evaluation of the hospital chief executive will be under the authority of the local board. This would be entirely within the traditional dimensions of the Joint Commission model. The alternative version that has not yet appeared in large numbers is the appointment of physicians and their privileges to system-level membership, entitling them to practice in any hospital in the system without further credentialing. Time may show that the system appointment approach is the most effective mechanism for true integration of physicians within systems and would therefore, require system survey by the Joint Commission.

A major item for further research on the governance of multihospital systems should focus on the relationship between governance structures and operational effectiveness and efficiency. The corporate model has the advantage of structural simplicity and clear lines of authority while holding company models provide for greater input and involvement at the community level. Further examination of the advantages and disadvantages of these approaches to system-level governance will become more important as the hospital industry in the United States continues to evolve under the influence of competition and managed care into more horizontal and vertical integration (Haglund & Dowling, 1993). But a multihospital system will never be fully integrated and will never have identical incentives until the physicians in some form of medical staff become as integrated as the corporate office is.

SUMMARY

Trustees or directors, as members of boards, bring to their job their own personal experiences as patients or with business relationships with individual physicians. When they assume their seats on the board, trustees are responsible for approving initial appointments to the medical staff, and then periodic reappointments. Perhaps, the trustee is familiar with members of physician groups who hold contracts to provide hospital-based services. Perhaps, also, new trustees bring to the board a community perception that doctors are the employees of the hospital and can thus be expected to follow the orders of the CEO or other managers.

Trustees bring their skills and experiences with them, including success with finance, bonds, land acquisition, law, human resources, sales, marketing, labor relations, management, philanthropy, and amassing of wealth. But none of them bring any previous experience or knowledge of the organized medical staff and how to deal with it. Boards must learn to work with the medical staff as an unincorporated association for self-governance with roles, rights, functions, responsibilities, political strengths, disunity, and lack of faith in almost everything.

Boards do not perform medical staff functions but must see that competent systems are in place. The real role of the board in the Joint Commission model is to exercise the duty of due care to protect patients, by treating the doctors not as employees but as independent contractors. Precedent court cases, such as Darling, have established that hospitals and their boards can be held corporately liable for the negligent selection or retention of physicians and their actions.

A particular issue for the future will be the existence, roles, and responsibilities of boards in integrated health care systems. Will each hospital in the system retain its individual board, and, if so, what will it be responsible for?

REFERENCES

Gassiot, C. O., & Starr, P. J. (Eds.). (1987). *Principles of Medical Staff Services Science.* Education Council, National Association of Medical Staff Services. Privately printed.

Goldberg, B. A. (1978). The duty of hospitals and hospital medical staffs to regulate the quality of patient care. *Western Journal of Medicine,* 129(5), 443–450.

Haglund, C. L., & Dowling, W. L. (1993). The hospital. *Introduction to Health Services (4th ed.)*. Albany: Delmar Publishers.

Ludlam, J. E. *Evaluation of the California Experience with the Medical Injury Compensation Reform Act of 1975 (MICRA)*. Unpublished presentation material.

White, C. H. (1983). *Responsibilities, Obligations, and Selection Criteria For Trusteeship.* Sacramento: California Hospital Association.

White, C. H. (1986). Differing perceptions on assuring quality care. *CHA Insight,* 10(2), 1–4.

White, C. H., & Green, J. S. (1988). Roles in assuring quality care. *Trustee,* 41(7), 14–17.

CHAPTER

15

Expectations from the Medical Staff

The board should expect open communication and timely, relevant information from the chief of staff. The board should not expect to get substantial portions of their information about medical staff self-governance backstage from individual physicians who have grievances or a special favor of self-interest to lobby. Boards should not tolerate unwilling or uncooperative secretiveness from the chief, acting in the role as the elected leader of the organized medical staff. The board delegated self-governance to the medical staff, but that does not mean that they have heard the last of it because it belongs to the doctors who do not want to share any of the details. Hospital and health system governance depends more than ever on working together in trust relationships. The 1980s attitudes of suspicion and hostility between medical staffs and hospital management/governance is a sure recipe for failure in the rapidly changing managed care environment.

CHIEF OF STAFF EXPLAINS ISSUES

The board should ask the chief to explain a number of concepts that will be both valuable and useful in understanding the larger health care system and for making wiser governance decisions. Chiefs should explain, for example, the provisional or conditional staff period when a candidate for membership is allowed to practice with full privileges, but with proctoring. The chief should then explain how the proctor is only an observer acting on behalf of the staff and is not responsible for assisting in case of trouble. Furthermore, the proctor is not being paid a fee by the insurer or the candidate and has no conflict of interest.

Another mysterious issue for the board, unless explained, is the concept of current clinical competence, where a medical staff member is reviewed and evaluated within each two-year reappointment period according to present practice performance, not according to medical school or residency training or even historical practice habits. There should be regular and periodic reports and explanations about the reappointment process being used in the hospital, along with descriptions and examples of what practice profile data is gathered and how it is being used.

There should be a quality improvement workshop each year, where the medical staff leaders demonstrate how the peer review, disciplinary, and judicial process programs are being used, along with their successes and failures. Some doctors will disagree with that recommendation on the grounds that what the medical staff does, if anything, is their business and is too secret to be shared with the board, forgetting that the only reason they are doing it at all is that it was delegated to them by the board.

Boards and administrations also need explanations and demonstrations of such public reports as Medicare mortality data prepared and presented by the Health Care Financing Administration (HCFA). Press and media stories arising from these and other patient-related data can focus attention on the hospital. Members of the hospital family should be instructed, informed, and prepared for interpreting press stories on the subject. Their friends and neighbors in the community will want to understand how their local hospital, which has offered care any time they needed it, could be called in glaring headlines a "death hospital," as some were when the first HCFA report was released.

A spokesperson should be appointed as the only contact with the press in these instances. For medical or clinical issues, that spokesperson should be the chief of staff or the VPMA/medical director, as appropriate. Do not delegate weekend responses to the junior member of the public relations department who caught the short straw with weekend on-call duty. That person will be no match for an eager reporter investigating a possible front-page story about a juicy doctor/hospital scandal.

Another completely mysterious subject about the hospital and its doctors is that of a Professional Review Organization (PRO), as those and other structures affect your hospital and, possibly, Medicare or Medicaid funding. First, make sure the chief or the vice president knows and understands the subject and can explain it coherently. Then have that person explain to the board whether any physicians from the staff have been criticized or punished by the review agency and how that will affect the hospital.

A board has the right to expect, and a medical staff has the obligation to provide, some other qualities of environment and atmosphere that will produce a better opportunity for high-quality patient care. There will be some medical staff hard-liners who will dispute that statement, alleging to the contrary that it is the duty of the medical staff to perform as opposition to anything the hospital wants to do. The hospital is the enemy, after all, they will say, and they will behave in that manner. The medical staff may not be clear on what it should expect from itself.

There is another constituency here besides the medical staff and their defensiveness. Honoring the dignity of those a person serves is a part of all service. Emily Friedman points out that "unless we are willing to submit ourselves to the scrutiny of the communities we seek to serve, and unless we demonstrate that we actually made a difference in their lives or their health, our claim of commitment to community care is simply a gimmick." It means that people are afraid of asking for the judgment of the community, as represented by the board of community leaders. She goes on to say that "being accountable is scary, but one cannot think of any other way to find out if we are doing any good" (Friedman, 1995).

The old attitude that the hospital is the enemy, although traditional with some physicians, is self-destructive in these days of rapid change and movement away from fee-for-service toward managed care. From the medical staff and particularly from the leadership, the board should expect at least the important aspects of professionalism and good citizenship as proposed by Spence Meighan and outlined in the next section.

EXPECTATIONS FROM SELF-GOVERNANCE

Present a Coherent Voice

Medical staff leadership, both elected and appointed, should represent the opinions and aspirations of the entire staff, not only the loudest voices. Leaders should have an opinion (or a range of opinions) regarding controversial issues. The medical staff cannot merely say no to everything.

Ensure Competent Able Practitioners

The medical staff must be made up of competent and up-to-date practitioners who are able to practice in the hospital and advise the board regarding the latest and most important scientific and technological developments.

Demonstrate Political Awareness

The medical staff and its leadership must recognize the political realities of modern health care and the reforms taking place. Medical practice is changing and much more is yet to come. The status quo will not survive any more. The hospital and its administration did not invent the changes taking place in the outside world and do not have the ability to control their outcomes acting alone.

Provide Help in a Crisis

The leadership and the senior staff should help to manage change and the crises that will inevitably arise. They will be needed to help untangle snafus that are, unfortunately, likely to occur. These are almost predictable when there are this many important issues and equally important egos all contained within the four walls of a hospital.

Continue to Bring Patients

There is an increasing tendency toward monogamy as physicians practice in fewer hospitals. The reason is not one of necessarily more loyalty, as board members would wish, but a very simple question of who has the contract that dictates patient terms of benefits and coverages. There are fewer physician choices about where to admit the patient, and fewer choices of physicians as well, because of who is a plan panel member and who has medical staff privileges at particular hospitals. But when there is a choice available, then loyalty becomes a variable.

Provide High-Quality Patient Care

The medical staff must take seriously the work of quality improvement and deal with problems as they arise, no matter who the doctor is. Sanctions must be applied when warranted in a timely and forthright manner. Clinical privileges must be granted in accord with education and experience and then limited or withdrawn when not merited, no matter who the physician is. That caveat presupposes that there is a competent quality review system that actually works the way it is supposed to, and the way it is described in the Joint Commission manual.

Complete Medical Records in a Timely Manner

There is a Joint Commission standard stating that incomplete and delinquent medical records can number no more than a certain percentage of the average number of admissions to the hospital. The medical records librarian knows what that number is. A reward from the medical records department or hospital administration is in order if the total is at or below the threshold. However, a better bet is that the number of delinquent charts is in excess of the limit, perhaps many times the limit. A medical staff cannot call itself an example of good self-governance as long as the physicians scoff at the requirement for completing records.

Usually, a successful program for keeping the number of delinquent records below the allowable threshold requires a notification system, a warning that a chief of staff and the executive committee are willing to uphold the law. Suspending one of the favorites or a major admitter takes guts. However, after the habit of completing records on time has been put in place, it will function more smoothly when the doctors discover that the rule is to be followed and applies to everyone. The records people will love it. The finance people will love it too, because they cannot bill for the services already rendered until the records are finished. Think of all the millions of dollars needed by the hospitals to pay salaries and expenses that cannot be collected because the medical staff will not complete their records. This is one of those medical staff situations that cannot be set aside no matter how much griping results.

Assist with New Physician Recruitment

The existing medical staff is the best recruitment force available to a hospital and board. New practitioners are always needed to bring the latest scientific advances and new procedures to the patients. While shopping for a practice location, new physicians will check around with their specialty colleagues or a friend of a friend to find out about the medical climate and business possibilities. If the local grumps are able to dominate the conversation, a promising young doctor will probably go somewhere else that sounds better. Although there should not be overstatement or deception, there are problems everywhere, and a candid assessment of the realities are what the medical staff, administration, and board should expect.

Assure Patient Safety

Constant vigilance by the nursing staff, with support by the medical staff, is a duty of care that must be upheld. Hospitals must be committed not only to high-quality care but to the prevention of accidents and the avoidance of claims or lawsuits. Nothing will reduce the confidence and morale of the employee staff as quickly and easily as the spectacle of bad medical care going undetected and unreviewed, or unacceptable behavior going unpunished. It is not nearly enough just to say all the right words, there must be immediate and overt action dedicated to doing all the right actions in the best interest of patient safety by the entire hospital family. Even the volunteers have a duty of due care toward patient safety.

Choose Good Leadership

The medical staff earns credibility for itself and respect for its success in self-governance by demonstrating its determination through the election and appointment of recognized good leaders who will foster productive working relationships and better quality patient care. No hospital or medical staff needs to have doctors elected to the executive committee who come there with an agenda to right all the wrongs of the past and punish all the enemies of one dissident group or other.

Participate in Strategic Planning

The organized medical staff through its leaders has an obligation to participate in the process of building a "vision" of a preferred future for the hospital. That vision will change from to time as the outside world also changes and evolves. The smart chief of staff also talks over those possibilities with a broad cross section of the staff, so as to have a pulse on what the doctors think and could support, in order to be able to report that sentiment at the board/medical staff planning retreat. The hospital should not involve only administration staff and selected board members in the planning process, leaving out the medical staff on the grounds that the doctors are not running the hospital.

Even better, the medical staff should have a planning committee of its own that works on the major issues as the year goes on so as to be able to participate fully with the board. The administration should play a major role in helping with this medical staff standing committee by attending meetings, supplying staff support and information, and, in general, helping with the process of working together as a team. That is the true meaning of partnership. Hospitals where the doctors and administration are enemies are not long for the world of managed care.

Accept Financial Responsibility

Medical staff physicians in general and the chief of staff in particular do not need to know all about the finances of the hospital, but they do need to understand and be willing to discuss the current constraints and limitations. Some doctors think of the hospital as a bottomless well of capital finances for their pet projects of new buildings and the latest equipment, but most hospitals of the mid-1990s are no longer in that fortunate position. An artifact of the world of the 1980s was that physicians on the medical staff could practice patient care in any manner they saw fit without interference or advice from the administration. It was the administration's job to see to it that there was an unlimited supply of money for each doctor's favorite expenditure. Now, with hospital census figures in the 50 percent range or even lower, rather than in the 80 percent range as they used to be, there is less capital for any reason. It is a cinch that under increasing pressure from managed care, there will be further limits on that former flexibility to increase hospital capacity. There will be few, if any, new buildings in a capitated world.

Resolve Conflicts

Medical staff leadership is expected by administration and the board to try to resolve internal medical staff squabbles without involving the entire hospital. Everyone accepts the fact that with so many bright people under so much pressure to care for extremely ill patients, there will be moments of rampant emotionalism or disagreement. Here is one of the toughest parts of the chief's job: to settle these issues by resolution, compromise, decision, or some other way, so that the business of patient care may continue. Nurses can relate how difficult it is to work in that environment and how much they want the chief to fix it.

Support the Nursing Staff

The medical staff stands alone in its duty to promote courtesy in the provision of patient care and the building of mutual respect among members of the staff. The administration cannot do this job because the administration does not control doctor behavior. The opponent of this productive workplace are those physicians who, for some reason, regard hospital employees as some sort of subhuman. The professional attitudes exhibited in a strong hospital are noticed by the patients and families, and it rubs off on them too. They will speak well of their hospital stay and tell their friends and neighbors that the hospital is a good place because people treat each other well. They may not know all about medicine as the doctors do. But, they know all about people as the doctors may not.

Being well regarded in the community is a thing to be desired and valued highly. Yet a hospital where doctors berate nurses and the technical staff, where doctors speak gruffly to families and refuse to explain care to patients, is not likely to be well thought of. Where that hospital is a contractor to a health plan, there will be employee resistance to going there. Consumer satisfaction is one of the products of the quality improvement movement. Cordial and professionally respectful relationships between the doctors and nurses has always been an issue and will be here to stay.

Be Aware of Regulatory Requirements

Although it is the hospital that is surveyed by the Joint Commission and inspected by state and local authorities, the most sensitive parts of these evaluations are usually focused on the medical staff. All too often, chiefs and department chairs pay no attention until the last minute. Then a frantic spasm may or may not produce enough minutes, notebooks, and reports to stagger through. Medical staff self-governance carries with it the duty and obligation to help meet survey and inspection requirements. It is not just a matter of helping the hospital, as some doctors always say. It is a matter of helping each other. Most of the time during surveys is spent with hospital employees trying to explain and demonstrate how systems work and how they comply with standards.

A goodly amount of that time is spent by medical staff services and peer review staff trying to explain and demonstrate how the medical staff systems work and how they comply with standards. Sometimes, it is painfully clear to everyone in the room that medical systems do not work and do not comply with standards. It could be that those systems were hastily put together at the last minute before the survey in the forlorn hope that the Joint Commission and other surveyors will be deaf, dumb, and blind. They are not. The medical staff leadership needs to make it clear to all concerned that surveys are important and that preparations should be made early, with training for chairs in what questions will be asked and how answers should be made. Here is where the value of a VPMA who has become a trained surveyor can be demonstrated. Even better is a pervasive attitude throughout the staff fostered by the chiefs and chairs that standards are something to live with all the time, every day in every way, and not just something to do grudgingly at the last minute.

A TRUE PARTNERSHIP

It is truly a partnership and not an analogy to the military, where the enlisted men and women are engaged in a perpetual tug of war with the officers (officers in this instance being represented by the administration and board and enlisted personnel by the medical staff). Passive resistance is not the hallmark of a partnership nor effective self-governance by a hospital medical staff. Being in medical practice is not an excuse for dereliction of duty to the community. Neither is it an artifact of science, that somehow medical practice requires forgetting the community that has provided a career and a good living all these years. As Stuart Davidson said, "one does not need to know all about the biosciences to practice medicine. Medical practice is not a science, it is the application of science for the benefit of patients (Davidson, 1995). The technologies of medicine are derived from science, but the practice of the profession and the care of patients is the art and the citizenship.

SUMMARY

The board should expect open communication; timely, relevant information; and the absence of unwilling or uncooperative secretiveness from the chief of staff and medical staff leaders. Hospital and health system governance depend more than ever on working together in trust relationships, because the opposite is a sure recipe for failure in the rapidly changing managed care environment. An annual quality improvement workshop should be held to demonstrate the successes and failures of the peer review/disciplinary/judicial review processes. The board should expect and the medical staff should provide qualities of environment and atmosphere in the hospital that will produce opportunities for high-quality care.

The ancient attitude that the hospital is the enemy, held by some doctors, is self-destructive and should be overcome by a number of effective solutions presented.

REFERENCES

Davidson, S. M. (1995). The metamorphosis of the modern physician. *Healthcare Forum Journal, May/June,* 66–73.

Friedman, E. (1995). If you really mean it. *Healthcare Forum Journal, May/June,* 9–12.

Meighan, S. (Ongoing). [Faculty presentations]. Estes Park Institute, Brighton, CO.

CHAPTER

Key Reports by the Medical Staff

The governance of the American hospital has always been elusive, amorphous, and confusing. Bewildered students of management have been able to find theories to fit the apparently headless enterprise and have dismissed the traditional hospital structure as an enigma. Hospitals have had to coordinate too many diverse parts and divergent interests to remain organizationally inexplicable, however, and have invented their own multi-legged organization. The traditional hospital governance structure was proclaimed to have three legs: trustees, administration, and medical staff. As Ray Brown (1970) said, that was magnificently designed to ensure that the hospital could move in three different ways without going in any direction.

INHERITED GOVERNANCE STRUCTURE

This awkward and fragmented governance arrangement of the hospital is an inheritance from its past. The hospital was originally conceived as an agency dedicated to doing good rather than doing well. It was little more than a home away from home for the sick poor. Doctors did not need the hospital in the beginning and the hospital did not need management. Money was almost the sole problem of these early hospitals, and that problem was easily solved by funds from the trustees who naturally, then, sat in the seat of governance over, essentially, their own money. But scientific medicine changed all that. So, also, did the evolutionary changes that have increasingly held the hospital responsible for the quality of the care delivered within its walls by the medical staff.

There have been repeated cries for the development of a more unified organizational structure for hospitals where the medical staff, governing board, and administration act as part of the whole and not as separate entities. Physicians have almost uniformly resisted any organizational form that appeared to give administration any sort of control over their medical practice in the hospital. Administration executives, trained in the principles of good business management, frequently find themselves unable to use that expertise. Boards of trustees can no longer measure their role and contribution to hospital success by donations and gifts. Instead, boards must evaluate how much of what they do contributes to the effectiveness of the organization, even if it is still separated differently than more controllable business structures. Boards in these perilous times must more closely examine their meaning and contribution to the ongoing activities of the hospital. It is the quality of the decisions they reach in determining the guiding policies that is the crucial ingredient of their responsibility (Johnson, 1979).

Business and industry is typically an economic enterprise with social overtones. Hospitals are a social enterprise with greatly increased economic overtones. Many medical staff physicians may not understand that hospital trustees most often see their role as requiring them to protect the public. Disagreements can arise when the medical staff believes that the board should see their role as protecting the doctors. Often neither of these understandings square with the perception of trained administrators who see themselves as being as fiscally responsible as other similarly trained business executive in the community. They may expect that this kind of ability should be highly regarded by both the trustees and the doctors. CEO/administrators, for the most part, can clearly see the interrelationships of fiscal matters to operating problems and are aware that if the wrong course of action is selected by the governing board in dealing with a current problem, the result could be a reversal in the financial state of affairs (Johnson, 1979). If the board is still thinking, in this early managed care era, that the hospital is a social enterprise with economic interests that are only overtones, real risk could occur.

VIEWS OF THE MEDICAL STAFF

Hospital executives often view the medical staff, because of their education and experience, as a part of the hospital operating structure, but not to be dealt with as are the other operating departments composed of hospital employees. Boards, from their perspective, often see the medical staff as an anomaly not usually found in the business world most trustees inhabit. According to Richard Johnson (1979), trustees recognize a hospital as a medical care institution; as a community activity; as a place where minimum standards for professional performance are enforced, where physicians make more or less free choice whether to use the facilities, and where the operating departments headed by the administration provide the support systems that permit these activities to occur. That is a different view than in the corporate world, where chief executives are clearly responsible and accountable for providing leadership, pushing for higher goals, and using corporate resources for attaining them. In the hospital setting, no one typically sees the hospital chief executive as the person who inspires and leads the medical staff. The administration is the head of a support system that is expected to do its job efficiently and responsively to medical care interests.

Physicians as individuals, and the medical staff as a loosely knit organization, see themselves in two ways with regard to their professional activities. They accept, though sometimes grudgingly, that they are part of a larger system of medical care when using the hospital and are willing, though sometimes grudgingly, to participate in medical staff activities. There is general recognition, if not full-fledged acceptance, of the need to abide by the adopted professional standards of the institution. In the office practice, however, a very different perspective applies. Here, they are individual entrepreneurs, solely responsible to themselves for the diagnosis and treatment of patients. This responsibility holds true whether in solo practice or as members of a group. Doctors believe the same degree of skill and autonomy should be applied and preserved in either setting. That belief is carried out when seeing patients in the hospital, where they should be left alone to do as they see fit. The doctors view the hospital as providing resources on a demand basis that are needed by them for treating patients, not as a control mechanism that decides anything for them.

As physicians find their lives hemmed in through ways over which they have less and control, their frustration level rises. The result of this inability to counter economic pressures and increased infringement on their ways of doing things is for physicians individually, and the medical staff collectively, to regard the hospital as the place they will make a last stand to protect their professional rights. The purpose of this resistance is to preserve the role of the physician in the hospital and the organizational relationship of the medical staff to the governing board and to administration in the future as it has been in the past. Any revamping of the hospital organizational structure to some sort of corporate model will not be easily accepted by physicians if it requires them to be accountable to the chief executive. The idea of a single, unified structure is not readily achievable in the present Joint Commission model of a medical staff.

REPORTING QUALITY-RELATED INFORMATION

Policy development and decisions needs to involve appropriate physician input at every step of the way, particularly related to the quality of medical care being delivered in the hospital. If the board is truly committed to its accountability to the community, which is the most appropriate role to play, then the act of seeking out and finding physician input and information becomes a crucial element in the continued struggle to make sense out of the hospital governance structure. In particular, the accountable body—the board—is obligated to respond to the community's need for quality health care services by monitoring the adequacy of the hospital's medical activities and closely coordinating with all sectors to achieve and maintain the required standards of medical performance (Harvey, 1978).

Hospital boards, left to their own devices, are not likely to know what they need to know, or where to find it. It falls to the chief executive to work in a collaborative fashion with the leaders of the medical staff to develop data systems and assign staff to collect that data. To that question, some hospital executives will respond that the data collection and preparation effort cannot be afforded. Medical staff reports on quality-related issues should be placed on the monthly agendas of the board's meetings. Some administrators will reply that there is no time to deal with such less important issues. There is both time and money available for everything that is valued. From the board's standpoint, their accountability to the community for quality of care dictates the actions to be taken.

There are a number of regular or periodic reports that the medical staff should provide to the board as a demonstration of the efficiency and effectiveness of self-governance. Some medical leaders will protest that secretiveness is preferable and that the board should be told as little as possible in order to reduce interference in the ways of the doctors. That attitude takes away from the opportunity both to perform well in the tasks delegated to the medical staff and to be able to show that success to the governing body that delegated self-governance in the first place.

History shows that there has always been an uneasy relationship between the relative effectiveness and efficiency of the personal health services system and the professional prerogatives of providers. Neither boards of directors nor payers, public and private, have ever really inquired into the details of servicing patterns or how or why providers make their diagnostic and therapeutic decisions. There is a general understanding that the utilization of health care by patients is predominately capacity driven, heavily influenced by the presence and availability of facilities, equipment, and personnel, independent of the "needs," however defined, of the populations served (Evans, 1991).

Practitioners have always argued that the "best" medicine was practiced by trained and experienced clinicians relying on their own clinical judgment. The threat of accountability to others, particularly local laypeople, who will draw on various amounts of statistical evidence in evaluating their performance, strikes directly at professional autonomy. For a number of years, researchers have been observing that there are large and unexplained variations between patterns of practice and servicing rates in the same regions, as well as between practitioners, that seem to bear no identifiable relationship to the needs of the populations served. These variations show up in the details of the structure of care, in particular procedures in addition to aggregate utilization rates (Wennberg, 1984). If there is evidence that inappropriate and/or unnecessary care is being provided in the hospital, that information is not proprietary only to the in-group of medical staff leaders. It is the legitimate business of the board to know. The ideal goal to be reached would be a better match between the needs of the population served and the types and numbers of procedures performed, as well as how successfully was that work done.

Patients trust their doctors and other professionals to make decisions on their behalf. The board trusts the medical staff to monitor and make decisions on its behalf. The evidence of Wennberg (1984) and others suggests that there is a good deal of identifiable room for improvement in this process. In the meantime, the hospital continues day by day to admit, treat, and discharge, and there are certain reporting obligations that the medical staff must honor in its good-faith dealings with the board and with itself.

WHAT TO REPORT

With each credentials report given to the board for approval, a brief biographical sketch of each new physician being recommended for membership and privileges should be attached. In some hospitals, a picture of the candidate is attached. It is the exceptional hospital where relationships are so strong that equivocal or even negative information gathered about a candidate for initial appointment will be reported to the board. A natural question for trustees to ask in such cases would be why the medical staff is recommending the doctor at all. If there are good and sufficient reasons to appoint the physician in spite of a less than a perfect pedigree, the board and administration are entitled to know them and have the right to disagree. Concealing important information is not acceptable behavior by the medical staff. What happens more frequently is that an unsavory past history is concealed by the candidate and those who provide recommendations so that the credentialing process proceeds without anyone at the new hospital being aware of a questionable application.

With each recommendation for reappointment should go a similar brief sketch of the physician's history at the hospital, including the record of service as a chief or chair or some other outstanding feature. Board members get acquainted with a number of the staff over time, but there are still many doctors they do not know. It helps with the process of blind approvals taken on faith to have a little bit of help. It also demonstrates that the medical staff is serious about productive working relationships and can be trusted to perform their work well.

Each month the chief of staff should present a report of selected quality indicators that will summarize the continual search for improvement of patient care. The administration and the medical staff must work together to develop hospital-based practice data on which cost-effective, medically effective choices can be made. Both participants in the care process must examine critically the real value of services in terms of both clinical outcome and cost. Data reports are difficult to put together, since longitudinal data must be gathered over time. Data reports can become lengthy and deadly dull, but that is precisely where the imagination of staff and leadership must find what the board wants to know that will assure them that the hospital provides good care.

Of course, what the board *needs* to know is quite different sometimes from what the board *wants* to know. Since the caregiving process is such a mystery to most board members, it is easy to spend most of the time at meetings studying financial reports. Hospital accountants use the same chart of natural accounts and then present their microreports month after month as if the audience is made up of other accountants. However, many trustees or directors are accustomed to reading accounting reports from their own businesses and find that to be more familiar ground than quality of care indicators. Chiefs of staff have been known to chafe impatiently during this part of the agenda, but the medical staff is not a helpless prisoner and can, after all, show the way to discussion and presentation of something else that is important also.

One of those important items is the process by which all parties in the governance structure spend an adequate amount of time and attention to examine critically the ways in which patients are managed, and which parts of the hospital's care patterns are medically effective and which are not. The object of having a hospital and being accountable to the community is to ensure that medically effective care is also cost-effective, so that there can be a win-win situation with good outcomes for all, particularly patients.

There should be a quarterly report by the chief of staff concerning the continuing work of the impaired-physician or support committee of the medical staff that supervises or oversees diversion programs for those members of the staff who have been directed to participate in recovery or rehabilitation activities. Here is another area where the tendency toward secrecy and confidentiality on behalf of the physician bumps directly into the need for protection of the hospital and the board members as a group and as individuals. The chief does not discuss names in an open meeting but does assure the board that the program is in place and is working to restore valuable human resources back to a more healthy and productive role as doctors and citizens.

On an annual basis, there should be an evaluation of the peer review process that sums up the cases reviewed by the committees, the relative severity assigned to these cases, and a summary of actions taken. For most of these, a letter will have been written, but when more than that was done, the board needs to know that. Once again, there may be a medical staff someplace that will not report this data with the explanation that there were no cases that needed to be sanctioned and that all physicians on the staff rendered perfect care and exhibited perfect behavior, and all are above average (just as Garrison Keillor would report about Lake Wobegon).

Also on an annual basis should be presented the report of the hospitalwide quality improvement (or assessment) program, which reflects the activity of the nursing service and the ancillary technical departments. Some medical staffs receive these reports at monthly meetings of the quality committee, and much valuable work is done that way. What can also happen is a "show and tell" mentality that consumes great amounts of time spent preparing and listening to such reports. If the board exhibits no interest in these matters, preferring to spend its time on financial and business reports, then it is no wonder that the medical staff functions independently—until something happens. Then there will be lots of grumbling about a lack of information.

There should always be regular and timely reporting of so-called sentinel events that call for prompt response and action. Boards need this information for risk management preparation. The administration needs to know to be able to respond to the media. The medical staff needs to know so that the peer review and quality processes can be set in motion for investigating the incident and for fact-finding. On occasions like these people find out how good the process really is and how good the cooperation and partnership really is. Closing ranks to deal with a problem does not mean pretending nothing happened. Rather, it means applying the scientific method and the quality improvement ethic in the best interest of patient care. John Ball, speaking from his vantage point at the American College of Physicians, described hospitals as the symbolic and practical battleground for the resolution of conflicts, both between physicians and the hospital and among physicians themselves (Ball, 1984).

Reporting CQI

Within the past few years, there has been a trend toward a focus on the impact of hospital systems and their interaction on overall quality of care. Borrowed from the manufacturing industries, this methodology has been variously termed *continuous quality improvement* (CQI) or *total quality management* (TQM). In such programs, the emphasis is not on individual failings but rather on analyzing and improving an organization's various systems and their coordinated activities, leading to improved functioning and outcomes for the organization as a whole (Davenport, 1993). CQI or TQM depend on the cooperative relationships of various technical and professional personnel toward a common end.

The goal of quality improvement, in comparison to quality assurance, is to improve patient outcomes and efficiency by coordinating and improving cross-disciplinary, cross-departmental processes. Success of the effort usually depends on both individual competence and team allegiance to the goal, if not necessarily to each other. By simply reapplying principles learned long ago about teamwork, quality improvement or management is of value only when it breaks down old barriers, trusting that when the system is fixed, quality will improve.

Now that the basic concepts of quality management and improvement have been applied and observed, there should be no reason why medical staffs do not participate fully in these activities and report their outcomes to the board, hospital employees, and the medical staff, particularly in the clinical department where the improvement project took place. Full participation may be more easily done by the hospital-based physicians than by those in offices, particularly in primary care. CQI team meetings take place, much of the time, during work hours when the doctors cannot come.

Perhaps the only major issue that has arisen is how CQI should interface with traditional medical staff quality assessment and peer review. Nothing about the newer focus on CQI/TQM relieves medical staffs from their ongoing legal and professional responsibilities to evaluate and monitor the clinical qualifications of each medical staff member and every person who is granted clinical privileges, says Davenport, (1993), stating the position of the California Medical Association. All traditional activity of a Joint Commission model—credentialing, privileging, reappointment, and peer review—should be maintained within the medical staff structure for self-governance, as should any other medical staff quality assessment activities that highlight problems connected with an individual physician.

However, medical staff doctors can and should serve on hospitalwide CQI committees. Sensitive peer review confidential information will not be jeopardized as long as the hospital committee focuses on systems issues rather than on individual physicians. Traditional peer review/quality assurance has focused mainly on the individual physician role. Good or bad outcomes were usually attributed to the doctor alone. This traditional approach emphasizes case by case review, rather than studying groups of cases that form patterns. Quality assurance has been to discover and deal with poor clinical care. Rarely has it ever recognized and rewarded exemplary care. The old way was to use the "bad apple" approach: catch and correct errant physicians. That way does not help "good apples" to improve. Most other physicians not being scrutinized by the committee were not called upon to be concerned with quality, just to stay out of trouble.

One of the differences between QA and CQI is that the first is strictly professional, while the latter focuses on pleasing the consumer/patient. Another difference is the emphasis that quality is everywhere in the organization and is the primary concern of each health care worker. Thus, effective quality improvement requires the involvement of each worker, not just those at the top or those assigned to enforce quality. The social and organizational change from QA to CQI requires high motivation, loyalty to the hospital and medical staff, and employee willingness to go beyond the normal job routine. CQI is based on the assumption that frontline workers are more likely to know about causes of problems and solutions than supervisors and top-level managers. Of course, this is a profoundly different management approach than the traditional top-down or "tell them how to do it" method.

As the institution tries to move from authoritarianism to shared responsibilities, it will be difficult to move away from the idea that quality problems are not the fault of inept or uncaring individuals; it is a nonfunctional system that is at fault. The new mentality must assume that high quality result from group, rather than individual, decisions and actions. There will be much confusion during such a turnover. Much training will be needed, though that money may be impossible to find during a managed care expense crisis.

However, quality improvement does appear to produce results of waste reduction, increased productivity, and cost controls, as well as some noticeable gains in staff morale. The implementation process requires time and unflagging dedication toward surmounting all the hurdles that will be presented. Both hospital executives and physicians will surrender some power and authority to CQI teams, but the new style fits perfectly into a managed care environment, if it has time to evolve (Zusman, 1992). The change process required means moving from an individual to a team focus with interprofessional relations and systems redesign that specifies group performance. The challenge is whether this system-directed approach can deal effectively with a problem individual whose basic difficulty is inability or unwillingness to adapt to the needs of the system. And, whether management and the medical staff can develop and support incentives for both individual professional improvement for physicians, as well as cooperative and effective improvement for management systems.

SUMMARY

The awkward and fragmented governance arrangement of the traditional American hospital is an inheritance from the past, but many have sought to develop a more unified organizational structure where the medical staff, governing board, and administration act as part of the whole and not as separate entities. Presentation of viewpoints and expectations by each sector are intended to provide greater understanding of the interrelationships and to point out clearly that the idea of a single, unified structure is not readily achievable in the presence of a Joint Commission model of a hospital medical staff.

However, policy input by physicians is essential to decision making, particularly related to quality of care. The board's accountability to the community must include monitoring medical activities and coordinating all sectors to maintain the standards of performance that it has delegated to the medical staff. The CEO works with leaders of the medical staff to develop data systems, assign staff to collect and array those data, and present them to the board at regular intervals, usually monthly. What to report is the subject of extensive discussion, but it should include credentialing information, quality of care indicators, effective patient care management, the work of the impaired physician or support committee (to be presented in a later chapter), a summation and evaluation of the peer review process, and a summary of actions taken, as well as the work and products of the CQI program.

REFERENCES

Ball, J. R. (1984). Credentialing versus performance—a new look at old problems. *QRB, March.* Reprinted in Darr, K., & Rakich, J. S. (1989), *Hospital Organization And Management: Text and Readings (4th edition).* Owings Mills, MD: National Health Publishing, AUPHA Press.

Brown, R. E. (1970). Strictures and structures. *Hospitals, 44–16 (August 16).*

Davenport, K. S. (1993). CQI (continuous quality improvement): Will it compromise medical staff confidentiality? *California Physician, August,* 68–73.

Evans, R. G. (1991). Life and death, money and power. In Litman, T. J., & Robins, L. S. (Eds.), *Health Politics and Policy.* Albany, NY: Delmar Publishers.

Harvey, J. D. (1978). Evaluating the performance of the chief executive officer. *Hospital and Health Services Administration, Spring.* Reprinted in Darr, K., & Rakich, J. S. (1989), *Hospital Organization And Management: Text and Readings (4th edition).* Owings Mills, MD: National Health Publishing, AUPHA Press.

Johnson, R. L. (1979). Revisiting "the wobbly three legged stool." *Health Care Management Review.* Reprinted in Darr, K., & Rakich, J. S. (1989), *Hospital and Health Services Administration: Text and Readings (4th edition).* Owings Mills, MD: National Health Publishing, AUPHA Press.

Lang, D. A. (1991). *Medical Staff Executive Committee Report, July/August.* Los Angeles: Hospital Council of Southern California.

Wennberg, J. E. (1984). Dealing with medical practice variations: a proposal for action. *Health Affairs, 3,* 6–32.

Zusman, J. (1992). From QA to CQI. *Medical Staff Counselor, 6(4, Fall),* 9–12.

CHAPTER

Hospital Leadership Duties

As things stand now, modern humans believe—at least with half their minds—that their institutions can accomplish just about anything. The fact that they will fall far short of that goal is due, they believe, to the prevalence of people who love power or money more than they love humankind (Gardner, 1968). John Gardner goes on to say that "a system that is not innovating is a system that is dying. In the long run, the innovators are the ones who rescue all human ventures from decay. Value innovators, and if you do not have any around you, you had better import some."

THOUGHTS ON LEADERSHIP

Although John Gardner wrote these words nearly 30 years ago, they seem particularly appropriate for the health care delivery system changes being wrestled with now. Today, people cannot afford not to take chances. It is puzzling to hear people who talk as though the advocates of change are just inventing ways to disturb the peace in what would otherwise be a tranquil community, such as the medical staff would like to think of itself: "We are not seeking change for the sheer fun of it. We must change to meet the challenge of altered circumstances. Change will occur whether we like it or not. It will either be change in a good and healthy direction or change in a bad and regrettable direction. There is no tranquillity. We can choose not to accept the challenge of change, of course, but it is less important to induce any particular change than it is to foster and nourish the conditions under which constructive change can occur."

On the subject of leadership, Gardner has always been particularly insightful, such as when he notes that the necessary attributes depend on the kind of leadership being talked about. In a single field there are different kinds of leadership that require different attributes. A good person is not good for everything. Few prominent people take a really large view of the leadership assignment. Most of them simply tend the machinery of that part of society to which they belong. A high proportion of the most gifted have been immunized against any tendencies toward leadership. The antileadership vaccine leads to the conception that the only kind of leadership encouraged is that which follows from the performing of purely professional tasks in a superior manner, such as the outstanding clinician. The world seems to be approaching a point at which everyone will want to be the technical expert who advises the leader, but no one will want to be the actual leader.

Refusal to Lead

People with lots of bright ideas frequently have no patience with the machinery by which ideas are translated into action. They will not take the time to understand the social institutions and processes by which change is accomplished. The medical staff is process oriented to a fault, which discourages many gifted clinicians from stepping out. There will never be effective leadership in social institutions, such as the nation, states, counties, and cities, until people can persuade the most able and influential members of the community that they must take personal responsibility for what happens in their world. Neither can they have effective leadership in hospitals, and particularly in the medical staff, unless the same principle applies. Trouble is brewing everywhere, and organizational evils accumulate while the patterns of society keep so many able and gifted potential leaders on the sidelines, unwilling to serve in front of their medical colleagues for fear someone might not like them or that they might seem not to be like everyone else.

One of the maladies of leadership today is a failure of confidence. The confidence required of leaders poses a delicate problem for hospitals, integrated health care systems, and the physicians who deliver medical care in those institutions. Falling under the leadership of people who lack the confidence to really lead is a clear danger these days, as the hospital system moves increasingly away from community hospitals toward ever larger corporate structures. There must be leaders, but it helps considerably if they are gifted in the performance of their tasks and have the confidence to persuade others to follow them toward what must be done. People do not need leaders to tell them what to do. They need men and women who will accept a special responsibility to advance the greater interest. They need such people to help them clarify and define the choices before them. And they need leaders to rekindle hope in the face of cynicism and disbelief, despite their own inertness, shallowness, and wavering resolve (Gardner, 1968).

CHANGES IN LEADERSHIP DUTIES

During the transition of the modern American hospital in recent decades, there have been corresponding changes in hospital leadership duties, brought on by changes in payment systems, the rise of consumer participation and, to a considerable degree, precedent court decisions. In earlier times, the medical staff appeared to have a role as free agents who came and went from the hospital as they needed to do. Their expectation level called for the anticipation that everything would be exactly the same the next time they admitted a patient as it was the last time. Due to the forces of change from outside influences, they have assumed some additional responsibility without wanting or asking for it. In addition to being providers of care, with their own personal liability, physicians have become "agents" of the hospital. From that standpoint, the expectation by the public that doctors are hospital employees may be coming closer to the truth.

The most common barriers to change are resistance by the doctors, and possibly the employees as well. A dysfunctional hospital or corporate culture can be the result, defined as one whose shared values and behavior are at odds with its best behavior. An organization might reward individual performance, such as bonuses for senior executives, even though the hospital or network owes its past and future success to the close teamwork of medical and nursing staff and the technical employees. Nothing will affect morale quite as drastically as to provide clear evidence that the professed desire for teamwork and partnerships really means that a few well-paid people at the top will now be paid even more while employee raises are cost of living or less. A more productive demonstration of leadership and reward would be to define and reinforce those aspects of the existing culture that are conducive to the hospital's business strategy.

New Corporate Cultures

Working with the medical staff, the administration and the board should find ways to forgive and forget the irrelevant or negative aspects of the previous single-hospital or stand-alone culture that need not be preserved. As hospitals become hospital chains and then integrated systems, they do not exist as a business organization to preserve the previous cultures of each individual facility. Particularly, they do not now exist to try to extend the culture of the largest or most well-known institution to all of the others. It should be the other way around. There is nothing sacred about a corporate culture, which can be good or bad, inspired or petty, freewheeling or authoritarian, gracious or mean-spirited. The point is that the members of the new organization subscribe to the mission and values that will be developed through new working relationships. An executive order to love one another and follow the plan will not quite cut it these days.

There is an obvious difficulty within the traditional hospital structure with its divided responsibilities and accountabilities that are like virtually no other modern organization. The medical staff directs the consumption of the major portion of hospital resources, as much as 80 percent by some estimates, but the individual doctors have no direct accountability for their actions. Ordering tests, imaging, pharmacy, or procedures are the doctor's prerogative and the order sheet cannot be questioned. As Bill Mohlenbrock says so pungently in his Iameter™ data system presentations, the most important piece of high technology is the doctor's ordering pen. The medical staff exercises its leadership duties by monitoring both clinical and professional behavior, as delegated by the board. Performance outcomes have become the focus of professional and legal assessments, particularly by the courts as well as the more familiar JCAHO surveys and the PROs reviewing Medicare claims.

The executive team of the administration has the duty to perform effective and efficient operations, including downsizing or right-sizing the organization when necessary to meet the market. That is one of the parts of the economic theory of marketplace competition that has never been well accepted by the health care establishment: there could be a marketplace, and hospitals could fight each other for market share, but that everyone would still have a job and nothing would change. In the move toward mergers and consolidations of previously independent hospitals, there has been a presumption that a consolidated organization operating under the firm hand of a single leader can and will respond with a unity of purpose. That newfound unity of purpose will allow it to increase the collective performance of once-independent organizations while outmaneuvering its competitors (Beckham, 1995).

Internalizing Mission

Beckham goes on to say that the experience of many modern organizations suggests that employees (or doctors) can be remarkably adept at ignoring the authority vested in a hierarchial power structure. Many CEOs, even good ones, have been brought to their knees by subversive organizations, which can definitely include the medical staff. Such recalcitrance requires more than a smooth and impassioned articulation of common mission and purpose. Too often, employees of the newly consolidated organization are hard put to make a connection between that purpose and their own self-interest. Beckham was speaking about employees when he wrote that, but it can be seen immediately that his meaning can apply as well or better to the doctors on the medical staff.

Of course the doctors will always say there are too many administrators who are the enemy, as are the officers considered by the enlisted personnel in the military services. A lot of doctors bring military griping with them to the medical staff where it can become very disruptive, because the doctors are not enlisted personnel any longer. Of course, they never were enlisted personnel since they had medical officer commissions. They just talk that way. But now they are powerful people in a community hospital who have a lot of control and leverage that enlisted personnel never have had and never will have. Enlisted personnel were not responsible for seeing the big picture and ensuring that the larger goals would be met, and sometimes some of the doctors also act that way.

Administration has classic textbook responsibilities for the management and coordination of organizational functions of planning, organizing, staffing, directing, coordinating, budgeting, and personnel review and evaluation. These tasks are right out of the management textbooks of the management-by-objectives school of thought, and they date from the fee-for-service/cost-reimbursement era. A better style for the managed care era is to exercise leadership by managing conflict instead of avoiding it. Diplomacy and sensitivity are assets of great value and served well during the doctors' workshop times. But so are honesty and the ability to deliver hard news, which seems to come so often these days. Many people, including specialty physicians, will be threatened by the new dynamics of an integrated or merged delivery system. They cannot and will not embrace it no matter how much involvement and support they are given. If happiness and harmony are the main measure of success, then the integration effort will fail (Beckham, 1995).

How can an administration acting alone plan for the future of the delivery of health care without involving deeply those people who deliver the care and can greatly assist with planning it—the doctors? The administration will never care for a single patient, but will plan for and manage the entire support structure that hopefully ensures good patient care. Clinical department chairs and medical directors are appropriate people to participate in organizing internal care systems and advising on the types and numbers of staff necessary to provide care. These medical staff leaders should not simply sit back and fail to participate in the planning process for their own reasons. Even worse is a refusal to share in management duties even when invited.

EFFECT ON THE MEDICAL STAFF

Chiefs of staff need to know the rudiments of the budgeting process, particularly the assumptions being used in estimating revenue and expense line items. The accountants are usually happy to have help and input from the doctors in calculating those budget estimates, but make no mistake, the budget will go forward and will contain assumptions and estimates whether or not the doctors participate. Medical staffs have long complained about the allocation of resources represented by budgets and must take a more proactive role and be sincerely helpful, if that situation is to be changed. And be changed it must in a managed care world.

Beckham (1995) reports that as a direct result of downsizing in hospitals, only 34 percent can show increases in productivity, and 45 percent show improvements in operating profit. At least 80 percent of those hospitals reported that morale among surviving employees has dropped. Morale among doctors has dropped also, although not measured by those same studies. Physicians know who are the good nurses and techs and who tries to keep the unit humming along in a productive manner. Physicians also know what the result will be when there are layoffs and terminations, all of which are not necessarily bad. Doctors should participate when invited and participate in a professional helpful manner. That is the way partners do it, and a better, more appropriately rewarded staff will be the result.

Obviously, governing boards have their own traditional responsibilities, including their personal duty of due care as a trustee or director. Boards have the fiduciary responsibility for ensuring financial stability and success, which is why they spend so much time on financial reports in board meetings. Some hospitals make a lot of money, many hospitals make an amount adequate for continuing to perform their mission, while a few lose a lot but continue keeping on. A hospital is a hard animal to kill, and the medical staff has both a role to play in ensuring hospital survival as well as to examine the care being delivered and the practice patterns of the doctors.

Medical Staff: Roll or Resist?

No hospital ever went bankrupt where there was active participation by the medical staff in reducing unnecessary consumption of resources and eliminating services that could not be done well and efficiently within the financial constraints available. Downsizing is an administration reaction to financial bad times by reducing the employee payroll. The medical staff's response is to study and evaluate variations in practice patterns and in physician ordering, which probably amounts to much greater potential savings than all the downsizing. Hospitals have gone bankrupt, however, when most of the medical staffs did not change practice patterns in order to help with preserving their institution. They simply went over to another hospital. The doctors did not go bankrupt just because the hospital did.

Boards are also corporately and personally responsible for the assurance of legal compliance with all areas of regulation, quality of care, antitrust concerns, and prudent policies and procedures. Maybe the military model would work better. Then there would be none of the divided authority, responsibility, and accountability that currently exists in the modern American complex tertiary care hospital. But there are the same tensions in the military model also, so maybe that is not the simple solution. Managed care financial incentives through capitation may actually be a better choice for getting together and furnishing better leadership. It seems intuitively reasonable that the principles of the CQI process apply to leadership as well as in patient care or self-directed work groups.

The administration will never care for a single patient, but the idea that the administration does the planning dates from the doctors' workshop era that is now, mercifully, passing on in favor of doctor/hospital working relationships that are better able to cooperate in the staffing plan, organizing and directing together the delivery of care. There are probably a few top administrators still around who believe that the budgeting process is the exclusive property of the finance department, but those dinosaurs are fading into extinction. Real unity of purpose is more easily built around a common commitment to mutual self-preservation and advancement, which is something the doctors can relate to. Less effective is a call to lofty notions of quality and quality continuums of care. One of the real tests of integration ought to be whether the preponderance of an organization's participants feel they have a stake in its success and in each other's success (Beckham, 1995). That is what partnership really means.

The medical staff has long complained about the allocation of resources in the hospital budget and now must face the responsibility to do it better by being an active participant instead of a critic who could enjoy complaining without having to face up to solving the hard problems. Chiefs of staff must learn how budgets are put together and what assumptions are used to arrive at revenue and expense estimates. Chiefs can do a much better job of arriving at some of those estimates than the accountants can, and to their credit, the finance managers welcome help of that sort. Medical staff department chairs and medical directors must take an active role in the review of clinical managers and staff when merit increases and promotions are being considered so as to ensure that the best staff can be recruited, retained, and rewarded.

There is a lot of talk about the value of honoring diversity and multiple opportunities when hospitals are being brought together in a merger, consolidation, or to form an integrated network. Organizations, particularly new ones without an agreed upon culture that binds them together, cannot stand too much diversity and conflicting incentives. It is a truism that a new health care delivery culture, if it is to be cohesive, dynamic and reinforcing, must exert the united leadership to stamp out some of the diversity that divides them in favor of some more real partnerships that will unite them. Work on what is possible, not just what is wrong.

SUMMARY

Leadership has always been important at every point in history. This is particularly true today in the health care enterprise. Following a period of success, high reputation, and financial gains, current leaders in medicine and health are struggling with the need for change and the threat that accompanies it. The medical staff likes to think of itself as a tranquil community that would continue along in peace with everything staying the same if it were not for administrators and insurers who are determined to change that comfort. John Gardner's thoughts on leadership seem more appropriate now than when they were written. Resistance to accepting leadership roles, refusal to step forward, personal lack of confidence in the ability to lead: these are the maladies that affect the members of the medical staff who could but do not step out in front of their colleagues.

The medical staff, management, and board need to find ways to forgive and forget the irrelevant or negative aspects of the former single hospital culture that need not be preserved. Moving to a new corporate culture for integrated health care systems will require moving away from the traditional hospital structure with its divided responsibilities and its turf guarding. Seeking a common mission and purpose requires much more than memos and exhortations from upper management to be partners. The medical staff can undermine or sabotage almost any plan to develop new structures, unless they are active and willing participants in moving toward the future. The administration cannot act alone without the wisdom of the clinicians, who, in turn, cannot refuse to participate or share in management duties.

A real test of integration is whether most of the participants feel they have a stake in the new organization's success and whether there exists the united leadership to stamp out some of the diversity that divides them in favor of real partnerships that will unite them.

REFERENCES

Beckham, J. D. (1995). Redefining work in the integrated delivery system. *Healthcare Forum Journal, May/June,* 76–82.

Gardner, J. W. (1968). *No Easy Victories.* New York: Harper & Row, Publishers, Inc.

CHAPTER

18

CME Revisited

This chapter looks again at the work load put on the medical staff, ranging all the way from being polite and helpful as the Boy Scout manual suggests to being relentless and merciless in the pursuit and punishment of the perpetrators of evildoing.

KEY ROLES

Among the duties contained in that work load are several key roles of the medical staff, whether or not they have been described in those exact terms.

Credentialing

Reviewing and recommending credentials of new staff is examined in depth in Chapter 5.

Reappointment

Reviewing and recommending privileges for reappointment was presented as an important issue for quality improvement in Chapter 6. Many long-time doctors still have the same privileges as when they first went into practice, in spite of the inroads of time, scientific advancement, and decreased stamina. One of the most unpleasant words in the granting of privileges is *grandfathering*. There is no such action as grandfathering when that word means that a physician can be granted privileges to do things to patients without being qualified to do it in the first place or without being qualified to do it now, defined as current clinical competence.

Corrective Action

Recommending corrective action or adjustment to practice or privileges when necessary is a subject discussed in detail in Chapter 7. Actions like this are almost more related to attitude than to technique, since there are many possible review systems of due process that could be used if the staff has the courage to face the unpleasant truth and take action when it can no longer be avoided. There is also the need to provide that corrective action once it has been recommended.

Bylaws

Regularly updating the bylaws, rules, and regulations is a subject mentioned several times before but worthy of repeating again here. Bylaws should be in a constant state of scrutiny and revision. An efficient bylaws committee should be constantly aware of the changing world and stay prepared to deal with it. Bylaws are not stone tablets that have been done once and never again. In a way, the bylaws can come to represent the hopes of the medical staff that the status quo will prevail.

Review and Evaluation

Development and use of a data-based evaluation of professional performance is a subject mentioned several times without suggesting exactly how to do it. There are a number of approaches to performance or outcome measures, some of them commercially available and others home developed by exceptionally clever staff. A word of warning: the staff had better make sure there is some form of severity adjustment involved or the system will not be believable to the doctors, each of whom will discount the program by saying in refusal "yes, but my patients are sicker." Every doctor's patients are sicker. No one has less sick patients, and so the system will be laughed out of the room. Be sure also that the accountants do not have the absolute choice about selection of this clinical data system because they will pick something that reports only financial data and is not severity adjusted.

Communication

Coordinated input to chiefs, the executive committee, the strategic planning committee, the administration, and the board should be given. The key word here is coordinated. It is not without some justification that the term *organized medical staff* has been called an oxymoron. Most input is usually griping and complaining, with too few helpful suggestions and ideas for a better way. Deliver regular and special reports to the governing board about medical staff activities, a subject covered in some detail in Chapter 16, which is usually the job of the chief of staff. Most rank and file members of the staff are unaware that the chief provides this information, and some of the chief's constituents will feel that too many secrets are being given away through this approach.

THE NEW ROLE OF CME

So far, this volume has not considered in any detail the responsibility of the Joint Commission model of a hospital medical staff to develop and provide continuing medical education (CME) to its members. In the majority of the community hospitals in the United States, there is a committee of the medical staff that has been assigned responsibility for the CME function. For the most part, that task has been attempted in good faith, with the presence of a CME chair who truly enjoys the role of educator. Why are the chairs of so many CME committees held by members of the pathology department? Are pathologists just naturally educators? When coupled with good staff work and a willing committee, programs can be put together that can be very helpful and useful over time, since CME goes on forever. If hospital-based CME has a generic fault, it is probably true that an overall or long range plan does not guide the selection of subjects and speakers.

When there is a requirement for some number of CME credits for relicensure of physicians, some of the hospital-based programs have attempted, with varying degrees of success, to try to meet as much of that requirement as possible. A familiar scenario would be the weekly or biweekly grand rounds featuring a noted medical school lecturer who describes the latest advances in a particular specialty field or, perhaps, the work underway in diagnosis and treatment of a disease entity. The researcher shows slides in the darkened auditorium and reads from notes that have or will form a journal article. Because most of the doctors who practice in hospitals are specialists, most of the audience for this presentation are the particular colleagues who are interested. Of course, latest advances are always useful. One of the indicators that should interest the chief of staff is whether there are any primary care physicians in the audience. Secondarily, the chief or the VPMA should be aware of what proportion of the CME programs offered by the committee concern primary care and its practitioners, particularly if that hospital, or the network it belongs to, is moving toward managed care and capitation.

Changing Hospital CME

Increasing attention is being paid to educational functions by the specialty societies in their annual meetings. It is now possible to earn some or all of the required continuing education credits at that level without depending on the local hospital programs for anything. The question for the hospital medical staff to reexamine is what kind of CME they are offering and for whom is it intended? Is there an evaluation process in place, and does that evaluation show general satisfaction? How is the attendance, and is it shrinking year by year? Are the programs exciting and interesting, or dull? Is a sign-in sheet used so that proper credit can be given for attendance? Does the sign-in process really mean that the doctor can sign and leave? Or, eat first, then sign and leave? Or sign for other doctors who are not present at all?

As a rule of thumb, participation in the programs should include a majority of the staff. The higher, the better. If a very high percentage of the members of the medical staff are not participating in the CME program, have questions been asked about why? Are the staff regularly assessed for suggestions about appropriate topics? Has anyone tried to determine the reasons why people do not attend? Is it the time or place? Is there some sort of convenience factor that is hampering attendance? Chances are the answer will be that the programs are not interesting any more and are not worth the trip, even for a free lunch. Maybe the chief needs to face the fact that the long-time CME chair has grown old and tired and is not putting on as good programs as in past years, or decades.

There should be a primary care component to most of the presentations, perhaps through the use of physician panels rather than the old-style research lecturer. There are so many newer techniques and multimedia available for use now that it is a true measure of status quo that the CME program lags behind all the other exciting developments occurring in medicine and managed care. One of the more exciting developments in CME is the growth of skilled professional staff who are trained as educators in addition to being coordinators and facilitators. They have professional skills and are connected with other peers and colleagues in the field, with the need to attend annual meetings and appropriate training sessions.

Changing Role

With a greater emphasis on primary care and a larger volume of services in ambulatory and outpatient settings, the hospital-based CME program will play a lesser role as the source of most information for the medical staff. More of that responsibility will be assumed by the medical groups, although many of the IPAs and even some HMOs still depend on the hospitals to provide that service. Indeed, some of the agencies that require CME credits for relicensure have realized the changing times and are now permitting the offering of other practice-related subjects in addition to the traditional clinical work.

Funding for CME has traditionally been provided as a subsidy by the hospital in the form of salary for the coordinator and the food at the meetings. Sometime, there has been a financial obligation on the part of the doctors, but that is usually minimal. More support has traditionally been provided by the drug companies and other vendors who are anxious to advertise and show the doctors their latest products. Declining markets and reduced profit levels have altered that pattern, and the vendors do not have as much of a CME budget any more. That could put a real crimp in the hospital's CME program if the drug company subsidy was the main support for the program. Now, in the days of capitation, it may not be very productive to ask the administration to pick up support for CME for doctors who are not happy about joining the managed care plans anyway.

There are demographic changes occurring in the medical staff that need to be taken into account as well by the education planners in the hospital. If the CME chair visualizes the staff as one composed of middle-aged white males, then some readjusting may be necessary. Between 1970 and 1990, the number of female physicians in the United States increased 310 percent. By 1990, one in five U.S. physicians was a woman, and the proportion is projected to increase to one-third by 2010. Women have tended to choose the specialties of family practice, pediatrics, and internal medicine, with much lower representations in the surgical specialties. Female physicians are also more likely than men to be employees and less likely to be self-employed (Braus, 1994).

There are age differences, too, in the doctor population of the United States. Women physicians are, on the average, younger than males. Because women began entering the profession in large numbers relatively recently, the age gap has widened over the years. In 1970, 51 percent of male physicians and 58 percent of female physicians were under the age of 45. In 1980, the percentages were 51 percent and 69 percent, respectively. By 1992, that gap had grown to 46 and 72 percent (Kopriva, 1994). How does the education planner factor in the changing pattern of gender and age, or are all doctors the same and the same CME will suffice for all? How many young women are on the CME committee?

Eli Ginzberg (1994) also notes that women physicians are more attracted to less entrepreneurial forms of practice arrangements and are more willing to accept salaried positions, which would seem to indicate that it will be possible to recruit them for new forms of organized practice arrangements involving managed care. He goes on to say that this development would enhance the rapid growth of these new modes of service delivery (Ginzberg, 1994). Obviously, rapid growth in new modes of service delivery is a definition of new modes of CME as well.

The steep increases that have taken place in the number and proportion of women physicians in obstetrics and gynecology help to explain the explosive growth during the 1980s in the number of hospitals and out-of-hospital settings that have established and expanded specialized services under the rubric of "women's health care." The growth of these centers points to their meeting a strong consumer demand. Apparently, clients believe that female physicians—and male physicians oriented to meeting women's conditions—provide them with better and more responsive care (Ginzberg, 1994). Likewise, there is a much broader range of CME efforts as well as patient and family educational opportunities that are being created.

WHAT KIND OF CME?

Is something different being advocated as the new paradigm for CME, or should it be the same as always—the researcher with slides talking about specialties? The answer is that the focus of the educational effort should be more internal, more focused on the care being given in that hospital or within that system, rather than in trying to bring to the hospital all the national standards and improvements. The purpose of the new paradigm of CME is to improve the quality and teamwork of the primary care–based managed care model, not a local imitation of medical school or residency. There should be attempts to bridge the generation gap, with encouragement by the leadership of the medical staff. Working relationships between the various medical groups that include members of the staff can more easily be accomplished through effective education programs than by some of the political negotiations that proceed endlessly. How many CME programs have analyzed the differing standards and benefits offered by the several health plan contracts being offered in the hospital? Does the medical staff work with the nursing staff in putting together programs like this that affect the hospital employees, so that all have a more clear understanding of the care required for each patient?

Education programs for delivering capitated care are valuable to offer, including manuals and handouts for the doctors' office personnel. Hospitals talk about managed care exhaustively—doctors talk about it in the lounge—but who explains to the office personnel how to relate differently to the hospital and other outpatient care? The office world is no longer so isolated from the rest of the continuum of care. What is the plan in a local integrated system for offering educational programs about the patterns of care across the network, with points of agreement on care patterns and on points of allowable individuality?

Joe Green has put together Table 18–1 to show graphically the changes that need to be made to move CME into the next world along with the rest of the health care system. Some of the changes are being forced on the health care system from outside influences, while others represent the appropriate responses of CME professionals (Green, 1994).

HOW TO DO IT

The principal change to be seen in this new philosophy of CME is that it is aimed more at teams than at individuals. It is no longer the role of the hospital-based CME

TABLE 18–1   Educational Philosophy

From	*To*
• Specialty	• Primary care/specialty
• Request driven	• Proactive change strategy
• Didactic	• Interactive dialogue
• Medical process	• Health care outcomes
• New techniques and procedures	• Cost-effective/ high-quality care
• Hospital based	• Medical group focused
• Physician as provider	• Physician as team member
• Quality assurance/ marketing	• Quality improvement

program, for example, to help a cardiologist become a better cardiologist. While that is a good thing to do, in the abstract, it is not the real mission of the hospital or medical staff any longer. A better approach is to help the cardiologist to become a more productive and effective member of the chest pain team, or to be a leader in the cardiovascular diseases service-line team. But if there is to be a clinical team, then there will need to be planned formal courses for teams instead of continuing to concentrate only on individuals, as before. The expanded content of the team approach can be best handled with problem-oriented educational sessions that will be very different than "latest developments" lectures for doctors only.

A good model that has taken hold in some places is that of the quality improvement team, which is dedicated to finding a problem and solving it. The purpose of CQI is not to find a guilty culprit so much as it is to find out why the system is not working as well as the people who work in it want it to. Using variations of the multimedia technology now available as well as traditional teachers, interactive formal courses should be aimed at the successful integration of patient care, professional consultation, and a CME vehicle to put everything together. Health care professionals can develop their skills at seeking information that is related to the specific case and patient being considered. Years of work have passed since earlier efforts focused on problem-oriented approaches, but the principle is still the same. What is it that is needed to solve the problem at hand, rather than to try to build a vast mental library of all the possible combinations that might be needed, if they ever are?

All of those approaches will require databases, which are seemingly never available when needed, because no one thought about it in time to store longitudinal data that bears on the problem at hand. The education department can put the training program together, but only the administration can provide the resources needed to build databases. If the administration is not convinced about the value of continuing and evolving educational interactions that will help to improve patient care, then this advice, while good, may not be able to be accomplished. The secret to this new generation of CME for care teams requires enlightened leadership and cooperation from management if it is to succeed. A quick fix it is not.

Meanwhile, the biomedical information and technology explosion continues unabated. Quality management moves on to new ideas and new successes. Information and educational technology bring out the best in CME professional staff, who are able to do many more things than they are allowed to do by the doctors or the hospital. One of the most important advances in the field is the increased understanding about how physicians learn and change and how they apply new medical science knowledge to the delivery of clinical care. Where there are real opportunities to match educational technology advances with medical technology improvements is in the move toward the practice-oriented approach to educational development. Practice-oriented approaches move further than the familiar research lecture approach, where the point was to let the doctor know about intellectual content that may or may not have any practical applicability to everyday practice.

CME in Systems

Although it is not likely to be an item of major discussion on the agenda of the upper management team of newer health care integrated systems, it should be, as a recognition that system integration is essentially an educational intervention. Just giving a command or exhorting people to "get on the train," while satisfying the CEO's ego, will not result in any measurable advances among the doctors. But education and training will. Business and industry in this country learned long ago to set aside some proportion of the budget, perhaps 5 percent, for education and training. In health care organizations, education is probably the first thing to be cut in a budget crunch. When there is a collaborative learning network of physicians and other caregivers in the hospital or health care network, then there will be more successful integration. More employees and more doctors will subscribe to the mission and values. They will identify with the incentives and the programs. They will show better attitudes toward the development of clinical pathways, algorithms, and guidelines, which are the real opportunity for improving quality and decreasing cost (White, 1994).

The system should put together a leadership training program to turn doctors into clinical managers. These new leaders need to learn communications skills, strategic management, marketing, some amount of financial management, and a basic knowledge of the current and future health care environments where they will be working in the future. Manager/doctors need to learn how to manage complex health care organizations. Since there never were organizations like these before, no one has a lock on how to do it. Learning to manage change will be an eye-opener to the physicians, who have had only the experience of trying to manage the medical staff, which is dedicated to not changing.

Quality management comes more easily to the doctors and nurses than to the administration, but they must work together if this talk of integrated systems is to be more than just nonsense to persuade the troops. Physician leadership training should be directed toward identified persons, including those who are in current positions in the organized medical staff, as well as those who will be the future leaders. In fact, it would be a quantum jump into the managed care world if a medical staff never again chose leaders who did not have that kind of training experience. Those who intend to offer such training should insist that the corporate executives take part as well, so there can be interaction and understanding of the decisions that were made and what the integrated system will face in the future.

The results will be immediately noticeable, particularly in the increased awareness of the communications problems facing all components in the network. Changes in the organizational structure will probably result and will be easier to facilitate with the nucleus of trained medical leaders who now understand the plan and their role in it. They will have the burden of explaining to their recalcitrant colleagues in the medical staff, but now they have some ammunition with which to do it. Integrating the physician network will take place much sooner and with better results, as well as shifts in attitude about the system and the people in it. There is a lot to be said about the growing of a new generation of physician-executives who will be expected to extend the early attempts at integration to new levels as the managed care noose grows tighter. The administration, management, CEOs, and corporate executives by themselves will not be able to grow and prosper in this kind of a constrained health care market without the leadership, guidance, and cooperation of the doctors. Anyone who thinks differently should get out the old resume and polish it up.

NEW CME GOALS

It should be the assignment to the new CME chair and the committee to develop a new set of goals for the next year and the next two years. One of the most useful goals in that plan would be to use the education program to assist in the transition to managed care and in transition to the integrated system. Some of the doctors will oppose that, since they do not want to see the ascendance of either managed care or an integrated system that involves their hospital. Here is the point where the Joint Commission model faces a threshold. Shall it continue with continuing medical education in the medical school model of adding memory information, or shall it move toward the future of practice needs of the members? Some will not want to hear information like this. Some will not want to listen to speakers at general staff meetings who try to unfold the next era and offer help in meeting it. Some will respond like the doctor who uttered the very last word in refusing to change when he said "don't tell us anything we don't want to know."

CME-Quality Link

The quality assurance/peer review program should be linked with the quality improvement program using consensus conferences, algorithms, and health care outcomes studies performed at the hospital. Peer review findings will then become the force for still other educational interventions based on local community practice. Medical groups should develop activities, based on their internal standards of performance, that will enhance the performance of their members, thus improving still more their competitive position in the marketplace. Team approaches such as those designed for product or service lines offer a real possibility for helping with the primary care/specialty care struggle that is taking place in hospitals. Feedback on variations in practice is the lifeblood of the medical groups and should be the major focus of the PPO organizations that suffer from lack of accepted incentives. Though some doctors will hate it, the real goal will be forced to be systemwide standards and parameters if there is to be most effective integration and enhanced market position. Integration is education, not command and control.

SUMMARY

The key roles of the hospital medical staff are reviewed again in order to place continuing medical education (CME) in its proper perspective, hopefully, with a long-range plan to guide the selection of subjects and speakers. Some hospital-based CME programs have attempted to supply enough credits to meet requirements for relicensure of the doctors. That has usually taken the form of presentations by medical school faculty or researchers who present their latest work. Or, perhaps, CME has been a review of the latest developments in some specialty field.

The problem with that traditional approach has been that it is specialty oriented, with little or no attention paid to the needs of primary care physicians. At the same time, the state or national specialty societies are likewise presenting latest developments in the field, so that it may be possible to not depend on the local hospital program for anything. Hospital-based CME programs should not be minature imitations of medical school or residency.

Changing hospital CME needs to be based on principles of teaching and learning, with exciting and interesting programs that involve the majority of the staff. There should be primary care input or application, with relevance to increasing services in outpatient and ambulatory settings. Reduced drug company sponsorship and funding forces the local leadership to be more innovative, although asking the hospital for money may not be innovative enough. An effective program of CME will take into account the changing demographics of the staff, age differences, organized practice arrangements, and should be more internal. It should focus on the care in that hospital (or in that system), should be based on data, and should improve the quality and teamwork of the primary care–based managed care model. The focus should be on delivering capitated care and on appropriate specialty referrals and aimed more at teams than at individuals.

REFERENCES

Braus, P. (1994). *American Demographics, 16(11, November),* 40–47. Reprinted in *Healthcare Trends Report, December, 1994,* 13.

Ginzberg, E. (1994). The woman physician. In Friedman, E. (Ed.), *An Unfinished Revolution: Women and Health Care in America.* New York: United Hospital Fund of New York.

Green, J. S. (1994). *A New Physician Educational Paradigm: Facilitating Integration and Change* [Faculty and consultant presentations]. Sharp Healthcare, San Diego.

Kopriva, P. (1994). Women in medicine. In Friedman, E. (Ed.), *An Unfinished Revolution: Women and Health Care in America.* New York: United Hospital Fund of New York.

White, C. H. (1994). *The New CME Paradigm* [Faculty workshop presentation]. American Osteopathic Association national meeting for CME coordinators and physician leaders.

CHAPTER

Hospital–Medical Staff Relationships

Early in this volume of advice and counsel, an organizational chart was shown that represented a frequent and customary view of hospital/medical staff relationships. That view was described as the way it looks to many doctors on the medical staff and some board members too: a hierarchy appearing as a military or corporate model. But Ken Mack (1993) cautions that woe is unto the hospital executives who swear that their success lies in controlling physicians, as suggested by the chart. He goes on to say that administrators who have lengthy tenures will testify that their success lies in cultivating excellent one-on-one relationships with individual physicians. Legal structures can facilitate collaboration, but partnerships only come from mutually beneficial relationships. There are no ideal models. Each organization must find its own best way.

Having presented that hierarchial view in the beginning as a starting point, the next chapters went about contradicting or challenging the hierarchical model. The medical staff model described by the Joint Commission as one of an unincorporated association for self-governance should be more properly portrayed as a two-wing model such as Figure 19–1.

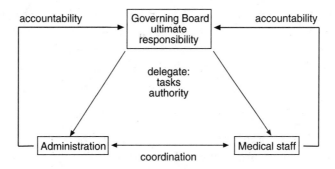

FIGURE 19–1 Hospital–medical staff relationship: Actual.
Source: Pointer, D. D., Ewell, C. M. (1994). *Really Governing.* Albany, NY: Delmar Publishers, p. 58.

It has been said by some administrators that the two-wing model in itself creates the impression of conflict, that there are two "sides" that must work together as partners, and if a visual image is created of opposition, then the partnership is hindered. That may be overly sensitive when the intent is to find some visual way of presenting what are the two delegations by the governing board: delegating managing responsibility to the administration and delegating the professional responsibility to the medical staff. Of course, there are alternatives to the Joint Commission model as will be seen presently. For now, the two-wing model is reality for the vast majority of hospitals that offer the traditional Joint Commission model of a hospital medical staff.

NOT THE ORGANIZATION, THE PEOPLE

Whatever it is that the organization looks like on the organizational chart, the real need is for physicians and the organization to accommodate each other. The intersection of clinical and organizational control is the battleground where actual relationships are forged. As seen in the previous chapters that describe the histories and development of hospitals and the medical profession, control has always been divided between these two authorities: doctors and managers. Physicians were primarily responsible for patient care, and managers were primarily responsible for organizational performance. Physicians have traditionally retained control of patient care and participated minimally in organizational control because they were not interested in it, lacked training and skills for it, and did not have many incentives to become involved in organizational issues. Besides, they did not see any need to be involved. As long as they brought paying patients, the hospital would do everything for them without argument or reservation.

Under the changing conditions now taking place, there is a wider and broader intersection between control over patient care and over organizational performance. Physicians still control patient care at the level of the individual or treatment, but, increasingly, they confront issues pertaining to organizational operations and performance. Managers still control organizational functions, but they confront patient care issues due to their decisions about resource allocations and the structure of the delivery process.

Patients Versus the Organization

Most health care organizations are interested in efficient resource allocation, cost control, planned investment, return on investment, and control of operations to attain budgets and predetermined financial goals. They are also committed to quality of care, staff satisfaction, patient satisfaction, and public service. Physicians are also concerned about all of these goals, but their professional value system gives priority to the hands-on elements of direct patient care. Consequently, conflict arises when the hospital, network, or integrated system emphasizes operating policies and resource allocations that intrude, or give the appearance of intruding, on this patient care delivery by the physicians.

There appears to be a growing tendency now for large-scale health care delivery systems to view doctors (and other staff providers) as units of production. In large systems of care the contribution by any single provider is less conspicuous and less important to the overall production. This frame of reference, that any doctor is the same as any other doctor, is reminiscent of an army mentality: any foot soldier with the rank of private is the same as any other foot soldier private. Arnold Relman described the changing role of the physician in despairing words. "What we are seeing," he said, "is the doctor simply becoming a cog—a unit in an enterprise that is basically a business. The central core of skills that doctors have is going to remain their monopoly, but that is not the essence of being a doctor. The essence of being a doctor is to serve the patient's needs, to be a good Samaritan. The doctor's master should be the patient, not a commercial interest" (Kent & Reichard, 1994).

By nature, by training, and by personal dedication, all doctors will declare that they are not the same and that they resent being thought of that way. As governmental agencies and business corporations have discovered over and over, large size and the discontinuities produced will probably create numerous dysfunctions between the quality of working life and reciprocity between the individual and the organization. Doctors want to be part of managed care, not pawns of managed care says Chris Nuland, Florida Medical Society (Kent & Reichard, 1994).

As power through financial control becomes increasingly concentrated in the hands of professional managers, physicians believe they increasingly overlook the implications for clinical practice of organizational decisions. That accusation may be more true as the transition to managed care and price competition in the health fields deepens. Doctors were unhappy enough in the past with the work of hospital administrators who were available in their offices most of the time and who intended to make a lifetime career working in the hospital setting. Now, as the corporate structure replaces more and more of the comfortable local community hospital setting, corporate managers are no longer trained in hospital management, or public health, but have business degrees and backgrounds not related to the provision of hospital care. They may not be very available and may not be very interested in talking to or listening to local doctors who practice in the hospital. They may think all doctors are the same, but the doctors do not think so.

How to Harmonize

It should be obvious that a harmonious relationship between physicians and the organization is preferable to acrimony. In the best organizational cultures, where there is open participation in defining goals, it is possible to promote excellence in productivity, quality of services, as well as maintaining financial solvency. Doctor/hospital relationship problems are a distinct impediment in creating such a culture (Burchell, White, Smith, & Piland, 1988). But how can that level of nirvana be reached? What is the magic potion that will resolve the problems, so that administration can go home earlier in the evening without all those late meetings and without getting all those nasty phone calls? Management needs to improve relationships by facilitating consistently open communication about vision and goals. Governance structures should be set up in such fashion that physicians have an opportunity for an equal say. The key to physician acceptance is control, said Ken Mack (1993).

Warren Bennis offered distinctions between leadership and management when he noted that leaders innovate while management administers. Physicians see themselves more in the former role, where they can be original instead of merely copying, as they believe management does. Leaders develop, managers maintain; leaders are people oriented, managers relate better to structure; leadership relates to trust, management to control. Leadership focuses on long range aspects; management on short range. Leaders are concerned with what things should be and why should they be at all, while, in Bennis' words, management's attention is on how to do something and when. Physicians fit into this distinction easily with their eye to the horizon rather than to the bottom line, with being their own person instead of a good soldier; with doing right things instead of things right (Bennis, 1989).

Physicians must decide about the extent of their involvement in the process of building and keeping good relationships and how much they want and need good relationships. Improvement should be measured by their accessibility to participation in the organizational dialogue that is the best civilized hope for resolving problems and resolving conflict. If physicians want to compete with insurer-owned networks, they should have to play by the same rules as the networks, according to Uwe Reinhardt (1994), unless, of course, the doctors do not really want good relationships. However, that might show a hospital or a network or an integrated system that probably cannot compete in the managed care market. A health care reform scenario that is based on a smooth melding of hospital/physician relationships will fail in a hospital like this, or else the market power will accrue to the insurers or the faster-moving integrated systems.

GET TOGETHER—WORK TOGETHER?

Jeff Goldsmith said that "given the heritage of suspicion between physicians and hospitals, it is a dangerous time for lay management to be working with the physicians." His point was that the changes taking place in the health care world have given rise to mingled feelings of fear, rage, humiliation, suspicion, and greed (Goldsmith, 1993). That combination makes it difficult to maintain any kind of productive relationships at all, much less a good climate for trying to meld these unhappy folks into "partnerships" or anything else. Goldsmith believes that most of the new organizations for delivering managed care will fail. They will fail because of "the inability of hospitals and doctors to set aside historic suspicions, and because of the poor interpersonal skills of the participants."

In the administrative suite, the leaders of the future need to be able to live and thrive on chaos, adapt quickly to rapidly changing concepts and organizational structures, be adept at improving internal systems, and be a builder of alliances and teams—and do all of this while making budget (Bowker, 1994). Loving uncertainty, ambiguity, and instability are not usually among the qualifications included in a job posting for an administrator. The headhunters also conveniently forgot to mention the impending reductions in census and capacity that must be effected immediately after starting a new job. Do many health care executives understand that their position will be eliminated in a few years as downsizing becomes more important than good relationships? Administrators come and go, but the doctors are generally lifetime members of the community who can have an effect over a long period of time.

Donald Berwick offers the viewpoint that the relatively clear hierarchial structure of the traditional community hospital is giving way to a complex web of relationships and that the administrative style of passing down directives will no longer work. He advises administrators to "shift focus from the minutia of financial reimbursement to providing administrative support for improved patient care and quality outcomes, and understanding their implications for the community" (Berwick, 1994). The traditional control style of management needs to be relinquished in favor of a collaborative, empowering style, if good relationships are to be achieved. There should be a shift from management to leadership. It is not enough to just lecture administrators and management about what they should do, as if they are acting in a vacuum. Medical staff–elected leaders and unelected but influential physicians also have an obligation to learn about these changing management/leadership styles. The doctors should learn to recognize enlightened and progressive behavior by administrators; they should want it and reward it when it occurs. Staying silent while someone tries to improve things is not acceptable.

On the subject of physician leadership and participation in the planning and decision making for the future of health care organizations, there are numerous references in other chapters. But, after all, this book is about doctors and their medical staffs and is dedicated to their past, present, and future success. So maybe the subject can stand another airing. It seems almost trivial to restate that new physician-leaders will be needed at every level in organizations and that physicians in solitary leadership positions, such as medical director or VPMA, often struggle in this new competitive environment. Jonathan Lord says this is because the skills they bring to the job—mostly quality management, utilization review, and peer review—poorly match the hospital's or organization's needs for organizing group practices, physician/hospital organizations, and the variety of other, more extravagant relationships evolving today between doctors and hospitals. Lord goes on to say that while new physician leadership may seem an obvious answer to many of health care's current problems, "the transition it entails is liable to produce chest pains for administrators and physicians alike" (Lord, 1994).

GROW YOUR OWN LEADERS

Members of boards of directors and administrators will readily agree that a fresh supply of these famous physician-leaders does not seem to be available at *their* hospitals, and they wonder where their neighbors, friends, and competitors are finding so many leader-doctors. The answer is, of course, that there are few if any leaders walking around the halls of the hospital, and it is almost a cinch that there are none in the doctors' lounge at this moment. Why is it not commonplace for the hospital or system to adopt a commitment within its statements of mission, purpose, and values to create such leadership? Why not develop an investment strategy for identifying and training those future leader-doctors? In Chapters 8 and 9, there were several specific suggestions and guidelines for the future of the leadership of the organized medical staff, in order to carry out the work of self-governance. Do the same thing with future medical business leaders, who may or may not be the same people as the medical self-governance leaders.

BARRIERS TO RELATIONSHIPS

In another of his pungent commentaries on the difficulties of promoting and improving relationships, Jeff Goldsmith (1993) described it this way. "Physicians crave order, but despise authority. Long deprived of their power to influence directly the operations of hospitals, physicians have resorted to guile and guerrilla warfare to win their battles" (as chronicled elsewhere in this volume). Many physicians selected the profession of medicine based upon their need and desire for autonomy and individual achievement. Some of their number have fallen prey to an illusion that medical school and residency training and their preferred place in society has endowed them with superior knowledge and judgment. Some have not, of course. But Goldsmith believes that "most physicians are incapable of submitting to the authority of anyone, even a fellow physician" (Goldsmith, 1993). That explains why chiefs of staff and department chairs find such difficulty in doing their jobs.

To continue with Goldsmith in an attempt to set the question of hospital/physician relationships in context, "many doctors lack the interpersonal skills or civility to function as a part of a larger enterprise. When physicians are unhappy, they whine—deafeningly." A favorite tactic is passive-aggressive resistance to initiatives that they cannot or dare not oppose, agreeing in public and subverting privately. One of the most puzzling characteristics of a general medical staff meeting is that the members are easily swayed by the last angry person speaking on almost any subject. Goldsmith states positively that doctors are terrible employees, and he recommends corroborating that with any medical group practice executive. Still, much of that behavior, while it is present, has no different effect on the conduct of business in the self-governance work of the Joint Commission medical staff.

Where it really matters is in the integration of a managed care delivery system or the formation and conduct of a provider organization. A sizable fraction of the current generation of private practitioners are poor candidates for participating in any health care enterprise, continues Goldsmith (1993). "The fact that physicians are in economic distress does not mean that they are emotionally prepared to surrender their autonomy or participate meaningfully in a larger health care business enterprise. Angry or depressed people make terrible business partners." This refers to the formation of partnerships here, not the medical staff doing credentialing and peer review, although that probably will not get done very well either by these particular people.

Does all of this gloom and doom, as Maynard Olson used to say, mean that managed care cannot succeed? Not at all, it is in reality an attempt to remind all players in the competition game, and the hospital medical staffs that furnish most of the doctor team in that game, that tremendous emotional and symbolic energy has been invested in the current world of health care delivery, particularly in hospitals. Its demise will not be orderly and the principal ringmasters, the doctors, will not go quietly into that good night of integrated systems, and framing new hospital/physician relationships will not be a pretty process. It may take a while.

SUMMARY

A typical hospital organization chart appears, at least to most of the doctors, as a military or corporate hierarchy. Actually, there is a more complex organization in existence that shows the delegations to administration for the supervision of employees and to the medical staff for self-governance. Each relationship demands collaboration and communication that may not show on the chart. But, whatever the chart, the real need is for physicians and the organization to accommodate to each other and find ways of turning that accommodation into high-quality patient care. The intersection of clinical and organizational control is becoming broader and wider.

In a managed care world, friction will occur when the organization—whether hospital, network, or integrated system—emphasizes operating policies and resource allocations that intrude on patient care delivery by the physicians. Doctors do not see themselves as units of production, each alike in the way each practices.

Obviously, a harmonious relationship between doctors and the organization is preferable to acrimony. The best advice available is to have consistently open communication about vision and goals. The members of the medical staff should decide how much involvement they want, how much they want to build and keep good relationships. Simply expecting the world (and corporate management) to come to them because they deserve it will no longer suffice, if it ever did. Traditional medical practice clinical skills are no help at all in managing the interpersonal skills needed to build collaborative, empowering organizations that shift from management to leadership. Growing a new generation of leaders is the challenge confronting medical staffs now.

REFERENCES

Bennis, W. (1989). *On Becoming a Leader.* Reading, MA: Addison-Wesley.

Berwick, D. M. (1994). Is hospital administration dead? *Eye on Improvement, 1(5),* 2–3.

Bowker, M. (1994). Health care leaders face future skydiving at ground zero. *California Hospitals, Sept./Oct,* 13–15.

Burchell, C. R., White, R. E., Smith, H. L., & Piland, N. F. (1988). Physicians and the organizational evolution of medicine. *Journal of the American Medical Association, 260(6),* 826–831.

Goldsmith, J. (1993a). Driving the nitroglycerine truck. *Healthcare Forum Journal, March/April,* 38–44.

Goldsmith, J. (1993b). Hospital/physician relationships: A constraint to health care reform. *Health Affairs, Fall,* 160–169.

Kent, C., & Reichard, J. (1994). Do doctors make better network bosses? *Perspectives—Supplement to Medicine and Health, 48(51, Dec. 19),* 1–4.

Lord, J. T. (1994). Clinical leadership in an era of health care reform. *California Hospitals, Sept./Oct,* 14–17.

Mack, K. E. (1993). Basic strategies lead to successful medical staff relations. *Report on Physician Trends, 1(8),* 8–9.

CHAPTER

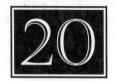

Things That Work

This chapter deals with tasks that work to help the medical staff perform its Joint Commission responsibilities, and will help the chief with the massive burden of duties (and the fun, too) that goes with the job. Things that experience shows are useful and productive will be offered here in the spirit of guidance and counsel without being proscriptive.

IDENTIFYING, SELECTING, TRAINING GOOD LEADERS

One thing that certainly is necessary and does work is to have a plan and a system for selecting chiefs of staff. There should be a nominating committee process, with a group of past chiefs and possibly other leaders who will offer questionnaires to the staff to discover who is interested in pursuing the leadership track. Ask promising physicians directly to determine whether or not they have any present or future interest in entering the leadership track. If a particularly bright or hard-working staff member expresses no interest, or perhaps, a negative attitude, make a good faith attempt to change that perspective in favor of serving. Ask whether a department chair has seen promising talent in the review process. Ask to find out who might be willing to become vice chair of a departmental supervisory committee as a learning experience on the way up the leadership ladder. Leadership is where people find it, and people may not find it without trying.

The nominating committee should meet about six months before the time of the annual meeting or election to identify a chief-elect, for the purpose of making a short list of likely candidates who might accept the position if asked. Each member of the committee should accept the assignment of personal contacts to reduce that short list to the eventual choice. The job is too important to hunt and peck at the last minute. Of course, there might be a self-professed candidate who might be the exact sort of person that is needed by the medical staff at that moment in time. Or, that volunteer might be the very worst person at the worst time for good medical staff self-governance. If the person is not right for the position, the nominating committee must have the courage to withstand that pressure and pick a better choice.

That will mean, of course, that members of the committee will be maligned in the doctors' lounge for their refusal to do the right thing, and the eventual chief will have earned a deadly enemy without having done anything wrong. It can also mean a revolt where there exists more deep-seated resentment than might meet the eye. All bylaws allow for nominations from the floor, and the best-laid plans of the nominating committee may go awry at that juncture. That has been known to happen, and the saving feature is that the surprise chief-elect is just that, a chief in training for the next two years, which will allow time to become familiar with the demands of the leadership role. Not to say that the chief in this example is not allowed to think differently or represent an interest group of the staff that may not have received what they think is an appropriate amount of attention and resources, but the duties of leadership and responsibility to all of the staff as well as to the hospital and its patients must, in the end, be more important than a private agenda.

In fact, it has been openly said that anyone who willingly volunteers to be a chief in these times either does not understand the position or has a personal agenda to pursue. In either case, that could very well spell trouble. The nominating committee must be able to evaluate, also, those candidates proposed by administration. The names may be the very best available doctors and may be exactly the same choices the committee would make. Or, the names might be administration favorites that would be deadly for self-governance and are not acceptable for that reason. Nominating committees almost never appear on organizational charts, but their choices for chief-elect are some of the most important good decisions made by the medical staff organization. Choosing a good future chief is a thing that works well every time it is done.

Leadership Training

Something else that works well is to have a leadership training program, which includes several components. At the very least there must be some sort of orientation for new chairs of committees to enable them to learn their jobs. For peer review chairs, there should be work sessions with staff to understand the process of selecting criteria against which to review. There should be sessions with medical staff services personnel to develop tracks for processing credentials materials. For all chairs and medical directors it is mandatory that there be training in how to conduct better meetings, how to accomplish more work in less time, and how to prevent porcupine politics from sabotaging efficiency. Doctors complain endlessly that there are too many meetings and that they last too long, but some of the same people who do all that complaining also refuse to learn the social skills that would relieve that unnecessary burden. It is almost totally unnecessary for meetings to be so long and unproductive. Doctors are willing to learn medical science but apparently not social science when it would help them immensely. Put together appropriate training programs and require attendance. Be better organized in preparing meetings, and do a better job of conducting them. Those are things that really work.

Another activity that works is to have a general training program for the information and education of staff members who are not yet in the leadership track but are thinking about it. These sessions are not so much how to do it but instead offer interesting and provocative speakers who will be able to stimulate thinking and create interest in offering service to the profession and the hospital medical staff. The output from these efforts, which cost some amount of money, whether paid by the hospital or the medical staff, is to attract future leaders, who will become department chairs and, later, chiefs. It takes a while to grow a good chief. They do not spring full-blown into the position two weeks before taking office just by being elected. The medical staff and administration, too, should agree that no untrained chief or chair should ever assume office. Making that pledge and reinforcing it by offering training opportunities will be some of the best-spent funds and the best investment in present and future success that can be accomplished.

Management Training

If resources and capabilities are available, another thing that certainly works is to offer a training program for medical staff leaders in becoming better at management skills. The object is not to produce M.B.A. degrees but to produce doctors who are capable of moving into administrative and management positions that will improve the organization with their perspectives. No major health care organization in these days of managed care will flourish without a physician perspective in high-level executive management positions. That statement may grieve some old-fashioned administrators, but if they are still erecting barriers to physician participation in decision making and partnerships, then those administrators are not long for this world, to say nothing of the next world of health care delivery. Those who are fortunate will have someone in the organization who will be good at putting together a training program like this. If not, find someone who can do it: the integrated system will be better for turning loose a bunch of trained tigers in its midst!

Send Teams to Important Meetings

Something else that works very well and has been the practice of a number of hospitals for a long time is to send teams to some of the good national meetings that are held for that very purpose. Teams formed of chiefs of staff, board members, and administration should attend together and learn together. Do not treat trips like this as a vacation or reward for simply being alive. If the teams really want to do it right, there should be some advance preparation to determine the individual interests of the participants and to make sure each session is covered. Then, if there really is intereset in making this a learning experience as well as a social outing for the spouses, get the team together for lunch or an early breakfast to discuss the ideas being presented to find out whether there is any applicability for the hospital. Whether anyone else does it or not, the chiefs should contact the leadership to check base each day to see if there is something important to learn more about.

These meetings are always held at wonderful locations, with scenery and fun things to do, but with a little preparation there can be some very helpful team learning as well. Put the cost of these trips in the budget and leave it there. Find something else to cut, because the working relationships and teamwork that results is worth any amount of money. Ask some colleagues at another hospital whether their trips have been helpful and productive. Their response is easy to predict.

VALUE OF MEDICAL STAFF SERVICES

Up to this point in the "things that work" section, all suggestions and recommendations have been directed toward physicians, but there are some other groups of people who need to be recognized. No medical staff organization is any better than the support staff who do the ongoing work, day by day. The medical staff services coordinator or manager is the single best friend any chief can have in the performance of the duties of that office. One of the great unknowns to most of the members of the medical staff is the volume and complexity of the job of the medical staff services office. From time to time, some administrator proposes that any secretary could do it, or that the secretaries in administration could fill in on a part-time basis rather than to hire another trained medical staff professional. Medical staff professionals are more than secretaries, with their required knowledge of the bylaws, the credentialing process, and how to put an agenda together and run a better meeting. They must also know about the National Practitioner Data Bank, about their state and federal regulations, and how to comply with Joint Commission requirements. Just as in the state capital or in Washington, the elected politicians come and go, but the staff go on forever, being loyal and working hard, no matter who is the present chief.

And they go on forever in a much better fashion if they are well selected on the basis of their qualifications and experience, including being a state and national member of the professional organization that has contributed to raising the level of preparation and performance: the National Association of Medical Staff Services (NAMSS). It should be in the position description for the hospital that a requirement for the job is certification as a medical staff coordinator (CMSC). Stand up to the human resources department people who do not understand what a medical staff coordinator is and how that job differs from the regular administrative secretary. The medical staff leaders will need help from administration on this issue, and the worst part is that administrators may not understand the requirements of medical staff services either. And then, always send a team to training, the coordinator and the chiefs, the medical staff services personnel with the department chairs. Include a little in the budget for the continuing training of the CMSCs at the NAMSS and other appropriate meetings.

Medical staff services coordinators are more than secretaries, and the chief may be forced to intercede and protect them when some overbearing doctor wants the staff personnel to stop working on credentialing, agenda preparation, or writing up the minutes to pick up his cleaning or her kids from school. They are not the same as the doctor's office people who work for that doctor. They are the staff who work for the medical staff organization, for all the doctors and not just the insensitive ones. This thing really works. Pay attention to it.

GOOD REVIEW STAFF IS ESSENTIAL

What else works is to have peer review staff who are also carefully selected and assigned to particular committees and departments. Usually, peer review staff are nurses who understand the clinical aspects of care and understand medical records, but there have been some outstanding performers who came from a medical records analyst background. It is entirely possible to have strained relations between the nurse review staff and the medical staff services people, brought on by turf guarding or status battles or by not understanding the true mission of the medical staff organization for self-governance. They cannot see the bigger picture. In that case, the chief, the medical staff executive, or the vice president for medical affairs must intervene to resolve the fuss. Make it all one department if that will help, but find some working agreement or compromise that will improve the process. Above all, do not fall victim to the doctor idea that the peer review staff are nurses, and doctors work with nurses, so they must be better than secretaries who only take minutes. Staff teamwork and cooperation make a dream world of that part of the chiefs' and chairs' jobs. Another thing that works is to be sure not to have a peer review coordinator who hates doctors and is in the position to get revenge. There are some people like that and they can do a lot of damage. That is something that does not work at all.

STAYING ALIVE

Things that work will help the medical staff and hospital to survive and continue to be on the crest of the wave of change. There are many more ways to stay alive, and no doubt the hospital and medical staff know what they are and have been using good ideas for improving the self-governance process. The point is: seek out and adopt things that will work toward the optimal development and perfection of the Joint Commission model. There are common problems concerning physician-trustee-management relationships and some solutions that will work, even though the solutions may be difficult. For example, the only solution to the absence of genuine mutual trust is to build with deeds, not just words, an improved and workable mutual trust relationship that will allow business to be done and the institution to survive (Leech, 1993).

In the hospital or system/network, there may be a historical pattern of the absence of candor in relationships that can only be improved to the point of becoming business partners, through honest, straightforward communication delivered in a consistent manner. One thing that is a constant source of irritation and suspicion is the constant reference to alternative partners or other secret negotiations underway. The other side in this kind of atmosphere has good reason to be skeptical about good faith bargaining. If there are contracts or arrangements, there should be an explanation about why and what the future plans are, even if exact details cannot be divulged.

What will undoubtedly be true in dealing with physician groups will be a widely differing assessment of the present situation and the likely future, as it affects the collective situation for doctors, trustees, and the administrative management. Clarifying the assumptions being used, sharing the assessments of strengths and weaknesses, and resolving the differences is the best way to resolve this perceptual difference well enough to allow further progress—if, indeed, it is possible to resolve those perceptual differences enough that any progress can be made at all with the players presently involved. Sometimes, the parties can only agree to disagree and go on looking for someone else to partner with.

The physician groups are more likely than the management groups to be unable or unwilling to acknowledge that there are absences of essential knowledge, competencies, and skills, although that caveat ought not to be taken literally as the gospel. Administration is just as likely as the doctors to be confused by the grandeur of ego, to the point that neither side can perform a critical evaluation of the needs and then be willing and able to secure them from the outside. Weak leadership from any party to this search for the right way to proceed will manifest itself next when, having reached a consensus on the assessment of the problem, opinions will differ on what to do about it and what strategy to employ. When that strategic direction can be agreed upon, then there may very well be an uneven commitment toward the support of that common strategy. Or, as frequently happens, the physicians' negotiating team will work out all the major strategic decisions, only to see those completely rejected by the members of their organization, who need to continue to use the hospital, the board, and the administration as the scapegoats for all past sins, and all sins that might ever be committed in the future.

What will work in this situation, if anything will, is to talk and act in a straightforward manner, without deception, with the offer of valuable incentives and the sharing of planning and governance. Plotting and conniving in the back room is a guarantee for failure, as is an infrastructure that is not skilled enough and flexible enough to handle the bumpy road that lies ahead. Meanwhile, Nate Kaufman's swift will be eating the slow.

SUMMARY

Experiential learning can be supremely valuable when in the presence of an art—such as medical staff self-governance—rather than a science. What doctors do is practice scientific medicine, but the medical staff has no access to similar resources, because there are none, until now. This chapter offers some useful and productive ideas that can and will make the job more doable, if not actually easier. The identifying, selecting, and training of good leaders should be ranked among the Joint Commission objectives and standards. Credentialing, reappointment, privileging, and peer review can and will be accomplished with good physician leadership. Conversely, in the absence of that skill and experience, there will be foundering and unsuccessful medical staff performance.

Leadership training should be a planned activity, given as much attention and resources as any part of CME. How to be a good peer review chair is a learned activity, aided immeasurably by the willingness to be there, instead of a grudging taking of the turn in an unpleasant job. Training potential leaders who are considering the role is a good investment for both the hospital, integrated system, as well as the medical staff. Offer management training as well, preferably with a university connection that will give credit toward a business administration degree. Medical school and residency is not the proper preparation for managing the affairs of a modern medical staff or medical group, or performing as the physician executive of a health care delivery system.

Something else that works, without which nothing else will work, is the insistence by medical staff leadership of a well-trained staff in the medical staff services and peer or quality review positions. As discussed in Chapter 10, the medical staff executive supervising an integrated department of medical staff employees is the best way. Either way, qualified, well-paid, well-supervised, and well-supported leaders are a must.

What else works is the presence of candor in relationships, true communication among business partners, offering valuable incentives, and the sharing of planning and governance.

REFERENCES

Leech, J. D. (1993). *The Future of Hospital-Physician Relationships.* Presentation at the American Hospital Association Trustee Forum.

CHAPTER

Things That Do
Not Work

A large number of things that do not work well in helping toward the success of medical staff self-governance have been mentioned in the previous chapters and do not need repeating here, but there is one important area that needs discussing. In most hospitals, the medical staff organization that is in place and functions as the Joint Commission model is the only vehicle available for solving problems and serving the members. As the years have passed, and the environment for medical practice and health care delivery began to change away from fee for service and cost reimbursement, the medical staff unincorporated association for self-governance was asked by physicians to do something it was never intended to do and cannot do effectively. That is, the medical staff organization, headed by an elected chief who is required to honor its bylaws, must play a new and active role, functioning as an economic entity that could somehow represent the personal financial and practice concerns of each of the members.

NOT AN ECONOMIC ENTITY

A Joint Commission model medical staff cannot represent the economic best interests of the individual physician members. A hospital medical staff performs credentialing, reappointment, peer review, and utilization review. It does not, and cannot, analyze contracts or act as advocate for individual physicians in their dealings with insurers or health plans. There was a considerable amount of hostility expressed against chiefs and executive committees a few years ago because, somehow, they were supposed to protect the physicians from changes in their practice brought on by outside forces. The hospital also felt those same anxieties and accusations. The hospital did not cause payment changes and cannot cure them. The medical staff organization did not cause the changes and cannot cure them, either.

The best solution is for the medical staff to adopt a policy that admits that sometimes the hospital must adopt a course of action that is in its best business interest; sometimes individual members of the medical staff must adopt a course of action that is in their best business or practice interests; and each must follow that direction (White, 1987). The organized medical staff does not dictate best business direction to the hospital board, although that board is composed of fools if it does not seek physician participation and guidance in important decisions. What is absolutely wrong is for the medical staff, in the form of its executive committee, to attempt to control financial decisions. One past president of a state medical association even suggested that the executive committee should vote on whether to allow the hospital to sign each particular contract. Of course, that is not a proper function for a medical staff.

What does work is for the medical staff to seek out and make available a counselor or advisor to whom the individual physicians can go for guidance when preparing to make decisions, at their own expense, of course. Those are individual interactions that are relevant to an individual physician's practice and are not the business of the other members of the staff. What can be done through the leadership of members of the staff is to go outside the formal medical staff organization and form medical groups or practice associations that fit the needs of some subset of doctors. No single group will serve all, and some physicians will not want to be associated with any group. That is the way it ought to be, and it is the reason the medical staff organization cannot represent the interests of all its members. Most likely, there will be several groups that will emerge, perhaps one or more IPAs (independent practice associations) that can enter into contract arrangements on behalf of its members exclusively. In a managed care world, there will probably emerge a primary care group, whether or not it is capitated and/or other forms of at-risk groups. Other organizational forms are emerging that will be discussed, such as foundation models. In any case, the formal medical staff has nothing to do with any of these coming-togethers and should not even try to play a role.

HOW NOT TO CONTROL COSTS

Another thing that Joint Commission medical staffs cannot do, and that will definitely not work, would be to try to use the existing structure for self-governance as a payment mechanism for physician fees. The idea to do such a thing was one of the proposals in earlier health care reform legislation. The proposal was intended as an incentive for hospital medical staffs to control the volume of services per admission provided by their colleagues. It would be used as a utilization review mechanism, carried several steps further, in other words. The proposal was based on the assumption that "the hospital medical staff is an existing organizational structure that can be used to facilitate physician collaboration in containing costs. No other structure universally exists for physician services" (Welch & Miller, 1994).

Conceptually, for such an approach to work, a medical staff would consist of all physicians practicing in a given hospital, which is the definition of a Joint Commission model. The medical staff would then be held collectively responsible for all Medicare physician services delivered to hospital inpatients. There would need to be a withholding of some portion of the physician payments to ensure that the appropriate limit was not exceeded. On the other hand, there would need to be a mechanism for returning money to the staff members, individually or as a group, if the limits were not exceeded.

All returned funds would be presented to the medical staff as a whole, not to each individual physician, and the organized medical staff would decide how to allocate the money among the physicians. Finally, in this greatly truncated version of the proposal, the executive committee of each medical staff would be required to select a fiduciary agent to receive the returned withheld money for distribution to individual physicians.

A much better arrangement would be for Medicare to return any withheld money directly to the individual physicians, leaving the medical staff out of it. The assumption underlying the whole proposal is false and not based on an understanding of the Joint Commission model. The hospital medical staff cannot and will not contain costs. It may be true that no other structure universally exists, but the self-governance model performs credentialing, privileges, reappointment, and peer review. It does not control physician services.

If, as proposed, the medical staff will decide how to allocate the withheld funds, that could mean even more trouble. Does that imply that the executive committee, the quality assurance committee, or some other medical staff component will allocate money that appears to belong to individual doctors on some other basis? Where in the Joint Commission manual does it describe how to take money from one doctor and give it to another? And would that be some sort of antitrust or anticompetitive action? Would there be any threat to quality of care by such a policy? Physicians would not profit individually from reducing services under the high-cost medical staff policy and might actually lose income, for which they could not escape blaming the organized medical staff that has now become their enemy. There would still be no practical alignment of hospital/physician incentives.

One of the suggested outcomes of the high-cost medical staff policy is that it would force closer attention to credentialing and acceptance to the staff. A policy like this is a direct encouragement to economic credentialing, which was discussed thoroughly in Chapter 5 and is simply not available to a Joint Commission medical staff as a strategy. Welch and Miller (1994) believe that where there is a variation in volume of services per Medicare admission, it can better be explained by the performance of individual physicians rather than by the medical staff collectively. They suggest this theory means that high-cost medical staffs are simply collections of high-cost physicians. That makes sense and is probably the result of many years of hospital interest in filling beds and encouraging complex services and procedures. It is not likely that most medical staffs would accept advice about being reluctant to reappoint these doctors, who are most likely the leading lights of the medical staff.

It is apparent that the proposal to limit high-cost medical staffs was intended to encourage physicians to practice medicine judiciously, with the global Medicare budget in mind. That may not be a very effective incentive at the level of the individual doctor treating a patient. The policy is correct in that it seeks to combine cost-containment objectives with a clear organizational structure that could be supported by utilization information that is severity adjusted. That theory is acceptable as far as it goes, but the Joint Commission model of a hospital medical staff is not the clear organizational structure that could accomplish that worthwhile purpose. A closed panel HMO medical group is perfect for such a policy, as are a number of the faculty practice plans in teaching hospitals.

Using medical directors to function as gatekeepers for Medicare hospital services would possibly succeed in those settings where medical directors have some sort of authoritative relationship to individual practicing physicians, such as some models presented in Chapter 27. But for most community hospitals, medical directors simply do not have that kind of control over the attending physicians who bring patients and treat them without asking permission to provide services. Congress and the Medicare program have every right, indeed, an obligation to develop cost-containment strategies. Everyone hopes they find some good ones. But trying to force the Joint Commission medical staff to take money from some doctors to give to others is not something that will work. Changing the medical staff to facilitate a high-cost policy would work. But then, there would not be need for a book on the Joint Commission medical staff.

SUMMARY

The foremost thing that will not work in the medical staff self-governance system is for the individual physicians to expect the Joint Commission model to function as a

244 • PART ONE • *Moving toward the Joint Commission Model*

defense mechanism for their practice difficulties. Some physicians have grown angry with their leaders and hospital administration because the organized medical staff did not protect them against the inroads of competition, managed care, and capitated payments.

Also presented is a critique of an idea proposed in health care reform legislation that would assign to the hospital medical staff the duty of collecting and parceling out fee payments. Apparently, the hope embodied in such a proposal is that the medical staff would function as a cost control mechanism, which it cannot do. As the discussion in Chapter 5 about economic credentialing notes, this is a mechanism that will work in a partnership or closed panel staff but not in a Joint Commission model.

REFERENCES

Welch, W. P., & Miller, M. E. (1994). Proposals to control high-cost medical staffs. *Health Affairs, 13(4)*, 42–56.

White C. H. (1987). [Faculty presentations] Medical Staff Leadership Conferences and Workshops, Grossmont Hospital, La Mesa, CA.

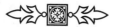

PART TWO

MOVING AWAY FROM
THE JOINT COMMISSION MODEL

CHAPTER

Medical Staff in Turmoil

Thus far in this analysis of the strengths and weaknesses of the Joint Commission model of a hospital medical staff, the emphasis has been concentrated more on what the model is and less on how well it works. It does work, and work well, particularly in a world of personal health services where there are fee-for-service payments to physicians and cost reimbursement to hospitals. Those payment systems encourage the training and practice of specialist doctors and the purchase and installation of ever improving medical technology for use in complex high-tech care delivered in hospitals by those specialist physicians. That is the personal health services system people read about in the Sunday supplement sections of the major newspapers: the personal health services system that can deliver medical miracles, no matter what the cost.

JCAHO MODEL CONTINUING TO WORK

The Joint Commission model, which has grown to be the traditional medical staff structure in nearly all hospitals, was created at a time when there was neither a competitive medical marketplace nor the degree of legal exposure now apparent. Today's world of hospital mergers and formation of regional health care systems for delivering personal health services demands closer working relationships between doctors, singly or in groups, and the health plan or system for reasons of economic survival, but the traditional model may not satisfy those demands. The historical medical staff structure is showing the effects of being buffeted by political, legal, social, and regulatory actions and growth in the health services enterprise. The traditional Joint Commission model may, in fact, have become an anachronism in some instances.

Personal health services have been embedded in an essentially private sector of the U.S. economy, a mixture of nonprofit and for-profit enterprises with gradually increasing government support and intervention. Odin Anderson (1991) describes the concept of intervention as a part of political jargon, implying that government intrudes in an otherwise normal situation. Most Americans, as well as the hospital industry and the medical profession, probably agree that it is all right for government to intervene by offering more money, just as long as there are no strings attached to it. Social and political values in the United States have manifested a great deal of ambiguity as to the responsibilities of citizens as freestanding individuals for their own health care and the extent to which they enter into collective solutions through government. There are essentially two different systems for delivering personal health care in this country, two different sets of doctors, two different groups of hospitals, and differing approaches to the use of the Joint Commission model of a medical staff.

PRIVATE PERSONAL HEALTH SYSTEM

In the earliest days in this country, health care was entirely a private matter, and people were expected to take care of themselves by obtaining services from private physicians and nurses when needed, purchasing medications from drugstores and chemist shops, and paying for all those services personally. As time went on, the society put together what has been described as *the* American health care system. In reality, *the* American health care system is that used by the typically employed, insured, middle-income individual or family. The most striking feature of this employed, insured, middle-income system of care is the absence of any *formal* system. Each individual or family puts together an *informal* set of services and facilities to meet its own needs. The system, therefore, has no formal structure or organization and is different for each individual or family. Further, each family's system may vary widely from time to time according to the particular situation in which it is being used. The only constants are the family itself, the service aspects that focus on and are coordinated by doctors, and the payment through personal, nongovernmental funds, whether paid directly by the consumers or through private health insurance plans.

For all of its looseness and lack of structure, the employed, insured, middle-income family's private system of health care allows for a considerable amount of decision and control by the patient. The patient is free to choose the physician, the health insurance plan, and frequently even the hospital where inpatient services are to be obtained. If additional care is needed, the patient can seek that out as well. If the patient does not like the particular care being provided, then the patient can vote with his or her feet, by finding care from another provider. As described, this system of care is a poorly coordinated, unplanned collection of services that frequently have little formal integration with each other. It can be wasteful of resources and usually has no central control or monitor to determine whether it is accomplishing what it should. Each individual service may very well be of high quality, but there may be little evidence of any "linking" taking place to ensure that each service complements the others as effectively as possible (Torrens, 1993).

PUBLIC PERSONAL HEALTH SYSTEM

A second system of health care in the United States serves those people who are not regularly employed, do not have continuous health insurance coverage, and often are minority group members living in the inner city. While the specific details may vary from city to city, the general outline is well known in all major cities across the country. It will be instructive to compare what might be the *worst* health care system in the country, that of the poor, unemployed, and uninsured or underinsured, with the previously described *best* system, that of the middle class. What is striking is that there are exact similarities, in some respects. The health care system of the poor, inner-city resident, like that of the middle-income system, has no *formal* structure. Each family must put together an *informal* set of services, from whatever sources possible, to meet the health care needs of the moment, with one major difference. The poor do not have the resources to choose how and when they will obtain services. They must simply take what is offered to them and try to put together whatever they are told they can have.

Most of these services are provided by agencies of the local government, such as city or county hospitals and local health departments. There is no real continuity of service with any single provider, such as the middle-income, employed person might receive from a family physician. The poor family is faced with an endless stream of health care professionals who treat one specific episode of illness and then are replaced by someone else (or no one else) for the next episode. While the middle-class family can establish some semblance of continuity by the ongoing presence of a family physician, the poor family cannot. Personal health services are provided, if at all, by the local health department clinic.

When ambulatory care services are needed, the poor family does not depend on the constant availability of the family physician for routine advice and treatment, but must turn to neighbors, the local pharmacist, the health department's public health nurse, or the emergency room of the city or county hospital. For many poor people, the emergency room *is* the family physician. The emergency room also serves as the entry point to the rest of the health care system. To gain admission to the outpatient clinics of the public hospitals, where the poor obtain many of their services, people must first go to the emergency room to be referred to the clinic. Once out of the emergency room, there may actually be more than one specialty clinic to which they are sent. Each clinic may handle one particular set of problems, but none of them will take responsibility for coordinating all the care the patient needs or is receiving (Torrens, 1993).

Collective solutions through community fund drives for hospital construction have had a long history and easy acceptance. Collective solutions through some form of private health insurance, on the other hand, have been adopted cautiously. For most people, insurance was considered a normal and prudent means for Americans to protect their own solvency. But medical care for the poor was once regarded as a responsibility of the noblesse oblige of the local physicians and the charitable tradition of the hospital (Anderson, 1991).

When inpatient hospital services are needed by the employed, insured, middle-income family, they will probably be provided by a local community hospital that is usually voluntary and nonprofit. The medical staff of that hospital is organized and functions exactly in the manner described in Joint Commission standards, and those hospitals are the backbone of the Joint Commission accreditation process. The specific hospital to be used for that family is usually determined by the institution in which the family physician has medical staff membership and privileges. The smaller, less specialized, more local hospitals will be used for more simple problems, whereas the larger, more specialized, perhaps more distant hospitals will be used for more complicated problems.

When the poor need inpatient hospital services, whether simple or complicated, they again usually turn to the city or county hospital to obtain them. Admission to the inpatient services of these hospitals is usually obtained through the emergency room or the outpatient clinics, thereby forcing the poor family to use these outpatient services first if they wish or need later admission to the inpatient services. That is a gatekeeper process. The poor may also turn to the emergency room, the outpatient clinics, and the inpatient ward or teaching services of the larger voluntary nonprofit community hospitals. Since these hospitals are frequently teaching hospitals for the training of physicians, they often maintain special free or lower-priced wards. It is to these wards that the poor are usually admitted. Since the care in the teaching hospitals might very well be as good or better than any that might be obtained at the local city or county hospitals, many poor are willing to become teaching cases in the voluntary nonprofit hospitals in exchange for better care in better surroundings. As Paul Torrens (1993) says, by and large, city and county hospitals, where they exist, carry the largest burden of inpatient care for the poor. Due to the understaffed nature of most of these facilities; their underfunding; the swinging door effect of patients entering and leaving the system; and the mixture of doctors that includes faculty, students, interns, residents, and local community attending physicians, there is a lack of any sense of cohesiveness and common past, present, and future of the medical staff that lends strength and credibility to the Joint Commission model. There might be a charitable tradition for the hospital, but there is probably not any longer a sense of obligation for the care of the poor in county hospitals by the doctors in the middle-class community hospitals.

EVOLUTION OF PERSONAL HEALTH SERVICES

It took over 50 years for the modern personal health services delivery systems to evolve from a general practice–centered to a specialty- and hospital-centered enterprise. In 1875, physicians and, to some extent, pharmacists were the sole dispensers of professionally recognized health services, two professions with long and prestigious traditions. On the periphery were recognized and unrecognized midwives who, by the turn of the century, were beginning to be replaced by doctors. A great deal of reliance was placed on home medication. Physicians and pharmacists were, as they still are, largely private entrepreneurs, presumably working within a code of ethics, standards, and services not strictly of a profit-making enterprise but undoubtedly influenced by the social atmosphere of nongovernmental involvement that characterized the United States in the later nineteenth century.

There were then as many physicians in relation to the population as there now (Anderson, 1991). They made a living by treating patients for fees and received very little income from government and philanthropic sources. No other country has been able to support as many physicians by payments from fee-for-service patients as has the United States. The same was true for pharmacists, who eventually established the familiar corner drugstore, because income from prescriptions alone was not enough to make a living. There were too many pharmacists because physicians frequently did their own dispensing from the relatively simple materia medica of that period. Once community hospitals became the focus for more complicated care and surgery, aided by advances in antisepsis and anesthesia, doctors received a free workshop in which some of them provided free care for some of the poor.

The United States has had a long tradition of voluntary self-help on a community level, and the voluntary hospitals have been a prime example of this tradition. Nurturance functions that had been a province of the family found expression in the voluntary hospital when the home became unequal to the technical demands and setting of increasingly high-technology medicine. Hospitals survived and prospered by serving the large and growing middle class for a fee. Approximately two-thirds of the hospital income came from fees paid by private patients, and one-third came from philanthropy, public funds, and other charities for the poor. In no other country but the United States have the general hospitals been able to survive on the income from private patients. Consequently, this country was able to mount a personal health delivery system for private patients, and the poor became a residual of this emerging industry, to be treated in the public facilities. Just the opposite was true in Europe, where the paying patients were the residual (Anderson, 1991).

Dentists paralleled physicians as private entrepreneurs earning their living from fees from private patients. Since the public perception of dental health earlier in this century were rather primitive, the services of dentists were hardly in great demand. The dental profession also benefited greatly from the development of anesthesia and antisepsis. In fact, it was a dentist who was the first to use ether for extractions, thus ushering in the widespread use of anesthesia. Health personnel came from apprentice arrangements, which later became university arrangements. Other types of health personnel, such as laboratory technologists, grew out of the advances in medical science and technology.

All of this took money, which became available as the economy boomed, and there was surplus to pour into the personal health services that people wanted and, at first, bought without governmental or insurance help. By the time of the Second World War, the personal health system as it is today was basically in place: voluntary community hospitals, privately practicing physicians and dentists, and private pharmacies. Stimulated by the enormous dynamics of medical science, technology, and ever increasing amounts of public and private money, the acute disease–oriented personal health services system was poised for an even more dramatic expansion: the emergence of a third party to pay for the day-to-day operating expenses of this monstrous structure, or nonsystem, as it has been called.

The salient point in this third-party development was that the existing infrastructure of health services was in place. It was accepted as a given, and the government and private insurance companies were concerned mainly with paying for it. In the case of hospitals, the concept was charges or costs, and the difference between those is still the subject of many debates in medical staff meeting. Doctors were paid by health insurers through fee schedules, or maybe no negotiations at all, since there were no contracts between doctors and payers. In retrospect, some of these financial arrangements and payment systems seem fiscally and administratively irresponsible. Insurance simply meant that the doctor sent a bill and received a check. Send a claim; get a check. But there was plenty of money in a rapidly expanding economy and health insurance as a collective bargaining benefit may have cost the employers less than take-home pay would have. Labor peace achieved through health coverage was worth the price. The supply of hospital beds increased and so did the number of doctors, and their specialization increased right along with it. Doctors were busy and prosperous. Hospital occupancy increased.

The only cloud on the horizon for this seemingly endless march toward perfection was a development that concerned itself directly with restructuring the delivery of physicians' services and, indirectly, hospital care. This was the emergence of group practice arrangements that began to attempt to replace the solo practice and fee-for-service type of medical delivery by engaging a range of specialists on a salary, providing a full range of physician services from curative to preventive, and serving a known population. Initially, the opposition on the part of the medical profession to these new arrangements was fierce. But over time, such programs began to take their place in the total spectrum of health services delivery types and began also to be regarded as options on labor-management negotiations for fringe benefits. There became intense concern with how to manage the health services enterprise so that buyers would know what they were buying and sellers would know what they were providing. The wide-open era of simply paying what the providers asked was seriously questioned. Then someone discovered that the payment system could be used to manage the delivery system rather than simply to write checks for bills received.

Attempts at rationalizing personal health services were expressed mainly in the group practice payment plans, which were not simply a means of saving money but one of providing high-quality and comprehensive services efficiently and conveniently. Saving money was recognized, but providing the most up-to-date scientific services was the major objective. Past experience and comparisons with other industrialized nations all seem to indicate that the upward trend of expenditures for personal health services is almost inevitable, given reasonably equitable access, continuing innovations in technology, and the aging of the population. As well, the public places a high priority on personal health services, especially when it is for them or their family members.

RAPID CHANGE MEETS STATUS QUO

In a newly competitive world of managed care, hospitals and health care corporations are attempting to develop a sense of teamwork with physicians whose training and experience clearly run counter to the characteristics of innovation and rapid change. The Joint Commission model ensures continuity and status quo, works best in the middle-class hospitals, works much less well in the public facilities that serve the poor, and serves as a real resistance to change, which was the most desired characteristic of a medical staff in a doctors' workshop hospital. Whatever other good things it will do in the way of credentialing and peer review, the Joint Commission model will not produce rapid responses to a changing world.

Thus, many members of traditional medical staffs encounter a real sense of trauma, resistance, and anger to the perceived inequity and unfair realities of today's health care environment. Sometimes the responsive behavior displayed by physicians on hospital medical staffs take on the features of the Kubler-Ross five stages of dying. During the denial stage, many physicians take out their crisis in spirit on administration, because that is the nearest handy target that cannot easily strike back. The crisis in spirit of today's practicing physicians is not restricted to older practitioners and transcends the bounds of age, gender, race, and specialty. Evidence for this phenomenon comes from *Rate Controls* (Silver, 1994), which states that managed care is driving physicians crazy! The Unum Corp., a major underwriter of disability policies, states that many of the physician claims in 1994 were for mental and physical disorders. Doctors are normally a robust lot, but that year claims rose by 60 percent compared to the year before. Unum blames managed care for sapping the entrepreneurial juices from physicians. The company wrote these policies during the fee-for-service era when there were few claims. It was such a good deal for the insurers that the policies were written to be noncancelable and now can never be repriced.

Physician morale directly affects patient care as that morale is affected by reduced hospital budgets that affect staff and the purchase of new equipment. Malpractice lawsuits or the constant threat of them weigh heavily on the minds of the more high-risk specialties. But what directly affects practicing physicians are the changes that have a direct effect on them, such as:

- declining income, whether from salary or simply fewer patients;
- loss of independence and change in patient base because of payer contracts that move in new patients or move out former ones;
- extraneous activities, the increased paperwork, the "hassle factor," which takes major amounts of time away from direct patient care or family life;
- criminalization of medicine, the increased scrutiny by licensing agencies, and fraud and abuse audits by public agencies;
- obliteration of some of the art of medicine and the freedom to make medical judgments by the increased encroachment of the numbers approaches to outcome measurements, length of stay guidelines, and prior-approval requirements;
- punishment of all for the sins of a few through such mechanisms as the National Practitioner Data Bank and the public release to the media of such data as doctor-specific and hospital-specific mortality rates (Meyer, 1989).

Declining Association Influence

In addition, there is the very real spectacle of declining influence by state and national medical associations in their ability to control the legislative agenda on behalf of their members. Although medical societies still are formidable in their abilities to deliver campaign contributions to candidates of both major parties, the amount of influence that goes along with those financial gifts is not as strong as it once was. County medical societies that at one time served as the restrictor to medical practice and sometimes even to membership on hospital medical staffs has declined steadily and may not have much of a future in some places. Paying dues to all of those organizations without seeming to receive benefits of protection against change will result in declining membership. And, in truth those associations cannot protect their member doctors against changes in medical practice and payment systems. What health care associations, both hospital and medical, now lobby about seems far removed from daily practice.

What is being discussed in the doctors' lounge are some of the same gripes and complaints that have always been there but with some new themes. The physicians' world has changed and many are fearful, angry, and dispirited. There is a lot of self-pity being expressed, and demands to be left alone can be heard more frequently. The old gripes against the hospital have a sharper edge because now the hospital is competing for patients, or even worse, hospitals sign contracts that take away private patients and then want help from the doctors in providing care.

Different Visions

The vision of the future for hospitals is no longer the same vision as the physicians. Doctors think the hospital is planning their future for them, probably without asking for enough physician input, which also makes the doctors unhappy. Services are being changed from inpatient to outpatient, which makes payers very happy and frequently serves patients better but can severely damage or even eliminate some physicians' practices. Physicians accuse the hospital of expecting them to help the hospital to get what the administration wants while not trying in return to help the doctor get what he or she wants.

In situations like that, the administration and the board tend to think of physicians as the entire group, as the whole medical staff, while the doctors think only of themselves as individuals. That may be a universal tendency: to think about what appears to be a homogenous group as if it really is a group, while the members of the group never think in group terms but only of themselves and appropriately so. The Joint Commission model imposes some group norms and standards of behavior within the hospital as it concerns the work of self-governance, but that has no relationship to medical practice outside the walls of the hospital, in the office or clinic.

Nonproductive Committees

One swift and sure reaction to these tensions is the accusation that administrators and employees get paid to sit in seemingly endless meetings while physicians do not. Indeed, as managed care increases, primary care doctors can make money only in the office and every hospital medical staff meeting can only take away from that necessity to process large numbers of patients through the office. A real improvement would be to build on that sentiment and reduce the number of dysfunctional or nonproductive committees that every hospital has. For people who talk all the time about how much they hate meetings, hospital staffs are notably reluctant to reduce the number of committees or spend less time and get more work done. There have been many eager chiefs of staff who went into office with the platform of reducing the number of committees during a term of office and then found themselves going out of office with more committees that they started with! Time wasting is a chronic disease of medical staffs and is one of the major causes of lack of respect and participation by some staff members. Even when times were good, the Joint Commission model witnessed unhappiness and complaining among the members of the staff. Now in an era of transition that promises to be less than good times, the traditional structure of the organized medical staff seems unresponsive and totally incapable of preventing that change from occurring.

SUMMARY

The Joint Commission model was created and flourished best at a time when there was neither a competitive medical marketplace nor the degree of legal exposure now apparent. Now, in an era of managed care, hospital mergers, and regional integrated health systems, the traditional model shows the effects of being buffeted by political, legal, financial, and regulatory action. To understand the depth and breadth of those effects and the changes that result, it is necessary to review the history of the two personal health services delivery systems in the United States, one private and one public.

What is usually called the American health care system is that of the employed, insured, middle-income individual or family that utilizes a set of facilities and services to meet needs. Then there is the public system, used by the unemployed or underemployed, frequently minority group members living in the inner city, who seek services from agencies of local government, wherever they exist. Medical staff self-governance in the different hospitals used by these two systems are very different, as are the services available and accessible. The history of the development of personal health services in this country parallels the story of hospitals and doctors presented in Chapters 1 and 2.

Rapid change is now occurring in these systems of care, where medical staff structures emphasize status quo and the absence of change. The Joint Commission model ensures continuity and a predictable future and will not produce rapid responses to a changing world. The result is unhappy responsive behavior by some of the members of the medical staff that affects behavior and morale as well as practice. The vision of the future for physicians may no longer be the same as for the hospital/health care system executives.

REFERENCES

Anderson, O. W. (1991). Health services in the United States: A growth enterprise for a hundred years. In Litman, T. J., & Robins, L. S. (Eds.), *Health Politics and Policy (2nd ed.)*. Albany: Delmar Publishers.

Meyer, C. (1989). *Minnesota Medicine, 72.*

Silver, A. (1994). *Rate Controls, 18(11B, November 30).*

Torrens, P. R. (1993). Historical evolution and overview of health services in the United States. In Williams, S. J., & Torrens, P. R. (Eds.), *Introduction to Health Services (4th ed.).* Albany: Delmar Publishers.

CHAPTER

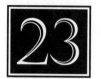

Wisdom from the Doctors' Lounge

The same negative mind-sets that infect some of the denizens of the doctors' lounge sound very much like typical armed services griping, such as insisting that the board is incompetent and should not be in charge, in spite of the fact that the physician doing the griping is also using the latest piece of million-dollar medical technology purchased by a trusting board anxious to see that patients receive the best care that money can buy. In this case, the best care that money can buy has been spent on capital expenditures that were recommended by the medical specialists.

ADMINISTRATORS ARE THE PROBLEM

The same turmoil mind-set would remind administrators that their roles are temporary and that the medical staff will be there long after that manager is gone from the scene. That is true, as a matter of fact. Some kind of organized medical staff will be there as long as there is a hospital, because that is what a hospital is. Doctors treat patients. Or, doctors write orders for other people to treat patients. Administrators do have a short shelf life, but as many a medical staff rabble-rouser has discovered with chagrin, the devil known is better than the devil not known! Sometimes it is better to keep the current administrator rather than to stage an uprising that will bring in someone even worse.

There are doctors that will say that physicians should be involved in decision making, and that is totally true. Whether the same individual physician making the accusations should be involved in planning and decisions is another matter altogether, but full partnership with hospital and physician involvement is a critical necessity in today's world of shrinking revenues and rising costs. The problem for a willing administrator and an enlightened board is to find physicians who are willing to participate in the decision-making process. Even more difficult is to find physicians who are not only willing but actually good at the decision-making process!

LAWYERS ARE THE PROBLEM

There are physicians who will say that all of the evils of the world are caused by attorneys and everything is their fault. Most of this attitude derives from plaintiff's counsel who are the litigation enemies of doctors whose pride and pocketbooks have been dented. Doctors will use lawyers in a hurry to help them put together partnerships and corporate structures, but it is still a matter of pride in the lounge to be able to tell the most scurrilous lawyer jokes. Doctors tell lawyer jokes. Lawyers tell lawyer jokes, too, and that is where most of them come from. There are not as many doctor jokes, because doctors are not usually funny. They take medicine so seriously that there is no room for humor.

One of the more serious sources of turmoil in the doctors' lounge is change and what it brings: the backlash of the loss of fee-for-service medicine and the rise of capitation and managed care, with control resting in the hands of the insurers or the health plans. The most available target for the frustrations of dealing with an economic world doctors did not expect to find is the organized medical staff that, for some deep, dark, conspiratorial reason, has not protected that individual from the loss of patients and accompanying loss of income and a previously orderly and predictable way of life. There are many doctors who will openly say that what is happening now is not the kind of medicine they expected to practice when they went to medical school, or when they graduated from residency. Is the tenured faculty in undergraduate medical education so entrenched in the past world of indemnity insurance, and is the residency faculty in graduate medical education so caught up in unlimited ordering ability that graduates today are turned out so unprepared as they say?

CHANGE IS THE PROBLEM

Or is the problem one of an accelerating rate of change as described by Donald Schon (1978)? People have always experienced change, but it has been a gradual and stable pace of change to which they thought they had learned to adjust and accept. What is new now is that for the first time in human history doctors are experiencing the accelerating pace of change, as evidenced by the knowledge explosion such as that in medicine; the technological revolution, so evident in medicine; the extension of the life span, so evident in the patient population; and the increasing mobility of populations (Schon, 1978). Malcolm Knowles adds that while the educational system has done a reasonably good job of helping people learn how to live with gradual and expected change, it has not yet discovered how to help people cope with the accelerating pace of change (Knowles, 1994).

Whatever the problem, it must be the fault of the chief of staff, who has gone over to the other side and now works for the administration and does not represent the doctors any more. That is a very frustrating thing to hear for a chief who has spent every day and most evenings in meetings trying to protect and help the doctors. Unfortunately, a few of the constituents are still totally in the dark about the issues and can find no other way to vent that anxiety and uncertainty except to rail at the chief. That is what makes the job of the chief more than honorary as it used to be, and that is why chiefs should be paid appropriately. The traditional Joint Commission model of a hospital medical staff is unequipped and ill prepared for dealing with change in the order of magnitude now occurring.

Donald Light has presented a chart shown as Table 23–1 that shows better than almost any other description why there is turmoil among the staff as expressed in the lounge (Light, 1991). The changes in doctors' practices and their lives are, in fact, so overwhelming that it is no wonder there is fear and loathing about the new and future world of medicine.

CONTRASTS IN PERSONALITY AND STYLE

One of the problems in trying to make sense of a hospital organization such as the Joint Commission model, which was never intended to do what it is now being called upon to do, is the essentially different personality types and decision-making approaches of physicians and administration. Allowing for the variances concealed in a generalization, there have been many presentations to demonstrate this point as an explanation for why neither "side" seems to understand the behavior and desires of the other. Perhaps Michael Kurtz shows us one of the most clean and simple versions in Table 23–2 (Kurtz, 1988).

This comparison is supposed to show that styles differ and that different roles demand differing styles. It always comes as a great shock to doctors turned administrators that they can no longer decide every issue by themselves immediately, as they can with their private patients, but must work with other people and give the management decision-making process a chance to produce a better indication for a decision. Some-

TABLE 23–1   How the doctors' world has changed

From	*To*
Provider dominance, a system shaped and run by doctors	Buyer dominance, as an effort to dismantle and reshape the laws, customs, and institutions established by organized medicine to allow buyer choice and competition
Sacred trust in doctors	Distrust of doctors' values, decisions, and even competence
Quality assured by the medical profession as high	Quality as a major focus of systematic review
"Nonprofit" guild mentality	Competition for profit, even among nonprofit organizations
Cottage industry structure	Corporate industry structure
Specialization and subspecialization	Primary care and prevention, with minimum referrals to specialists
Hospital as the "temple of healing"	Home and office as equal centers of care
Fragmentation of services as a byproduct of preserving physicians' autonomy	Coordination of services to minimize error and reduce unnecessary and inappropriate services and costs
Payment of costs incurred by doctors' decisions	Fixed payment, with demand for a detailed account of decisions and their efficacy
Cross-subsidization of the poor by the more affluent, of low-tech and service departments by high-tech departments	Cross-subsidization seen as what it is: cost shifting, a suspect maneuver that imposes hidden charges on buyers and is frequently a hidden subsidy for underfunded government programs

times good decision making means allowing time to see whether there really is a problem that needs solving. Whether these characteristics of personality and style are a product of self-selection and training or are job related, the point is that there is disagreement,

TABLE 23–2   Contrasts in personality and style

Physicians	Administration
Doers	Designers
Problem-oriented	Process-oriented
Proactive	Reactive
Immediate	Long-term response
Deciders	Delegators
Autonomous	Collaborative
Independent	Interdependent
Patient advocate	Organizational advocate

unhappiness, and plenty of blame from a medical staff in turmoil, who may have neither the time or the inclination to ponder the meaning of life.

This is not to say that some of these issues and complaints are new or that they have not been stated before by others during the long history of medicine and the somewhat shorter, but equally trying, search for hospital/physician relationships. Competition is not just a brand new discovery by self-important managed care experts in the 1990s, as witnessed by this example:

> I scarcely know if it would be worth my while to allude to the base competition of trade which affects the interests of our profession in California to a ruinous extent. Underbidding and undermining are bad enough when they are induced by sharp necessity. But they are perfectly excusable when prompted only by a spirit of rivalry or ambition. It is in the power of a single medical practitioner in a city or county to reduce the gross income of the members of the medical profession by one-half or more; while the sacrifice of position and character in the public estimation is a much greater loss.
>
> Often our most successful and eminent physicians are guilty of this injustice.
>
> We have four classes of patients to deal with. The first have money without honor; the second honor without money; the third neither money nor honor; the fourth, both money and honor. At present, it is only in the most fortuitous conjunction last named that we have any chance of getting paid at all.
>
> The lawyer demands his fee in advance and gets it. But then his services are more highly prized than ours. He has to do with property while our concern is only life, and everybody knows that in California the latter is of little moment in comparison with the former. (Grant, 1986)

That statement seems so pithy and reflective of the feelings and attitudes of modern-day physicians that it is always instructive to ask who said it and why. The answer is that the remarks were made by Henry Gibbons, M.D., first president of the new Medical Society of California, in his keynote address at the first annual meeting in 1858. Many doctors would say now that Dr. Gibbons speaks for them on the subject of a modern-day competitive marketplace in health care. The more things change, the more they stay the same.

SUMMARY

Unhappiness with the current state of medical practice among some physicians can be blamed on the actions of health care corporate executives or the law profession, but the real problem is the accelerating pace of change. Gradual and predictable change has always been present and can be accommodated, but the Joint Commission model of a medical staff is unequipped and unprepared to deal with the magnitude of upset occurring now. Changes in the doctors' worlds are bringing to a sharper focus some of the differences in style and issues that may have always been present but seem so divisive now.

REFERENCES

Grant, P. N. (1986). [Unpublished dissertation]. Harvard University.

Knowles, M. S. (1994). Predicting the future of higher education. *The Network, 12(2, Fall/Winter),* 23–25.

Kurtz, M. (1988). Cited in Sheldon, A. Physician-administrator cooperation in the postprofessional era. *Physician Executive, 14(5, Sept./Oct.),* 2–7.

Light, D. W. (1991). The restructuring of the American health care system. In Litman, T. J., & Robins, L. S. (Eds.), *Health Politics and Policy (2nd ed.).* Albany: Delmar Publishers.

Schon, D. (1978). *Beyond the Stable State.* New York: W. W. Norton.

CHAPTER

The Consequences of Competition

The cause of all that turmoil in the doctors' lounge is a decided change in the fundamental health care delivery and payment systems in this country. Normally the fountainhead of all the accumulated wisdom of the medical staff, there is doubt and confusion in the lounge in the middle 1990s, about where medicine is headed. Not only does the individual practice of medicine that can be under the control of each physician seem so unsettled, but there is great uncertainty and grave concern about where the health and medical system of the nation is headed in the future.

THE HOT BREATH OF REFORM

For the first time in the history of the country, health care reform rose to the top of the national political agenda, and a president was elected with a clear intent to reform health care. Reform to the practicing physician means changes in the way life is organized, the way care is delivered, the number and kinds of employees in the office, the way claims are paid (or not paid), and the volume of paperwork that may be required. Changes have always meant bad news to the prophets and visionaries in the doctors' lounge, forgetting for the moment that other, similarly earth-shattering changes were responsible for their becoming successful and prosperous in recent decades. But it is more fun and more colorful to talk bad news along with gloom, doom and dire predictions that the whole hospital is going to hell, especially the inpatient unit where the speaker's patients are in beds. In that unit there are probably not enough nurses, or the ones who are there are not as good as nurses used to be, as the doctor remembers it.

The forces in favor of health care reform show unusual persistence in their efforts to put together health care legislation and find some sort of political compromise that would enable it to be passed by Congress. Their persistence remained in spite of continual time delays, opposition from within the president's own party as well as the expected disagreements from the other party. Eventually, the 1994 session of Congress was completed without reform legislation being passed, and control of both houses of Congress changed from one party to the other. Maybe this time, after a number of false starts toward health care reform by other presidents during their terms of office, something different will happen and the health care system will actually change, showing another lurch in a different direction, as has been the case so many other times. The path of history is never a smooth line of progression from one era to the next but moves more in fits and jerks, no pun intended. The possibility of change is presented in a two-scenario form in Chapter 30.

And then again, maybe there will not be a major overhaul of the patchwork quilt of complexity that seems so unmanageable some days. It is also entirely possible that even if far-reaching legislation at the federal level is never passed at all, there is so much momentum at state levels and in the private sector that the health care system will continue to evolve all by itself. There may be too much energy already unleashed to turn back now to complete fee-for-service medicine for the doctors and full beds with the latest technology for the hospitals. There does seem to be a recognizable trend toward political acceptance of health services coverage for all citizens, including noncitizens. The providers and insurance payers, however, definitely want to unburden themselves of the uninsured who are unable to pay enough or at all.

EVOLUTION LED TO REFORM

The health care reform movement in the 1990s is the direct product of health care delivery system evolution in the 1980s, which was another period of rapid change that also upset the denizens of the lounge. They complained as bitterly then as they are complaining now. The outcomes of that decade of evolution have set the stage for competition, managed competition, managed care, cost containment, universal access, portability, and all the other buzzwords that accompany this latest (but hardly the last) wave of change.

The very important and apparently generally accepted concept of competition in the marketplace, between various types of HMOs and the fee-for-service system trying to cope with its relatively new competitors, is still not yet well understood. Employers are complaining that HMOs are not lowering costs as much as they expected, while premiums continue to rise. There are no standards yet to measure what is a reasonable level of premiums to be paid or a level of expenditures by the public or private sectors. Economists who promote price competition do not appear to really understand the nature of the health services market as compared with other goods and services. They are mystified by the continuing rise in expenditures and premiums. It is likely that health services are not regarded by the public as a commodity like automobiles and refrigerators. Instead, health services are a basic need and right, regardless of cost (Anderson, 1991). There is some speculation about, after years of experience, whether competition lowers prices, makes care more available and accessible, or actually results in the destabilization of the very complex hospital/medical industry that requires mutual trust as the major variable in being able to function.

Price competition may result in the offerings of competing delivery systems becoming quite similar because of the inherent extensiveness of the health services involved and the insistent demands for them. Competition may then become based on softer, less objective rationales than advanced medical sciences, such as convenience of access and quality as perceived by the public, including better parking, pleasant receptionists, doctors' offices that run on time, and less cash paid out of pocket at the point of service.

There is a prevailing view that the traditional fee-for-service insurance coverage and open choice of physicians will disappear as the HMO concept and its varieties reach more and more of the population (Anderson, 1991). The traditionally wide-open system of "unmanaged care" and reimbursing physicians on the basis of usual, customary, and reasonable fees, as well as retroactive reimbursement of hospitals, may be a thing of the past. Yet the tenacity of that style should not be underestimated in a country with the free-enterprise, consumer choice mentality of the United States. As more and more Americans experience the restrictions imposed on them by the limited choice and closed delivery systems as represented by staff and group model HMOs, an appreciably large minority might very well be led toward selection of more open system like IPAs, which are the medical profession's response to the competition of closed system model (Anderson, 1991). Can the profession group itself together in a not-necessarily self-serving manner to deliver an open choice system at a cost approximately the cost of the closed system model? How will the hospital medical staff be able to function in the traditional Joint commission model when there are all those conflicting care systems, payment systems, and wildly conflicting incentives?

Health care in the 1980s also saw the advent of much greater patient involvement in decision making about matters of care and treatment. The consumer movement in retail purchasing moved to medicine, where it was met with varying degrees of acceptance and resistance by physicians in their many different practice styles and settings. Patients showed more interest in their care and exerted more effort to share control of their treatment.

Malpractice suits, dramatically higher liability insurance premiums, and multimillion dollar settlements and awards accompanied growing impatience with the disciplinary procedures of state medical licensing boards during the decade of the 1980s. All of these outside forces created some amount of increased awareness among the insiders sitting on medical staff peer review committees that business as usual might be changing and that it might be more useful to pay more attention to the actions of their colleagues. Cases like Nork, where the medical staff did not seem to pay enough attention early enough, made it clear that the self-governance requirements of the Joint Commission model involved more than just lip service and a perpetuation of the existing order.

Effects of Inflation in Costs

For years, health economists were fond of saying that "there is no price competition in health care" or "there is market failure" in the health care delivery system. Economists filled their journals with these arguments and showed data to prove their contentions. Some experts argued that the solution to steadily growing costs of health care was the establishment of marketplace competition, while others favored state or federal regulatory approaches such as rate review or single-payer systems.

These solutions to ever increasing health care costs that seemed to defy all attempts at control are opposed to each other, of course. Regulatory approaches can only be implemented by federal or state governments. There has been a move within the liberal wing of one major party for more than 60 years to put in place a national health insurance program that would offer available, accessible health care to all citizens within a framework of controlled prices and fees for payment to health care providers for their services.

Several states during the 1980s experimented with less comprehensive efforts to control costs by focusing only on setting hospital inpatient payment rates, for the most part without dealing with many other aspects of the system.

States that tried regulation had little or no success to the point that the programs were abandoned while costs continued to increase. A federal or national approach was never able to aggregate large enough support to even be taken seriously. Private sector approaches continued to receive lip service as the favored way to control costs, but how exactly to do it was not clear. People did not fully understand the causes and they would not face up to the solutions that were proposed during the early and middle 1980s.

People learned only slowly that the major causes of cost increases—first-dollar insurance coverage together with cost-based reimbursement schemes—were highly inflationary. They also provided incentives for more providers to give more services to more patients with ever increasing cost shifting to private sector payers and the providers themselves. Provider behavior is on the supply side of the economists' theory. Third-party coverage and cost reimbursement also offered massive incentives on the demand side, leading more patients to want all the technological services that modern medicine could provide, no matter whether it would be proven useful or not, no matter what the cost, since it was someone else's money paying the bills.

People never seemed to learn the lesson from defense contracting that basing payments and profits on provider costs was an open ticket for enlarging those costs. They never learned the same lesson in health care, while all the time complaining about inflation in spending, by both public and private sectors. It was the system that was responsible for good things and bad, for making doctors wealthy, raising insurance premiums, and threatening to bankrupt some state treasuries from paying entitlements.

Beneficial Effects of the Growing System

It was inflationary, but those incentives also led to a wonderful era in which to go to medical school and residency, to practice medicine, to train specialists, to do research, to perform procedures, and, particularly, to buy and use ever changing and improving medical technology. The U.S. health care system is widely recognized and acknowledged as the finest in the world by doctors, medical school deans, and politicians. All of that is the legacy of the 1980s passed forward into the 1990s. And, in the doctors' lounge, even the most pessimistic and acerbic will agree with that assessment of modern American medicine. The finest in the world at treating sickness and disease and a golden era of development, expansion, and prosperity.

It was a golden era that promised never to end. Medical practice in the United States was never so good, so fulfilling, so exciting, so limitless, and so financially rewarding. Hospitals were built to serve as workshops for hospital-based medical specialists, and the medical arms race was exciting and rewarding to manufacturers and salespeople as well. Organized medical staffs in hospitals saw only a limited view of their role in having a watchdog effect on the medical practices of themselves and their colleagues.

The quality of continuing medical education (CME) in hospitals was good, with lots of drug company subsidy. Drug companies marketed directly to the doctors and prospered well during the years of increasing costs. CME is one of the obligations of the organized medical staff and was aimed for the most part toward the hospital-based specialists who practiced there. Drug companies paid for the specialist speakers who brought news of the latest developments. Not many brought news of the latest developments in primary care, so there were not may primary care physicians in the audiences. Maybe some came to hear the speaker talk about cardiology or cancer research, or maybe some came for the free lunch and the CME credits that applied toward relicensure.

The price of this world is high, because third-party payment is inherently unrealistic since the consumer of care is shielded from its costs. A la carte medicine (sometimes referred to as fee for service) is inflationary and serves to fragment any attempt at coordination of services. Patients and doctors together pushed the system along. Patients sought out their own specialists, frequently complaining about how difficult it was to move about within the medical care system by themselves. Medical specialists became even more subspecialized and treated very well increasingly smaller portions of the whole patient. Separate payment and delivery systems cause cost shifting, because after all, it is someone else's money that is being spent. The financial incentives operated in favor of seeking out more specialists to perform more exams and studies, do more procedures, and prescribe more pharmaceutical products and medications.

One regulatory approach tried during the 1980s was to create statewide rate review systems to control hospital budget and expenditure growth. Hospital control, not doctor control. Rate review was not successful in downsizing the health care delivery system because it attempted to control only the hospital supply of care, without any impact on the doctor and hospital supply of care and patient demand for care.

CHANGING INCENTIVES

Both supply and demand will be affected by a change of incentives. Since doctors both create demand and provide supply, any changes in incentives in either direction will inevitably affect their practice lives with resulting efforts on their duties in the organized medical staff. These changes in incentives, or the threat of change, is the reason for such emotional harangue in the doctors' lounge.

Rearranging the cost/payment structure within the private sector to rearrange incentives involves changes of behavior for each element and self-interest group in the health care delivery system. For patients, changes in the 1980s meant more personal involvement in the financing of health care through co-payments and deductibles. Based on economic theories of value in investment, it is assumed that when patients pay out of pocket for care they will be more careful about utilizing medical resources. Besides, patient participation in co-payments and deductibles provide relief for the employers and insurers paying the rest of the bills. Increasing marketplace incentives were created for preventive care through more healthy lifestyles, to seek less costly care when they must, and to help pay for it so they will understand cost relationships.

Co-payments in the 1980s paved the way for large-scale entry into managed care in the 1990s. Patients became accustomed to paying a share and began to choose health plans on the basis of a lower premium. To that extent, at least, price competition had come to the health care system.

Paving the way for changing physician incentives to suit managed care also derives from the 1980s. Major departures from medical practice patterns that stress high-tech science, specialty training, and hospital-based equipment are necessary for managed care to succeed. Outpatient is better than inpatient in a managed care world. Changing emphasis to primary care based in physician offices or medical group clinics is becoming the foundation for the new system. Physicians have always competed fiercely among themselves for medical school admissions, grades, residency slots, and patient referrals. The competition that takes place in managed care by having access to patient populations through health plans is a different form from the one patient at a time approach of fee-for-service plans. In a managed care world, patients come and go in blocks. The situation is decidedly either/or. If the doctor belongs to the plan, new patients can choose or be assigned. If the doctor is not on the plan panel, there are no patients.

In a managed care system such as that being proposed by health system reformers of all parties, physicians must compete not only against each other but against hospitals, insurers, plans, and the government. All of this changing of the status quo is for competing for a piece of a smaller pie of dollars to share with younger doctors who are comfortable with working for HMO salaries and using the latest high-tech computers and medical science.

Doctors see their 1990s incentives as an opportunity to compete fiercely for the chance to make less money, see their image tarnished, exercise less and less control over their medical practices, and be less satisfied with their careers. Two things worry physicians in practice these days: one is that things may never get back to normal, and the other is that things are back and what they have now is normal.

New incentives for hospitals in a competitive system include implementing more effective management by downsizing or right-sizing manager groups and by reducing operating costs due to reduced census figures. Trying to see into the future is not easy at all. Certainly, trying to do strategic planning now is directly opposite to the incentives of a cost-based reimbursement system that emphasized adding new equipment, new programs and staff, increasing new technology, and luring physicians into bringing patients for in-hospital admissions. Dramatic changes are occurring that change the balance of power between hospital management and labor, and between hospital administration and the medical staff.

This book will focus on the traditional roles and relationships between and among doctors as individual physicians who apply to and become members of organized hospital medical staffs; doctors as a group performing as the organized medical staff doing self-governance; and the relationships between and among the medical staff, hospital administration and boards of directors. It will not venture into the realm of management/labor relationships, important as those may be, leaving that field for others to till.

Other Payment Systems

There are several other ways to pay hospitals for services performed by employees, using technology equipment and supplies bought by the hospital but ordered by physicians. Ways other than cost reimbursement, that is. During the 1990s, the health care world is exploring per-case payments, per-diem rates, fixed price arrangements, and, particularly, capitated or prepaid health plans. Capitation is increasing rapidly, while cost reimbursement is vanishing rapidly. For many hospital-based physician specialists, cost reimbursement can now be looked back on as the good old days. In those parts of the country where managed care is increasing, the Joint Commission model is undergoing severe stress. In nonmanaged care, non-HMO areas, the Joint Commission model still prevails in the grand old manner. The work of self-governance in both places is essentially the same, but the attitudes of the physician workers is not.

Per-diem selective contracting such as the MediCal program California has used, shifts financial risk to hospitals through daily limits but has virtually no effect on physicians or their practice patterns. MediCal payment rates have a great effect on physician practices and on medical staff governance, but that is another story. For per-diem patients, there is little or no discernible difference in the quality or style of inpatient care. Per-diem patients usually show a pattern of high-cost first hospital days with declining use of technology and procedures as the days pass. Hospitals lose money in the first days, hoping to make it up in later days. For physicians, there is the possibility to bill for each day. Per-diem contracting attempts to limit hospital supply of care, but is not directly aimed at reducing doctor supply of care.

DRG, or per-case payments, offer the exact opposite incentive for hospital managers. Daily cost is not the point; it is the total cost of the hospital stay that matters. Reduced length of stay becomes the object that could change physician visit fees. The DRG system has clear goals: reduce the number of surgeries, shorten lengths of stay, and reduce utilization of ancillary services. All of these are intrusions into the fondly remembered nostalgia of fee-for-service, physician-controlled practice and have heightened tensions between hospitals and doctors. This approach is a direct attempt to limit the doctor and hospital supply of care through utilization review and other mechanisms. Anything that affects the relationships between hospitals and doctors comes home to roost in the organized medical staff as it performs self-governance.

Growth of Contracting for Services

Negotiated discounts with payers that occurred in the mid-1980s and afterward could use either per-diem or per-case payment methodologies or some combination of both, but all served the same purpose of creating further contrasting hospital/physician relationships through differing responsibilities and incentives. Usually those contracts were enacted by the administration trying to bring more volume of business to the hospital to fill inpatient beds. Filling beds is a cost-reimbursement behavior that is almost directly opposite to managed care behavior. Usually those contracts were enacted without physician knowledge or participation and could have either good or bad effects on relationships. Usually those contracts, coming in the era before managed care, allowed any member of the hospital medical staff to act as the attending physician for contract patients and permitted primary care doctors to use their usual and customary referral patterns. All parties acted out behaviors drawn from and reminiscent of the fee-for-service era.

Doctors still had a lot of flexibility about diagnosis and treatment, including sometimes the ability to choose to which hospital to admit the patient. That was the period before exclusivity, which came along a few years later. Exclusive contracts were a sudden change, because doctors with privileges at several hospitals were no longer able to play the whipsaw game as easily and the administration was not quite as vulnerable to their pressure tactics as before. Nonexclusive contracts continued to preserve and encourage the traditional Joint Commission model of a hospital medical staff. Moving toward exclusive contracts changed the mix. Some doctors suddenly had access to new patients, while other doctors lost parts of their practice. Their enthusiasm for and participation in the activities of medical staff self-governance waxed and waned accordingly.

Payer contracting was the result of new militancy by the health insurance industry, which is not new to their health care scene, but has more recently achieved newer and larger political clout. Tired of being at the end of a cost-shift "crack the whip" effect, insurers were forced to find ways to reduce premium increases for their subscribers in order to succeed in their own competitive world. Contracts bring new patient volume that sometimes results in forced changes of providers. The tables are turned when hospitals, through contracts, bring patients to the doctors rather than the time-honored opposite pattern. The medical staff organization is also affected by new applicants for membership from the medical groups serving those contracts. And, gaining or losing contracts can very well result in changing the practice profiles of large admitters and heavy utilizers who have grown accustomed to some of the perks and privileges previously based on their volume and revenue streams. What a shock to the hospital industry and the doctors to discover that admitting patients and filling beds were the very worst things that could happen, depending on who the patients were!

The major new players during the 1980s were the large employers and, to some extent, their employees who collectively bargained for new health care benefits. Some of the benefits in new labor contracts were retractions of previously held coverages. Because of pressures from health care cost increases, the business sector is now the most important and powerful influence on government and the effort to reform the health care system. Employers have adopted refinements from the other major payer sources (government, insurers) and will produce the most important and long-lasting effects on the health system. The private sector is now more than a political match for the provider associations that formerly exercised the primary influence with governmental bodies in the public sector. The associations continue to be leading contributors to political campaigns and political action committees but do not win all the important votes as they once did. Politicians are not as afraid of them as before, and will take their money, but vote against them without fear of retribution.

PATIENT RESPONSES

What may be even more interesting than any approach by organized payers was the unorganized but unmistakable reaction of the American public during the 1980s. People responded to wellness incentives and paid attention to fitness, diet, exercise, smoking less, and weight loss. Part of the reason for those changes was a general feeling of responsibility for personal lifestyles, but there was also a conscious awareness of the importance of being fit in order to spend less on health care. For the growing number of employed but underinsured Americans, the object was to spend nothing at all on health care, or, if possible, going bare on insurance. For a growing number of people, access to the health care delivery system became a matter of trying to qualify for Medicaid or county assistance or seeking care on a no-pay basis from hospitals and doctors. Uncompensated care placed new and troublesome burdens on hospital medical staffs, particularly with respect to such mandatory duties as emergency room backup.

Spending less on health care became the motive for providing patient care in a continuum of less costly settings, from inpatient hospital care to ambulatory settings, subacute or skilled nursing, or home care. As capitation began to emerge on a larger scale, the scene for an increasing volume of care shifted from inpatient settings to physician offices and medical group clinics. As first-dollar coverage ended, patients, employers, and payers found more reasons not to seek health care, or at least, to seek it in less costly settings. Both of these trends were consequences of various "competitive" approaches that affected hospital medical staffs as a subset of the medical care system. Medical staffs were affected as doctors in their individual roles as caregivers, and in their collective roles as organized medical staffs performing self-governance.

SOW COMPETITION; REAP THE CONSEQUENCES

What if the economists are right? What would happen to the health care system, particularly to hospitals and doctors? Would there be changes in the delivery system and practice patterns, and what would those changes be? In theory, marketplace competition based on price should strongly emphasize a movement from inpatient to outpatient services, with resulting impact that has not yet been clearly documented and reported.

"consequences of competition" were more or less predicted by advocates of a marketplace in health care, but those were largely theoretical, since there had never been a marketplace before. Now that researchers have seen some of the actual effects, it is possible to identify and enumerate those real-world changes affecting doctors and hospitals that are no longer just theoretical. In addition to political changes that lessened the ability of provider associations to control public policy, there were payment system changes, more sharing of risk, growth in the number of health plans, new patterns of incentives, and contracts based on competitive pricing. All of these forces combined produced at least the following operational consequences for inpatient care that have been witnessed and noted (White, 1991). In fact, this could almost serve as a how-to manual for hospital managers moving into managed care.

Impact on Hospitals

Hospital utilization and delivery of care will never be the same again, due to:

• lower census figures
• shorter lengths of stay
• fewer admissions and patient days
• more empty or closed beds
• increased shift to ambulatory/outpatient care
• more subacute units
• higher average acuity for inpatients
• higher average acuity for outpatients

Changes in Services

The hospital delivery pattern will be different as these effects occur:

• less surgery
• fewer tests
• fewer x-rays
• fewer ancillary services
• fewer nursing hours per patient
• fewer days in intensive care
• reduced changing of bed linens from daily to every other day, or less

Reduced Employment

As hospital utilization shrinks, so will the numbers and kinds of employees, as well as how their jobs are structured. Downsizing or right-sizing mean the same thing to one of the victims of a layoff, such as:

- fewer hospital managers
- fewer registered nurses
- more nursing assistants
- more physician extenders
- less overtime and weekend work
- more per-diem and call work

Other Hospital Effects

Reverberating through the hospital or network will be such effects as:

- more uncompensated care
- more accounts receivable
- more hospital finance department workers
- more marketing staff
- more cost shifting
- higher insurance premiums
- lower profits
- higher losses

Impact on Physicians

Many of the changes that have occurred during the ebb and flow of hospitals through the past three decades have skipped over the doctors, but not this time, showing such dramatic changes as:

- lower physician incomes
- change of medical practice patterns by reducing elective procedures
- elimination of standing orders for presurgical or predelivery workups
- reduced preadmission testing
- more utilization review
- more medical necessity scrutiny
- more services ruled inappropriate
- increased demand for primary care physicians
- decreased demand for specialist physicians

Physician Practice Changes

In their office or clinic practices, doctors will notice these effects:

- more need to hire office practice clerks, billers, and insurance workers
- more physicians trying to join medical groups

- more physicians refused by medical groups
- more medical groups
- more practices sold or closed
- more physicians responding to surveys by stating that they would not go to medical school now if they had it all to do over again
- more and faster transition from fee for service to contracts to capitation

Effects on the Medical Community

These changes in practice patterns and payment systems are not going unnoticed, with parallel developments including:

- fewer new doctors entering solo practice
- fewer doctors staying in solo practice
- more women in medical school entering classes
- more women graduating from medical school
- more new doctors, both male and female, willing to work for groups or HMOs because of positions that offer regular salary and regular hours
- more former specialists thinking about providing primary care

Effect on the Medical Staff

The organized medical staff cannot escape these tensions and alterations that affect its members and the hospital where they practice. They will see such forces as:

- more tension between medical staff physicians and their elected leaders
- more tension between medical staffs and hospital administration
- more tension between individual physicians and hospital administration
- more apparent need for severity-adjusted data systems
- more resistance to installing quality data systems
- more need for clinical pathways, guidelines, and algorithms
- more need for the spirit of cooperation and quality improvement that encourages pathways, guidelines, and algorithms

Health Care System

In the larger health care system, at both state and national levels, there will be some other, more generalized changes occurring as consequences of this move deeper into price competition, such as:

- reduced demand for care
- reduced supply of care
- more focus on prevention and wellness
- more incentives for cost conscious behavior by doctors and patients alike
- more pressure on public hospitals
- more hospital closures and mergers
- intensified growth of regional health care systems and networks
- more not-for-profit hospitals becoming for-profit

And finally, to cap off this list of painful complications, there will be a manifest increase in the occurrence of moral/ethical dilemmas about withholding or withdrawing of care.

More Consequences of Competition

All the while, during the period of time when these events are actually occurring, the beat goes on as medical staffs perform credentialing, privileging, reappointment, and peer review. As new doctors continue to apply to the staff, they proceed through the same bureaucratic process as always, which never seems to move any faster in a competitive world than it does in a fee-for-service world. Eventually they are (or are not) approved for membership and privileges by the governing board. The Joint Commission model of a medical staff is alive and well, still in place and still doing its job in spite of all of those waves of change crashing about its ears. There may be the sounds of gloom and doom in the doctors' lounge about change, but the work goes on uninterrupted.

Looking back from the vantage point of the mid-1990s, the picture that can be seen of this evolutionary process during the decade just past is that it was necessary to go through those changes. It is clear now that competition did work somewhat, but it did not work completely or on a widespread basis. It is clear now that cost increases can be slowed or halted altogether by price competition and managed care, just as the economists have said. It is also clear now that more fractionalization of the system will be produced, and there will be repeated entreaties for physicians to become "partners" with hospitals.

In the end, cost increases will continue to occur on a piecemeal basis unless a universal application controls all, not just some, of the U.S. health care delivery system. Medical practice was changed forever by DRGs and other payment reforms during the 1980s and so were hospital/medical staff relationships. The competitive systems of the 1990s will see, and even force, still more dramatic changes in those relationships as larger and still larger integrated health care systems flourish and prosper. Jerry Brown, as governor of California from 1974 to 1985, frequently said in his political speeches that small is better, but in the next iteration of the health care system, big may be better.

/er, the combined growth of HMOs, discount employer contracts, government er-diem or per-case payments, and preferred-discount private payers together
constituted a concentrated attack on the 80/20 or Pareto principle of insurance theory
that has been the foundation of all insurance payment systems for decades, including
health insurance. The significant few (20%) utilize more services than the insignificant
many (80%), but each premium payer paid the same rate whether they used insurance
services or not. The 80/20 principle had allowed a few, very ill people to have the cost
of their care spread across a wide base of well persons in a cost-shift approach that was
recognized, approved, and marketed. That particular cost shift has been socially acceptable and politically correct for centuries.

Segregation of the patient market is the outcome of competitive systems where
healthy, middle-aged working adults are ideal customers (low-dollar, low-risk). These
patients, when in the private sector, have always been the source of support for subsidy
of public patients through cost shifting. Competition sorts out the high-tech, high-risk
patients that no payment systems wants to sponsor, resulting in patient dumping or ever
greater amounts of uncompensated care absorbed by private hospitals and doctors.

Competition also short circuits any charitable inclination to care for high-risk social
unfortunates, thus creating a moral, ethical, legal, and financial dilemma for taxpayers.
Heart-rending stories of incredibly ill patients who need medical miracles become sta-
ples for TV anchor people who seek help and support during one segment of the evening
news broadcast, while in a later segment station management rails against the high cost
of health care during the editorial. For this problem of high-cost patients, sponsored or
not, the situation will certainly get worse before it gets better. Being forced to care for
unsponsored patients is a strong source of friction within the medical community and
within the medical staff, where a staff member faces the same disciplinary consequences
for inappropriate care of an unpaid patient as any full-pay patient.

Of course, quality of care *should* be the highest possible goal for everyone, but isn't
that an incentive to try to evade such patients? That is exactly what happens more and
more often with E.R. backup. Backup problems are one of the most frustrating and
intractable tensions between the medical staff and administration. Backup problems set
the recalcitrant physicians against the chief of staff and forces that officer into the camp
of the administration on this issue. The chief is sworn to uphold the bylaws and rules of
professional behavior contained within. So are the members, of course, but that agreement, signed on the medical staff application form, may get lost in the shuffle.

One of the consequences of a cost-based system is that there is no limit on the development of new services and procedures, but there can be considerable debate on the reasonable cost of a service. In a competitive system, it is necessary to consider whether the
service should be offered at all. The theory of a gatekeeper approach by a primary care
doctor is based on delaying or denying of services by specialists unless strongly indicated. It is not so much that the patient does not receive the service, but it may now be per-

formed in the primary care office instead of a hospital specialty unit. The primary care gatekeeper now decides whether a specialist is needed, not the patient or the specialist. Specialists do what they were trained to do, and have all of the package of incentives in the fee-for-service system to recommend themselves and their specialized services for treatment of the patient's condition.

Cost reimbursement rewards and encourages specialty medicine and use of more training and technology. Departmentalization of the medical staff is encouraged for closer professional relationships and protection among the specialties. Growth of new professions and their societies is stimulated. All of this calls for more advanced training, higher degrees, more certification, more barriers for entry into the field, higher pay, greater incomes, bigger houses, foreign cars, and capitol-based lobbyists to ensure access to legislators and protection from competitors.

Downsizing

A competitive environment works against each of these characteristics by forcing hospitals to consider what services can be provided within revenue limits. Inevitably, as competition grows more managed, hospitals will move away from the 1980s cost-reimbursement model of full service and will become more specialized as financial margins shrink. A specialized hospital, one that does fewer things well, probably for fewer patients, also means an inadequate volume of work for fewer specialized physicians, relating to fewer professional staff, with less total technology and more generalized procedures. Certainly, it means reduction in the manager group, fewer bonuses for executives, a medical staff that has fewer physicians giving less service to fewer patients in the inpatient setting because of lower census figures brought about by shifting to outpatient settings. That is what downsizing means, and it has a profound effect on medical staff self-governance.

The most important skill for a hospital administrator to have in a world like that is to be able to fire people and still sleep at night. Especially helpful will be the ability to fire those assistant and associate administrators who were recruited and hired only a few years earlier at great expense. Downsizing or right-sizing also has profound financial impact on an institution that needs financial improvement by reducing quickly the expenses of personnel salaries and wages, particularly in a purge of those middle management/technical experts who worked hard and probably have given the hospital its unique character and culture. But achieving success through working hard with a lot of devotion, working smart, and showing a good work ethic can become a recipe for termination when the salary gets too high in the world of managed care of the 1990s.

Terminating middle management is only a quick, one-time fix that does not address the more costly long-term issue: a medical staff that is still practicing old-time, every man for himself, fee-for-service medicine that utilizes resources in a far greater volume ie middle managers ever dreamed of. Downsizing affects the total numbers of medical staff membership by reducing the range of hospital services provided, which leads to reductions in the number and kinds of new applicants and what privileges they request. Downsizing reduces supply by decreasing the total volume of services provided. Downsizing reduces the mix of professional and technical staff who act out physician-order sheets. When patient and service mix are changed that much, it is not the same hospital any more. That is the way it must be in moving from a hospital world of cost-based reimbursement and fees for service to a managed care, primary office/clinic-based delivery system. Most of all, downsizing affects the tenuous relationships between hospital and medical staff as those feelings are reflected in the performance of self-governance work (White, 1991).

MIDWAY THROUGH THE CHANGE PROCESS

The U.S. medical care system is midway between the cost-based, fee-for-service world just left and the reform world of total managed care, which may (or may not) lie directly ahead. Doctors and hospitals, as well as many patients, are in the middle, with many of them trying desperately to cling to the old against the tide of the new. The swift are, meanwhile, trying their best to eat the slow. It is truly an ungainly process, watching the system as it seems to be lurching crabwise toward reform that seems destined to be based on theories of managed care and risk sharing between doctors and hospitals or health care systems. The 1995 delivery system exists as a mixture of points of service, including:

- physician and other provider offices
- clinics
- hospital inpatient facilities
- hospital outpatient facilities
- subacute facilities
- skilled nursing facilities
- board and care facilities
- home care

These services are provided by a wide variety of caregivers, supported by personnel and employees as well as some volunteers. They are paid (or not paid) for by some mixture of public, private, and personal payment systems that include:

- federal tax funds
- state tax funds
- county tax funds

- insurance payments
- self-pay
- no pay

Why does this health care system cost so much? Everyone shares the blame: consumers, providers, insurers, other payers. All suffer from unreasonable expectations.

Consumers have shown that they want top-quality comprehensive health care services whenever needed but do not want to pay the necessary amounts of funding support that is required. That means *increasing demand.*

Hospitals have amply demonstrated that their leaders want top-of-the-line technology, equipment, and services that will continue to attract physicians, patients, and payers. That means steadily *increasing supply* through capital expansion.

Physicians have expressed that they want relief from regulatory and competitive restrictions, return to fee-for-service practice, and to continue to have the ability to use multiple hospitals by choice. Practice overhead and total office expenditures have grown under either system in excess of any measure of inflation, and there appears to be no way solo or small group practices can reduce that overhead with the income from capitated patients.

Insurers want to stay in business by controlling costs, keeping premiums from increasing, maintaining market share and profits, and, as far as possible, accepting only low-risk patients.

All of these conflicting demands are compounded by more recession; more downsizing by business and industry; a declining defense industry; and more unemployed, more uninsured, and many more employed but underinsured patients. AIDS, environmental hazards, and other economic pressures have increased tendencies to cost shift health care expenses to what few paying patients remain. At the same time, federal costs for uncompensated care have been shifted to the states, from state governments to counties, and from counties primarily to private doctors and hospitals.

No system is perfect. No system will provide state-of-the-art medicine to everyone who demands it without someone paying for it. One way to reduce overall costs would be to reduce both supply by providers and demand by consumers, but there have been no offers yet by either group to voluntarily reduce their portion of the supply/demand equation in health care.

EFFECT ON THE MEDICAL STAFF

At any point in time, the world is a product of its accumulated history, and so is the hospital medical staff. Reform and restructuring of the U.S. health care system is currently gathering speed, affecting medical practice. The demographic shift brought about by increasing numbers and political power of the elderly added to the volume of demand for services with accompanying increases in total cost. Many services provided to the elderly are provided through in-hospital care by specialist-physicians, thus extending the traditional nature of the Joint Commission model.

Meanwhile, medical technology continues its relentless advance, adding more possibilities for medical miracles at heroic costs, along with the gut-wrenching ethical/legal problems that accompany those increased choices. Bioethical issues can only increase as more choices must be made between cost and caring. Patients show greater willingness to explore promises of nontechnical or nonphysician healing services. That represents a greater volume of total services, but at a lower per-unit cost and fewer hospital admissions, unless of course, the patient becomes seriously ill, which will mean emergency department treatment, a stay in the intensive care unit, and possibly no payment for any of it.

More active patients will pay attention to preventive activities and habits, changing lifestyles, diets, exercise, and endorsing wellness concepts. Science and payers will devise more and better ways to measure and compare health outcomes and utilization, seeking to know better how comparisons between volume of high-risk procedures and success measures such as mortality rates can be used for better effect. Specialist-physicians will feel more pressured by studies of severity-adjusted length of stay, infection rates, and returns to surgery and complications, particularly as those indicators are used for economic credentialing by medical groups and health plans.

As well, there will be increased scrutiny of the behavior of some of those doctors whose verbal or even physical abuse will no longer be tolerated, no matter how many patients they have customarily brought to the hospital. Some of these outbursts are for the same reasons they existed in the past: a mean and nasty personality that was tolerated by colleagues and hospital managers, particularly if the guilty party was a heavy admitter. But similar outbursts by some usually reasonable good guys can be caused by feelings of anger at loss of control, loss of income or referrals, or invasion of their "territory" by utilization review nurses or by the identification of out-of-pattern utilizers through outcomes-measuring systems that would dare to trample on physician judgment and individual practice patterns.

The problem lies in trying to persuade people to change who do not see any need to change. Things were doing very well and the world was a predictable place. They do not want to change. Perhaps George Washington said it best in his Second Annual Address in 1789:

> One of the difficulties in bringing about change in an organization is that you must do so through persons who have been most successful in the organization, no matter how faulty that system or organization is. To such persons, you see, it is the best of all possible organizations, because look who was selected by it and look who succeeded most within it. Yet, these are the very people through whom we must bring about the improvement.

Remember, at some point in the future, some people will look back and call these the good old days.

SUMMARY

The cause of all the turmoil is a changing health care delivery and payment system in the 1990s. Both the individual practice of medicine and the health and medical system of the nation seem to be up for grabs, with an uncertain future. Health reform legislation ebbs and flows with more piecework modifications but without a major overhaul, yet. Prior periods of reform and change brought about the stage setting for competition in health care, managed competition, managed care, cost containment, universal access, portability, and other buzzwords. It is still not clear whether price competition in health care lowers prices, increases availability and accessibility, or actually results in the destabilization of a complex hospital/medical industry that requires mutual trust to be able to function.

There is an experiment going on to see whether HMO concepts of managed care will replace the traditional fee-for-service insurance coverage and open choice of physicians. It is also not clear whether that open choice model can deliver care at a cost approximately the same as a closed system model. Inflation in costs spurred the economic argument that there was no price competition or a market in health care and that first-dollar insurance coverage along with cost-based reimbursement schemes were the cause. Those incentives for higher volumes of highly specialized services helped to create an era of high technology, high quality, and financial rewards, where consumers of care were shielded from costs.

Rearranging the cost/payment structure will affect both supply and demand for care, as well as involve changes in behavior for both providers and consumers of care. Prominent among these incentive-driven changes is downsizing or right-sizing, either or both of which means firing employees. As price competition grows, there are consequences to anticipate and consider, including, of course, the movement from inpatient to outpatient care. Other effects that are detailed in the chapter are a chronicle of the events that could occur when a hospital enters this new world, which is not necessarily brave.

REFERENCES

Anderson, O. W. (1991). Health services in the United States: A growth enterprise for a hundred years. In Litman, T. J., & Robins, L. S. (Eds.), *Health Politics and Policy (2nd ed.).* Albany: Delmar Publishers.

Washington, G. (1789). Second Annual Address to Congress. In Flexner, J. T. (1970). *George Washington and the New Nation (1783–1793)*. Boston: Little, Brown and Company.

White, C. H. (1991). The consequences of competition. In Dunlap, H. E. (Ed.), *Fifty Years: An Anthology by Ten Contributors Who Helped Shape the History of California Hospitals*. Glendale, CA: Bright Publishers.

CHAPTER

What Is
Managed Care?

Probably the most dramatic realignment of the nation's health care delivery system in recent years has been the development of managed care plans. Managed care is a generic term that has evolved over the past few years to encompass a variety of forms of prepaid and managed fee-for-service health care. But, exactly what do people mean when they use those words?

Under managed care programs, the fundamental incentive structure of traditional fee-for-service medicine is dramatically altered to encourage greater control over the use and costs of health care services (Williams & Torrens, 1993).

The concepts incorporated into managed care programs involve restructuring the delivery system for health care services; providing appropriate incentives and barriers for providers and consumers to contain costs; imposing an administrative structure with various components relating to managing the enrolled population and its use of services; and facilitating the paperwork required on the part of consumers (Kongstvedt, 1989).

Managed care represents a serious challenge to both consumers and providers in their traditional approaches to the provision of health care. The underlying concepts of managed care hold promise for allowing more comprehensive services to greater numbers of people while providing significant incentives for providers to contain the use and cost of those services. The risk concept that is so much a part of managed care threatens financial ruin for the providers if those goals are not accomplished and the dislocations of changing plans and doctors again for consumers. It is essential that the structure and implications of managed care systems be well understood by everyone involved in providing and using health care. It is equally essential for those same elements to be well understood by policymakers before and during their efforts to reform a health system that, much of the time, does not want to be reformed.

While managed care has been evolving over the years, many of its underlying concepts have already become institutionalized within the delivery system. These principles are likely to remain in place, in one form or another, regardless of the further evolution of managed care and potential legislative or regulatory reform of the health care system itself. It would be helpful to pose a definition that can summarize all of these concepts into one statement that can be used for quoting and dissemination.

Managed care is the organization, management, and direction of

- the expenditure of *finite resources*
- by a *defined* group of *providers*
- to an *identified* group of *enrollees*
- for prevention, treatment, and amelioration of disease and its consequences
- against *explicit standards* of care
- in the most *efficient, effective,* and *economic* manner
- for the health and benefit of both the *population at large* and the *individual* served.

It will also be helpful to compare and contrast some similarities and differences represented in the movements in the health care delivery system now taking place, in order to explain in as few words as possible what managed care is and is not. The basic underlying concepts of change in large-scale social or organizational structures involve moving from one pattern of structure and behavior to another, or in the favorite buzzword of the 1990s, a paradigm shift, such as Table 25–1.

Day-by-day details of medical practice are affected by each of these changes, both in the way care is paid for and in the ways that physicians relate to their patients and to each other. Another way to look at the paradigm shift would include the characteristics shown in Table 25–2.

A workshop presentation by Frederick Porcase of Des Moines was helpful in assembling these contrasts between practice and payment styles. Similarly, workshop and training material by Jacque Sokolov present a point of view about the evolutionary

TABLE 25–1 Delivery system changes

From	*To*
Acute inpatient care	Continuum of care
Treating illness	Maintaining wellness
Caring for an individual patient	Accountable for health status of groups
Product	Value-added service
Market share of admissions	Covered lives
Fill hospital beds	Care provided at the appropriate level
Manage an organization	Manage a network of services
Manage a department	Manage a market
Coordinate services	Actively manage quality

process between and among what he labeled "generations" of managed care, shown in Table 25–3.

To further contrast the changes represented by the evolution of managed care through Sokoloff's construct of at least three generations so far, here is another pictorial representation presented in Table 25–4.

TABLE 25–2 Medical practice changes

From	*To*
Fee-for service	Capitation
Retrospective payment	Prospective payment
Cost based	Price based
Individual focused	Population focused
Episodic	Continuous
Intervention	Prevention
Revenue generation	Resource conservation
Retail	Wholesale
Procedures	Relationships
Aggressive	Conservative
Cost shifting	Risk shifting
Autonomous	Interdependent
Decision maker	Facilitator/team player
Spend money to make money	Spend money to save money

TABLE 25–3   Evolution of managed care

First generation managed care	• Benefits limits • Utilization review • Second surgical opinion
Second generation managed care	• Benefit differential • Provider networks • Utilization management
Third generation managed care	• Quantitative quality measures • Patient care management teams • Advanced physician selection and monitoring

The paradigm shift, or the evolution of managed care, or whatever it is being called is not a smooth and easy path. Profound and major change never is, because, as George Washington noted, it is the very people who have been most successful in the old system who are being asked to voluntarily change to the new system, knowing perfectly well that things will not be as good for them. There are a number of obstacles that confound and bedevil the best laid plans and good intentions of the planners and architects of change. All advocates of competition or managed competition or managed care speak in the same language about the need for partnerships between physicians and someone else, depending upon who it is that wants them to join the club and participate, whether willingly or not. These same advocates who want the doctors to change will agree that there are formidable difficulties that must be overcome if, indeed, there are to be formations of these physician/plan or physician/system or physician/hospital partnerships. The systemic or organic reasons why physicians as individuals, and the hospital medical staff as a participatory democracy, find it hard to move away from what they liked to what they fear they will not like are usually expressed as shown in Table 25–5.

TABLE 25–4   Contrast with the current system

Today's approach	*Third generation*
Large preferred provider network	Highly selective network
Providers rewarded for volume	Providers rewarded for performance
Bureaucratic Administration	Customer-driven administration
Fragmented patient care	Coordinated health management

TABLE 25–5   Partnership barriers

- Revenue vs. cost culture
- Specialty-controlled medical staff
- Weak primary care leadership
- Ignorance of the business of medicine
- Lack of trust
- Primary physician time constraints
- Lack of board understanding
- Conflicting economics among
  - Hospital
  - Specialists
  - Primary care
  - Ancillaries

In the indemnity insurance, fee-for-service system there were incentives for patients to want all the medical care they could get, and incentives for the doctors to provide all the services they could give, because it was someone else's money. The whole point of managed care is that now, it is the patient's money and the doctor's money!

DELIVERING MANAGED CARE

The fundamental concepts of managed care—prepayment of services or discounted fee-for-service arrangements for defined, enrolled populations—has a rather extensive history, and has actually existed for quite some time. To most people, however, managed care means HMOs. For more than 20 years, HMOs have been expected by their supporters to deliver the United States health care system from the problems that have plagued the fee-for-service delivery system. These problems include:

- runaway costs
- episodic care
- overuse of high-tech care

HMOs

Politicians and policymakers from Nixon to Clinton have featured HMOs in their versions of health care reform at the federal level. Numerous state programs have moved in that direction also. The idea particularly appeals to politicians, because it puts the onus for retarding cost increases on the private sector, sparing them the kinds of fights over regulatory cost controls that inhibit campaign contributions from the providers whose ox has been gored. The largest and strongest vote of confidence in HMOs has come from the employers, who view prepaid capitation as the best available means for ensuring quality while managing costs. Some employee benefits managers and human resources professionals have staked out a position that HMOs are the *only* hope for restraining the mammoth cost increases in recent years that have had such a profound effect on corporate prices and earnings (Kent, 1994).

The recent origin of today's managed care programs in the United States dates from the inclusion of health maintenance organizations (HMOs) in federal legislation during the Nixon administration as an approach to reorganizing health care services to facilitate cost containment and to control utilization. The intent of promoting prepayment plans that incorporated both the group practice model and the independent practice association (IPA) model was to strengthen private sector medicine through self-regulation, while at the same time incorporating some incentives for containment of health care costs. It is one of those interesting bits of strange arrangements that occur in politics, that a Republican president fostered a program that was such anathema to so many of the members of organized medicine and the hospital industry who made campaign contributions and voted for him. The legislation was passed, but no one will ever know how strongly the Nixon administration would have pushed creation and adoption of HMOs as a form of health care reform, because Watergate got in the way and attention was not refocused on health care reform.

Prepaid group practices, such as HMOs, got off to an early success in providing comprehensive and acceptable quality health services for lower total costs than the fee-for-service sector. One of the provisions of the federal legislation that helped develop HMOs included the dual choice requirement under which certain employers had to offer an HMO health care option to employees. This established the precedent for employer endorsement and introduced, perhaps forever, the twin concepts of co-payments and deductibles that were not a usual feature of first-dollar indemnity coverage. Many employers now offer as the only choice some form of managed care plan as the fully paid benefit. In that case, employees may choose an IPA or fee-for-service arrangement as their choice instead of a prepaid or capitated plan but at a much larger out-of-pocket cost to them. One of the problems that emerged for the new HMOs were difficulties in attaining financial viability, which may have been the result of federal program requirements that included offering a full range of services as well as a period of open enrollment during which anyone could join without concern for preexisting conditions. Of course, there was some poor management that caused part of the failures, both early and late.

The most successful prepaid groups have generally been the larger, better capitalized plans or those serving populations with high levels of insurance coverage. Staff model group practice plans were the HMO type that fit the federal prototype. These group practices provide prepaid, rather than fee-for-service, care through intermediaries that enroll consumers and assume responsibility for all covered care. The characteristic of these plans has been to provide incentives to both providers and consumers that are intended to reward the ensuring of access to high-quality care while also containing costs (Williams & Torrens, 1993).

IPAs

When HMOs were originally proposed, consideration was also given to allow forms of prepaid health care that could be provided by community-based physicians, rather than by just the closed medical staff group practices. A second organizational format, the IPA, was formed by affiliations of independent practitioners in the community who, in addition to their fee-for-service patients, contract to provide care for prepaid, enrolled individuals. In this format, the IPA sells the insurance product as a prepaid program with a set monthly premium for all covered services. The IPA organization, usually formed and run by physicians with some professional management help, signs up community-based solo and group practitioners and provides an opportunity for participation in prepaid health care delivery by physicians who are not part of closed panel programs. It is not at all unusual for these IPA physicians to be quite hostile toward the closed panels, particularly to the point of considering them as the major competition.

It was not uncommon for the early IPAs to reimburse physicians using an open-ended, fee-for-service fee schedule, while the plan itself collected revenues on a prepaid basis, in contrast to the salary arrangements of the closed panel plans. One of many characteristics these IPA plans had in common was an initial capital investment, donated by the participating doctors who were determined to strike back at the group practices. Donate was the right word to use, since the bankruptcy of many of these plans meant that the original investment was never recouped, and neither were the outstanding bills for services already rendered. Chances are that if the plan failed, these claims were never paid.

Another feature was physician management, as the doctors wanted to prove to everyone that they could do a better job than the administrators. But the real problem was the failure to control the use of services and resources by the doctors, whose incentives continued to be those of the fee-for-service system. Increased use, more volume, and more procedures rewarded the specialists but not the plan, and so they failed. That constitutes the worst of both payment system worlds (fee-for-service utilization, and prepaid or capitated payment). It cannot be done. IPAs were an expensive bath for some physicians. From the standpoint of the hospital medical staff, IPAs were just more of the same practice styles the members were accustomed to rendering, and it was not really a partnership with the hospital or the emerging integrated system. Other than the source of the reimbursement checks that came to the doctors' offices, the medical staff continued down its familiar Joint Commission path.

PPOs and EPOs

While managed care experiments were taking place, another concept not too dissimilar to the IPA occurred in many places. The preferred provider (PPO) organization combines the aspects of fee discounting with IPA membership concepts. A PPO sponsor can be an insurance company, an employer or some other entity that contracts with participating hospitals, doctors, medical groups, and other providers to offer services to plan members or enrollees. The usual characteristic is for the doctors to be reimbursed on a contracted fee basis using an established fee schedule for specific procedures or on a defined, negotiated discount on usual and customary fees, established in advance. Some PPOs also included requirements for utilization review and other quality controls, whether or not these have been as strongly focused as similar programs in the closed panel group practices. Where controls lean more toward IPAs, there will be leakage in the system. Where they lean more in the direction of the closed panels, there should be more functional monitoring.

Patients who enrolled in the PPO agreed to use only contracted providers to obtain maximum benefit under the plan. Thus there was some loss of access and freedom of choice for the consumers. Patients could always obtain care outside the contracted network, but with a substantially reduced level of coverage and correspondingly increased out-of-pocket expense. Typically, PPOs require 30 to 50 percent co-payments, based on allowable charges, for care by nonparticipating providers. These numbers are in comparison to the usual standard deductible and co-payments of 5 to 10 percent of allowable charges for covered services provided by doctors who are participants in the plan. The message to the consumer patient is clear: stay in the plan, and use doctors who are on the panel.

Most payers now offer a PPO option as well as an HMO choice. Few offer any kind of indemnity option any more, although there are still some prophets in the doctors' lounge who remain convinced that indemnity, fee-for-service medicine is coming back and that all this managed care stuff is crazy. Another extension of the PPO is the exclusive provider organization (EPO). EPOs are usually more restrictive for consumers' access and choice than PPOs. These plans reward providers by channeling patients, usually in groups, thus reversing the old role where doctors brought patients to the hospital.

A closed panel, staff group practice model of a managed care provider organization forms itself by selecting physicians to be members of the group. IPA and PPO panels must also form themselves, but they usually do it by developing networks of community providers who are less related in a formal structure. Provider networks have both solo practitioners and groups. Each provider signs contracts with the managed care sponsor and agrees to the specific terms and conditions of the plan, including such important items as fee schedules, discounts, and whatever utilization review requirements exist.

Whatever are the terms and conditions, they do not include a mandate that the doctor must only treat patients from this contract or plan, leaving the physician free to join others as well. The decision making here is the most important factor. In closed panels, the leadership of the medical group negotiates and signs contracts, and the members of the group are bound by them. In the other models, each doctor still reserves the right to sign one contract at a time, thus preserving more options for the physician, as well as preserving the feeling that what is occurring is not really managed care but is just a latter day extension of independent practice, even if it is not exactly fee-for-service.

EFFECTS ON PHYSICIANS

An important and practical issue, in regard to physicians and their practices, is the effect of having both fee-for-service and prepaid or managed care patients. That is a practice choice of the individual doctor. Hospitals can enter into managed care contracts with or without members of the medical staff. A hospital could contract independently, which could cause problems if the physician members of the panel are not members of the staff. The credentialing process will not be short circuited or made easier in order to accommodate these "intruders."

As Williams and Torrens (1993) point out, the managers of group practices or hospitals participating in a managed care contract will want "their" physicians to regulate and control their use of services for enrolled plan members or patients, particularly with regard to inpatient hospital care. That attitude is from the managers' standpoint. From the doctor's standpoint, it only makes sense to increase fee-for-service revenue by enhancing use of services and procedures, including lab, pharmacy, imaging, and specialty referrals within the group or the regular referral patterns. This conflict in incentives places the hospital or group and the administrators in the position of sending signals to the doctors that are direct opposites. Managed care plans and their managers want less service and fewer hospital patients, and so do the hospitals sharing risk in that same contract. Both the doctors and the hospitals benefit from the cost shifting available in other types of insurance coverages and more generous payments. There will be a noticeable difference, also, in the approach to utilization review, with more focus on use rates than on quality indicators alone. The Joint Commission model is decidedly anachronistic in its ability to mediate this sort of puzzle.

The doctors will resent the degree of control and interference that necessarily results when a group practice that serves both fee-for-service and managed care patients tries to determine how to reimburse for both types. Within each physician's practice there could then be conflicting incentives provided to the doctors to enhance use by fee-for-service patients and reduce the utilization by managed care or at-risk patients. Most doctors and their office staffs are really not good at, and not very interested in, trying to offer two standards of care based on a patient's payment source.

Other concerns of physicians in solo practice in networks or contracts include the sudden assignment of a large panel of new patients. The same thing is also true with groups. New patients always require the opening of new files, the making of initial appointments, and initial efforts to determine health status. Both group practice doctors and those in solo practice are concerned with the risk of adverse selection, particularly when there is open enrollment. Physicians in control of their own practices are usually able to limit the total number of patients for which they have assumed responsibility by screening beneficiaries based on clinical criteria. But contracts, especially those having no restriction on preexisting conditions, carry the threat of adverse selection. The group or the solo doctor can be at a substantial level of liability if there is a high degree of risk sharing in the contract. Stop-loss insurance does offer some amount of protection.

Entry into the world of managed care contracts also brings along another essential that may be relatively foreign to the doctors, the concepts of risk management. Hospitals have employed people called *risk managers,* who had more to do with setting up notification systems that would give early warning in the event of a possible liability claim or lawsuit. Now, the doctors must become accustomed to the entire panoply of binding arbitration, positive patient relationships, more productive doctor-patient interactions so as to reduce complaints, and the ever present utilization review. Good risk management also includes careful attention to the terms of contracts, fair and accurate bidding on those contracts; monitoring systems of the doctors' practices to indicate use patterns and costs, generally called *resource allocations.* There will be a variety of quality assurance systems and mechanisms that may be the same as the peer review described in Chapter 7. Or, as in some of the more sophisticated groups, there may be quality improvement mechanisms that go far beyond the traditional Joint Commission medical staff standards. The difference is that now most of the members of at-risk contracts are truly protecting themselves from each other, and the traditionalist attitude no longer applies.

Risk management also includes some insurance concepts that most of the doctors will not be interested in or not be good at, such as adequate underwriting and stop-loss protections, malpractice coverage, adequate capital reserving, and opportunity to reopen the contract for renegotiation at specified terms.

Networks do offer the consumer more freedom of choice and access than the closed plans, by making available a wider geographic spread of primary care physicians (PCPs), hospitals, and other providers. As specialty care providers become integrated into systems such as these, there begins to be greater control exerted over use and costs, and the resulting rigidity is exactly what the doctors who went that way were trying to evade. As control grows, so does the dissatisfaction of some of the doctors, and the lounge erupts again in the same type of turmoil that happened a few months before. "I told you so," becomes the rallying cry, because it must be the administrator's fault. The Joint Commission model is spectacularly ill equipped to deal with dissension and practice differences such as this, but the organized medical staff is the only vehicle available for expressing concerns and unhappiness. The chief of staff did not cause the growth and constricting control of the plan or the provider network, but that person will be blamed for it and be expected by a few to fix the problem or be accused of not representing the staff.

Even in their early developmental years, HMOs were viewed by economists, employers, and governmental policymakers as a practical and viable alternative to traditional fee-for-service medicine and one that would help to stem the apparently rapid and uncontrollable escalation in health care costs. HMOs gained employer political support and consumer credibility in some states, while failing to penetrate other states at all. There were HMO failures, just as there were IPA failures, due to the same reasons: managerial incompetence or, sometimes, downright fraud.

CHARACTERISTICS OF MANAGED CARE PROGRAMS

There are a number of operational characteristics of managed care programs that are designed to affect both the operation and structure of the health care delivery system as well as the use of services by patients or consumers. These concepts are intended to affect and change both supply of and demand for services and have an impact on quality, access, cost, consumer choice and satisfaction, doctor-patient relationships, and the role of insurers.

Gatekeepers

Among the most important of these concepts about how to perform managed care is the role of the primary care physician (PCP) as a gatekeeper. The gatekeeper concept is that one individual physician—usually a PCP in family practice, internal medicine, or, in specific instances, pediatrics or obstetrics/gynecology—is responsible for all primary care for the patient. The PCP also determines when referral to specialists is needed and provides an oversight and coordinating role for all the patient's health care needs. The gatekeeper concept is designed to manage the patient's use of resources, to reduce the self-initiated use of specialty services, and to ensure overall coordination, not duplication, of services (Williams & Torrens, 1993).

Gatekeepers can function in two different ways that could affect the care of the patient with a resulting effect on the medical staff. Patient care management and coordination of services can go very smoothly, but those are mostly outpatient or office based in nature. As such, these services are unknown and invisible to the hospital and the medical staff. Gatekeepers can also be a barrier to access to specialty services. Since most of these are performed by hospital-based or related doctors, hospital utilization and the performance of procedures can be dramatically altered. The PCP may underrefer to specialists, depending on practice patterns and the particular financial incentives built into the plan. It is not as likely that PCPs will overrefer to hospital-based specialists, since it is now "their money" that is at stake, with no deep pocket to bail out the PCP. The gatekeeper concept has received large doses of conventional wisdom that it will work well to be cost-effective while still improving quality of care, but there is little real evidence to prove it. That gatekeepers will work well to provide coordination of care seems much more intuitively acceptable and easier to demonstrate through patient testimonials. Another real question is whether there are enough primary care physicians whose training and experience is good enough so that these doctors can function as effective gatekeepers. It is certain that the generation of doctors practicing now were not taught a class on how to be gatekeepers at the time they attended medical school or residency.

There is another worry about the gatekeeper concept: whether the ethical base of the traditional physician/patient relationship still exists. Of course, for patients who did not have a personal physician, there never was a relationship. But critics still will say that inherent in all cost containment, such as that represented by managed care, is limited access to services. Thus, the only really successful cost control is not delivering services at all. So, if the gatekeeper oversees the entire care plan of the patient, balances cost and quality, serves as a filter for need and appropriateness, then the gatekeeper is in the business of rationing services. That is the ethical dilemma: balancing profitability of the plan against the health care needs of the patient.

Physician Payment

Various managed care programs or plans pay physicians using a number of mechanisms. In the closed staff model, group practice HMO, doctors are paid on a salary basis with some incentive compensation, usually distributed at year end based on the overall profitability of the plan and the productivity of the individual. This approach seems, at face value, to be more of an apparent partnership arrangement than those the hospitals dangle before physicians on the medical staff. Maybe they are not really different, but it seems more likely and more obvious to the doctors that they could be partners in a financial arrangement that might resolve in their favor with other doctors, rather than with their ancient enemy, the hospital.

In some other managed care arrangements involving PPOs, the participating community-based physicians may be reimbursed on a fee-for-service, discounted fee basis, or they may receive capitation payments with bonus or additional incentive payments if there is any money left over at the end of the year. These arrangements do not carry with them the same degree of feeling about being partners, either with the other doctors or with the hospitals. There is not the same attitude that without the attention to utilization control of each doctor, the plan will suffer financial hardship. For some doctors in this sort of plan, there is a cynicism that there will not be any money remaining at the end of the year to give them a bonus anyway.

Most managed care programs reimburse hospitals on a predetermined basis, after negotiations. Sometimes older methodologies such as per diem will be used, sometimes negotiated discount rates, and, in a growing number of instances, a capitation arrangement will be put in place. The partnership game is hard for the hospital managers to sell to the medical staff when it is per-diem or discounted rates, because those are familiar and a continuation of the traditional tug of war that has always occurred. When both doctors and hospitals are capitated from the same pool of funds, there is the opportunity for a real partnership to be forged and given a chance to work. That is probably the only partnership that will work to mutual advantage, if that is what both sides really want. As long as there is a feeling of still needing one-upsmanship, there are no partners. For example, if the costs of emergency room care comes from the doctors' risk pool, there will be noticeable reduced usage. But if emergency room care is paid by the hospital risk pool, watch the utilization go up from the attendance of patients sent there by their doctors.

Reduced Hospitalization

As was shown in Chapter 24, there are profound implications for the structure and performance of hospitals in the managed care era. All of these changes also affect members of the medical staff, who see their incomes fall as their referrals change, brought about by the movement of patients on and off plans and by the influences of gatekeepers. For decades, there has been a conventional wisdom that there was too much capacity in the hospital system that needed to be reduced. A number of approaches were tried by federal and state policymakers without notable success, but the competitive era did that job for them, to some extent.

Historically, most prepaid plans have achieved their lower costs for health care services that could be competitive in the marketplace through hospitalization rates that were lower than those in the fee-for-service sector. As a result, ambulatory care use has been generally higher in managed care plans or HMOs as services have been increasingly shifted from inpatient to outpatient settings. One of the peculiar features of the indemnity insurance market, as expressed in fee-for-service payment plans, was the insistence that patients must be treated in hospitals rather than outpatient facilities. Managed care simply reversed these incentives, stimulating growth in the outpatient market while decimating hospital occupancy.

There are a number of other mechanisms by which prepaid group practice systems have also rationed services. Rationing is a nasty word, preferably left unspoken or unwritten. But that is the practical effect of the use of waiting times to obtain appointments, encouragement of self-care, and triaging of patients to provide care first to the more seriously ill. Another successful tactic has been the use of physician extenders such as nurse practitioners and physician assistants to see patients rather than doctors. These latter methods are the only real demonstrable differences in managed care, besides the significant and undeniable reductions in hospital admissions and length of stay, that can show evidence of cost control.

Williams and Torrens (1993) point out that there is little evidence that managed care providers offer any specific service, such as a doctor's office visit or pharmacy prescriptions, at substantially lower cost than fee-for-service providers. Multiple studies and publications by the California Hospital Association during the 1970–1980 era demonstrated many times that HMO hospital costs per day or per stay were as high or higher than any other hospital, once the patient finally reached the HMO hospital (White, 1988; White & Ariey, 1978; White & Morse, 1979–1986).

Utilization Control

Utilization review is an integral part of managed care, and some will say that control of supply of medical care is the secret of competitive success. The concepts of utilization review revolve around monitoring the use of services and determining the appropriateness of the care that is provided (Romeo, 1988). Utilization review, when done thoroughly, occurs at several levels. Surgical or other procedures must be authorized in advance by the provider organization. Bedside care is reviewed, sometimes daily, by on the scene nurse reviewers, to see that estimated lengths of stay are being observed. Managed care contracts from payers or insurers almost always now stipulate the utilization review program to be carried out. Variance or unwillingness to follow the program will bring quick repercussions, even to the point of canceling the contract.

Most traditional and usual utilization review focuses on either the use of expensive inpatient hospital services or referrals to other settings for complex secondary and tertiary care that is, perhaps, even more expensive. But even that much is not enough. To be optimally effective, utilization review must also include analysis of physician practice patterns and individual physician behaviors within the contractor organization, because it is not unknown for doctors to practice differently depending on the plan. The purpose of this approach is to detect, on a patient-specific basis, whether there is inappropriate use or abuse by either patients or physicians (White, 1988).

In either case, utilization review is not an outstanding gem of enthusiasm for the Joint Commission model of a medical staff. In the fee-for-service system that fostered that model, more use was better for all, referrals to as many specialists as possible was good, and the hospital benefited from the occupancy and use of technology, equipment, and personnel. Utilization review is the worst enemy of all of those incentives. Think of that for a moment. Most members of medical staffs are specialists, and the utilization review nurse and medical director are asking these doctors to deny themselves the opportunity to practice well and enjoy the good life.

Risk Sharing

Partnerships in managed care have a more meaningful form when there are risk-sharing pools. Although they are increasingly important, and are of more interest as time goes on, there are many varieties. No alternative has proven to be the single best or optimum choice. The general definition of a risk pool involves the establishment of a designated sum from which certain services are to be paid throughout the year. The obvious incentive for participants is that the funds remaining at the end of the year will be divided, either between doctors and the hospital (or corporation), or between providers and the insurer. Most commonly, risk pools are established for primary care providers, not including specialized referral physicians, who have been used on an as-needed basis and paid on some sort of modified fee-for-service or discounted fee arrangement.

Obviously, the purpose of risk pools is to provide a powerful incentive to reduce utilization, particularly hospitalization and specialty referrals, which produces the consequences noted in Chapter 24. The jury is still out on whether risk pools will be effective in general or whether the successes so far are just due to exceptional managers. Similarly, there is a nagging concern that risk pools and the whole concept of managed care will result in underutilization and denial of needed services. Some of those results may require 20 years before researchers will know them. But, there is general agreement that risk sharing in some form, between payers and providers, will be necessary to ensure containment of costs and utilization. That is the real definition of partnership, and the Joint Commission model is not very good at fostering and working with these arrangements.

Insurers cannot be blamed for trying to obtain the best possible prices from providers, but those payers also have an equally powerful incentive to be sure that providers are not backed against the wall so much that they cannot stay solvent and reasonably happy with the contract. Commonly now, insurers accomplish these twin objectives by sharing risk in another way, by providing reinsurance for the provider organization or medical group. Stop-loss insurance built into the contract is the mechanism that has worked best in guarding against the unavoidable catastrophic case that could bankrupt providers. The insurer also needs to find ways to preserve satisfaction among patients and plan members since they are, after all, the customers who can vote with their feet and walk away to another plan at the next open enrollment period. Patients are also risk sharing, since they are greatly affected by this restructuring of the system. For the most part, patients are silent partners in risk sharing, having no access to risk pools but taking the gamble on the provider group in return for lower premiums.

EFFECTS ON CONSUMERS/PATIENTS

In return for lower premium payments that favorably affect the patient or consumer, or more likely, favorably affect the employer that chooses one HMO or integrated delivery system over another, there is a decided amount of control applied over consumer behavior. In the fee-for-service system, patients chose specialists and other aspects of their care, including choice of hospital. Patients had access to the entire world of doctors, picking one over another through word of mouth recommendation from friends and family. If, as rarely happened, the patient was dissatisfied with the doctor, then just get another. Physician referral systems were helpful with this action. Most of those choices disappear when enrolled in a plan. The insurer, the plan, or the integrated network now makes most of the choices. If a long-standing personal physician is not a member of the plan, then choose another. Some patients find that very difficult, and the fear of loss of physician choice has been a powerful political force against health care reform plan.

Gatekeepers are created in order to control and guide the behavior of consumers. In return, the patient receives coordination of a pattern of care that was almost certainly lacking before. Gatekeepers channel patients, as do HMO administrative organizations, by creating funnels for appointments, procedures, admissions, pharmaceuticals, and so on. That is why it is called managed. Early HMOs were successful in avoiding patients with preexisting conditions or those with severe illnesses and expensive care needs, although to their credit, when an existing patient became seriously ill, care was likely to be as good as or better than what could be put together in the fee-for-service system.

In the competitive era of managed care, the newer form of patient control and channeling is through the use of case management. When done well, an experienced case manager with knowledge of the resources available to the hospital or network monitors the care provided to the patient and determines whether the care is necessary and is being provided in the most cost-effective setting. Case managers also serve a vital function in the coordination of services and the education of patients and families. Case management may involve bringing to bear specialized resources within the network or hospital system, including home health, hospice, and other unique opportunities that the patient could never put together acting alone. Nurses have made patient care plans for many years, but this is a quantum jump past that technique. When case management is combined with newer techniques such as clinical pathways for the patients and nurses and algorithms for physician decision making, then there is a real possibility for quality improvement. Research has not yet proven that case management is an effective force in reducing costs of care, but there is no doubt about the support and assistance that is provided. Peace of mind and awareness of the care process must be worth something.

Consumers/patients/plan members benefit in other ways that are not clinical, such as pathways of care. The benefit packages and administrative coordination of most managed care programs are generally an advantage to the user and are frequently much more convenient than a system where the patient was forced to seek out care without much guidance. There are conveniences for the doctors, too, in being relieved of administrative responsibilities and office costs. Each needs the other. As James Rice (1994) said, "We need to do everything within our capacity to empower the real customers, our patients. When they have sufficient information they will know what they need. We need them as active partners in the health care debate."

Most of the major managed care contracts and the HMOs that service them offer a more comprehensive package of benefits than did many of the traditional indemnity plans. Covered preventive services often include, at little or no cost to the patient, routine physical examinations, including vision and hearing screening, well-child care, and patient education services. Coverage for reproductive health needs, such as infertility diagnosis and treatment, may be more extensive in managed care programs (Williams & Torrens, 1993). Reimbursement of services provided by contract allied health professionals may be provided by the plan, and access to those may be more lenient than offered by indemnity plans that placed so much emphasis on inpatient hospital care and so little emphasis on outpatient care.

Administration and management of managed care plans can be a blessing for both doctors and patients when things work well. In most plans, paperwork for the consumer is virtually eliminated, with the exception of some simple co-payments and prescription slips to the pharmacy. There are no claims or bills to be prepared or submitted to anyone, since the plan has already been prepaid for the care. Doctors are supposed to be relieved of all of the paperwork in the outside system, except for those elements of actual clinical care such as medical records, writing prescriptions, and the like. There are to be no more bad debts and collection problems. All of these administrative efficiencies should result in lower costs for the plan, and the assumption is that lower costs will mean a more competitive position in the marketplace, and the possibility for more profit. Everybody is supposed to share in the profit—payers, doctors, patients, stockholders.

Most managed care plans are doing a greatly improved job of providing consumer activities to improve health and minimize total dependence on the acute care system. Making it easier to change primary care physicians, offering diet and weight loss classes and smoking cessation programs, handling plan member complaints, and using mandatory arbitration are risk managing and cost reducing. All of these are quality improving measures that may very well be a lot better than anything that was available when doctors controlled the fee-for-service system.

The quality of information being given to plan members is also worth noting. For example, one member newsletter offers as practical and useful a definition of managed care as any now available: "Managed care is supervision of utilization, quality and claims using a variety of current cost management methods. The primary goal is to deliver cost effective health care without sacrificing quality or access" (*Highlights,* 1994). The Sharp Health Plan calls managed care the most effective form of health care, addressing escalating costs while meeting the plan members' needs for top-quality care. It will be an essential that plans, payers, and medical groups take pains to inform their consumer/patient/members so that they thoroughly understand how their plan works, what it will do, and what it will not do. Likely, it will only be then that all can be active partners in utilizing benefits properly to be successful in maintaining high quality at an affordable cost. The educated consumer has always been the goal of the reformers who recommended managed care to people as a better way. Being active and responsible in health care decisions will be as important to consumers as any of their other lifestyle decisions.

What would rain on this parade would be restriction of access on choice of providers, but sometimes that happens when the doctor refuses to join the plan and the patient has no choice but to get a new doctor. Plans sometimes refuse to pay for treatment of a catastrophic illness, a financial decision that might earn them a place in the TV news spotlight or a well-publicized court trial. There are so many plans being put together that may not be managed well enough, or not capitalized well enough, so that they will fail. Then the consumer must change plans and get a new doctor all over again. As Fortune magazine said: "The most crucial reason of all for why companies fail is that they follow the crowd instead of leading it" (Silver, 1994).

Some large medical groups have decided that the best way to bypass intrusive insurance companies or integrated network managers while taking control of their futures is to completely seize control of both the clinical and business sides of their practices. By assuming the central role in the management of risk and utilization, the doctors think they are now in the catbird seat. Capitation allows groups to grow, because of spreading the risk that individual physicians cannot take. However, it is still possible that full risk contracts will not be successful unless the physicians who participate in them have an understanding of both costs and of the natural history of the diseases that they are agreeing to be gatekeepers of. To at least one observer, "total reliance on primary care gate keepers may not solve the problem of controlling costs for the sickest and most expensive patients, who often reside in ICUs and consume a much higher percentage of resources" (Gipe, 1994).

Bruce Gipe goes on to say that "gatekeeping for these patients must be done by specialists who understand the natural history of the disease states that occur at the high end of acuity. That raises the question whether physicians who are not regularly involved with managing critically ill patients will be able to manage the risk associated with their care in the ICU." But there may not yet be any security in these advances. The balance of power among insurers, hospital systems, and medical groups is constantly shifting. As

Nate Kaufman said, "being large does not mean being safe. The large won't eat the small. The swift will eat the slow " (Cunningham, 1994).

Another real possibility for the future of managed care that will affect consumers is the lack of long-term financial viability for physicians (singly or in groups), hospitals and other providers that have been excluded from integrated systems and networks. Where there is large scale physician dissatisfaction, where the hospital is not competitively successful, where the utilization review controls seem excessive, where there are more constraints on practice patterns, where the financial effects of continued deep discounting have finally squeezed the slack out of the system, there you will find turmoil in the doctors' lounge that the Joint Commission model will not fix. Most of the self-governance work of the organized medical staff takes place in the sunshine of success. A real feeling of despondency and "what's the use" does not encourage scrupulous attention to credentialing, reappointment and peer review.

SUMMARY

The generic term *managed care* has been used frequently to include a variety of forms of prepaid and managed fee-for-service care. The fundamental structure offers incentives to contain costs and provide more continuity of care and a continuum of services while maintaining quality. Assumption of financial risk by the doctors and hospitals or systems moves the emphasis from retrospective payment for episodic interventions focused on the individual to prospective payment for continuous, preventive, population-focused, team management concepts. All advocates for competition speak about the need for partnership with the physicians, many of whom know perfectly well that the future will not be as good for them in that partnership.

Indemnity, fee-for-service care offered incentives for patients to demand all the care they could get and for doctors to supply all the care they could give, because it was someone else's money paying the bills. In managed care, it now is the patient's money and the doctor's money. Barriers to true partnerships are inhibited by many factors, not the least of which is the inability of the specialty-controlled medical staff organization with weak primary care leadership to change fast enough to matter.

To most people, managed care means HMOs in the prepaid model with closed panel medical staffs or groups. There is a demonstrable track record by some of these organizations in providing comprehensive and acceptance quality health services for lower total costs. Other organizational formats, such as independent practice associations (IPA), or preferred provider organizations (PPO), have combined features of fee discounting with open physician membership. In any form, there is a loss of control and increased interference in physician practice, but there may no longer be enough local alternatives to be able to opt out altogether. Hospitals sign contracts or join plans that may or may not match the preferences of the doctors on the medical staffs, particularly the specialists.

The ascent of primary care gatekeepers creates tension by being a barrier to access to specialty services. In any form, there is more utilization review and control and reduced hospitalization.

REFERENCES

Cunningham, R. (1994). Perspectives. *Medicine and Health, Nov. 14,* 1–4.

Gipe, B. T. (1994). Vencor Hospital *Newsletter, 2(2),* 1–2.

Highlights, Vol. 4. (1994). [Sharp Health Plan Member Newsletter, San Diego].

Kent, C., & Firshein, J. (1994). Perspectives. *Medicine and Health, August 29,* 1–4.

Kongstvedt, P. R. (1989). *The Managed Care Handbook.* Rockville, MD: Aspen Publishers.

Rice, J. L. (1994). Editorial: Whose patient is this, anyhow? *San Diego Physician, November,* 3.

Romeo, S. J. W. (1988). The economic effects of utilization review in prepaid care. *Medical Group Management Journal, 35 (3),* 54–6, 60.

Silver, A. (1994). Why do bad things happen to good companies? *Rate Controls, 18(10B, Oct. 31),* 2.

White, C. H. (1988). From utilization review to utilization management. *Healthcare Computing and Communication, October,* 5–7.

White, C. H., & Ariey, M. (1978). *Hospital Fact Book.* Sacramento: California Hospital Association.

White, C. H., & Morse, L. (1979–1986, annual). *Hospital Fact Book.* Sacramento: California Hospital Association.

Williams, S. J., & Torrens, P. R. (1993). Managed care: Restructuring the system. Williams and Torrens (Eds.), *Introduction to Health Services (4th ed.).* Albany, NY: Delmar Publishers.

CHAPTER

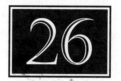

Medical Staff in Competitive Times

The characteristics of a Joint Commission model of a hospital medical staff became what they are now during the past two decades and are the product of those times. The medical staff would probably be different than it currently is had there been some other kind of health care delivery system and other forms of payment. It is very useful to compare several characteristics to show exactly what is different and what will need to be changed if the hospital staff is to become, in effect, a closed medical group that delivers nothing but managed care. The Joint Commission model allows any physician with appropriate training to enter the staff without regard for the numbers of doctors already in that field or specialty, and exhibits the following features.

JOINT COMMISSION MODEL

1. It is clinically divided by specialty as demonstrated by most medical school faculty departments. Each department is a club of similar practitioners joined together for

mutual protection and advancement, with the added value of useful continuing education.

2. There is voluntary leadership with nominal political elections without real campaigning or platforms for advancement of the specialty as a group or the medical staff as a whole.

3. There is annual or biennial turnover of leadership without long-range planning or goals other than to try to preserve the status quo in a changing world.

4. There is an entrenched aversion to resource management as a concept and outcome systems as particular mechanisms for bringing about that management since it promises to challenge individual judgment.

5. There is professional autonomy without any allegiance or loyalty to the staff as a whole, preserving all the best and worst features of medical staff participatory democracy and its one-person, one-vote approach.

6. There is short-term focus without a vision of where the hospital is going in the world and what actions will be needed to help it get there. Instead of this sort of future planning, most medical staff members assume that the world will stand still, that the hospital will continue to be what it has always been (except that it will buy the latest technology as soon as available), that their medical practice will continue along the current line, with the same staff, with no new training needed, and that the revenue stream will continue to meet and exceed expenses.

7. There is an inefficient committee structure that lives on in perpetuity and in defiance of any semblance of good sense. Through the years, the typical medical staff response to any new Joint Commission requirement or identified need was to create a new standing committee, which took on a life of its own. Committee chairs are reluctant to endorse change in their world even when it means eliminating a worthless or nonproductive committee. The Joint Commission wants to see the medical staff perform functions and does not require that a separate committee must perform each of those functions. It is a catch-22 situation. The doctors gripe about the time demands of committees, and they are quite right about time-wasting. But when a chief proposes streamlining the committee structure, constituents come out who want that particular committee to protect them from their competitors.

One of the most noticeable features of the Joint Commission model of self-governance is the democratic decision-making process where each member's vote counts the same. The result of this approach is frequently the standoff that occurs when the hospital and the medical staff leadership are interested in a change that is intended to help all parties but can be blocked or stymied by those members who do not practice at the hospital very much (if at all) but who keep getting reappointed every two years with full voting privileges. Their resistance and organized sabotage of practically everything that smacks of progress becomes a real millstone around the necks of the leadership. There may be solutions through communication, using every vehicle available such as meetings (though no one will come except those already knowledgeable and convinced), newsletters (but no one will read them), or word of mouth through departmental colleagues. Most of these efforts need to be conducted in a good faith effort to share information, but there should be recognition of the worst-case scenario that it is not an information gap that needs closing. There is a real gulf, not a gap, and the gulf war is about change and its possible effects on the practice routines of the member doctors. They may not know for sure that the change will hurt them, but they will not even take the chance.

The net result of a medical staff organization created and operated according to the Joint Commission model could be the presence of good work done to credential new members, good attention to peer review, and attention to quality improvement. Self-governance in this model looks inward toward itself and the maintenance of predictability. The bottom line is status quo.

COMPETITION MODEL

1. The competition model uses a package price for all clinical services, arrived at through careful cooperative work between the clinicians and the finance types. A real cost-finding system is needed, one that can isolate each component of the care being delivered and can therefore produce the ability to compete on carefully calculated prices. These abilities are not universally available in hospitals, but they should be. A package price subjugates the individuality of the physicians involved and removes a lot of the variance in practice that is so confusing and frustrating to insurers and payers.

2. Its high-risk leadership recognizes the changes in the world and willingly move rapidly and decisively to meet those challenges. This will probably mean that a different type of leader should be chosen for the medical staff, perhaps not even elected at all, or, if elected, certainly not for a one-year term. Many, if not most of the physicians who have served as chiefs of staff would not now be appropriate for this modern-day executive position. Chiefs in this model, if they are called chief at all, will not be honorary positions, and there will be no more taking turns. This model is serious business, with an emphasis on the business aspect.

3. Its active and effective resource management is the most basic of tools in this model of an integrated medical staff, where idiosyncrasies of practice styles are no longer to be admired and encouraged. Instead, best-practice examples will be emulated based on practice guidelines and clinical pathways. Cost containment in health care has been a bumper sticker slogan for years now, but simply reducing the ranks

of management is not the final solution. What will reduce costs is to reduce the supply of care being ordered and delivered by the doctors and impeccably accurate utilization data is the only way to do that.

4. This model has strategic plans for the short- and long-term future that contemplate further tightening of the payment system and more emphasis on contracting that involves risk sharing and profit incentives based on reductions in utilization. A competitive model medical staff cannot operate in a vacuum as did the Joint Commission model and must be interlocked in partnerships with hospitals or health care networks. Plans are not the unilateral possession of either side in this model. One of the most difficult things for the doctors to learn is that there are no longer "sides": "We are us," so to speak. Planning involves all parts of the integrated organization, but planning skills are not part of the medical school curriculum, so some fast training is needed.

5. Rapid strategic decision making is the hallmark of a successful corporate structure, which is what an integrated health care system must be to succeed. This does not refer to a hospital system with individual approaches and preservation of the unique culture of each institution, but a top to bottom unified and integrated organization formed for business purposes where everyone buys into the mission and purpose. Doctors will find that very hard to do. They want to reserve the right to change their minds or to keep some other options open. That attitude will not mesh well with the corporate business types.

6. Professional interdependence in a competition model will be a major and abrupt change away from the Joint Commission model. Individual, solo practice, fee-for-service physicians will need to face the issue of giving up their own offices in favor of joining a group. The most pronounced change will be that of directly opposed incentives. Rather than working toward survival as an individual, the doctor must turn attention toward survival and success as a group, with some individuality foregone. Groups will never practice the same way as most of the group members would if they were doing it by themselves. Group success depends on working within guidelines and practice patterns that will contribute to making annual targets and ensuring success for all specialties. The specialty war taught in residencies must be set aside and cooperation emphasized.

7. Intensive, goal-focused leadership is the principal identifiable characteristic of successful medical groups and the same pattern must be adopted by a hospital medical staff intent upon forming and acting as a competitive model. Honorary leaders assume their office in the Joint Commission model based upon past performance and recognition and an assumption that the status quo will prevail. A competitive model is based on the assumption that the past is past and that the future is all that counts. A competitive staff must move forward with rapid strides, reacting to the

outside world and adjusting to it. Members of a competitive model do not exhibit the hallmark of a Joint Commission model in that all applicants are not appropriate and all members are not to be accepted just because they have appropriate credentials of training and experience. Long-term, continuous leadership with management training and skills and a clear understanding that the staff is a business venture will be the key to success for this model.

8. Delegated decision makers will be routine in a competitive model. The organization will look and act as a corporate structure with contracting authority lodged in the medical staff executive office without question. The individual doctors do not need to be asked about business decisions and do not have a vote in the conduct of business affairs. Doctors practice medicine in the corporate model and doctor-leaders practice business on their behalf. There are not many examples of the corporate model of a medical staff available for study and emulation, but if a new hospital were being formed, with no medical staff yet in place, it is a model worth considering seriously for life in a managed care world. Actually, it would work well in any other kind of a payment world, since most of the weaknesses of the traditional way of performing as a Joint Commission model have been corrected.

The result of forming a hospital medical staff as a competitive model will be the ability to make rapid change without clumsy democracy and foot-dragging resistance getting in the way. Participatory democracy has worked well to safeguard the rights and protect the turf of individual-practice doctors as they carry out self-governance, but that is not the only way to do it. Forming a team, with all the clichés commonly used in talking about team sports, can also apply to the medical staff for those physicians interested in working in that environment. There will be many who dislike every aspect of a competitive model and want no part of it. To move a hospital medical staff from an existing typical Joint Commission model to a competitive model would be traumatic for many people, notably the board, but it can be done, if that is the plan.

Other Features

It is possible to predict some other features of a competitive model of a medical staff with reasonable certainty. For example, there will still be credentialing, reappointment, and peer review no matter what model is being used. It will still be necessary to identify who the applicant is, what training there has been, and whether clinical competence fits the privileges being requested. Looking at it from that standpoint, the Joint Commission model from the past has simply become the new Joint Commission model, only now it will be applied to a selected or chosen group of doctors rather than to self-selected individuals.

There will be more paid medical directors and department heads chosen by the executive leadership rather than by election in a competitive model. There will be many fewer committees. More of the JCAHO functions will be done by employee staff, with medical oversight. There will be more line authority by appointed leaders who have budget and hiring-firing responsibility as well as financial targets to achieve. The goal of the competitive medical staff will be to compete successfully, rather than to have a participatory democracy.

There will be more movement toward integrated health care systems that will replace multihospital ownership systems. These organizations will increasingly take on the structures and attitudes of major business and industry, with less of the warm and fuzzy nature of former community hospitals. It will become very difficult to make a lifetime career in one of these vertically integrated systems, and administrative personnel will come and go in a revolving door fashion. Good people will be thrown away at the drop of a hat, or more likely, at the drop of a census.

DEFINING SYSTEMS OR NETWORKS

Steve Shortell and his associates (1993) defines this newer model as a network of organizations that provides or arranges to provide a coordinated continuum of services to a defined population and is willing to be held clinically and fiscally accountable for the outcomes and health status of the population served. Former hospital-ownership companies are becoming more broad-based community providers on a geographic pattern of coverage that offers primary care, wellness, home health, long-term care, hospice, and other related components of a continuum of care, in addition to the more familiar inpatient hospital acute care and ambulatory services, whether in the hospital or clinics. They will not all be the same, since systems will combine the organization, financing, and delivery of health care in ways that respond to the demographics and economics that prevail in the different regions of the country.

The real measure of success will be the extent to which these systems are somehow able to achieve integration of clinical services. That means the extent to which patient care services are coordinated across the various personnel, functions, activities, and operating units of the system or network (Gillies, Shortell, & Anderson, 1993). There are functional integrations that can be coordinated across operating units, such as financial management, human resources, strategic planning, information management, and quality improvement. These mergers and consolidations from individual hospitals to the corporate office can add benefits from economies of scale and provide greater overall value.

However, the real key is physician-system integration, or the extent to which doctors identify with the system, use the system, and actively participate in its planning, management, and governance (Shortell, Gillies, & Anderson, 1994). Physician-system integration means that the doctors identify themselves and their practices with the mission and values of the system. The relationship is so close because there is a management leadership structure in place that can allocate resources to strengthen clinical integration. There is also a medical leadership structure in place that offers credible explanations and reasons for changing the doctors' practice patterns. Physicians in top leadership and system management positions are essential to integration, as is the participation by more doctors with all or the majority of their practices in system-owned or affiliated facilities. Doctors would move from having membership and privileges in only one hospital to a network or system allegiance. Doctors who practiced in nearby but competitor hospitals would be faced with the need to align only with the system.

The most difficult part of changing from a single hospital mentality to an integrated regional system will be to change the attitudes and interests and to expand the outlook of the medical staff. Becoming a vertically integrated, regional medical staff with privileges to practice anywhere in the system is a pattern that is recognized by some organizations, being promoted by a few, and being accomplished by almost none. Changing from single hospital practice to system practice will be difficult to sell to most physicians as long as they are still in solo or small group practice because of the increased competition and opportunity to feel mistreated by the corporation or by administration. That will be their fear, and they may have historical reason for those feelings. Doctors stay in one place and one practice much longer than most executives stay in one job.

Read again the previous discussion about a competitive model for a single hospital medical staff and then transpose those ideas onto a larger screen. Make an integrated hospital staff into an integrated system staff. But that will mean there are too many doctors, more than will be needed for managed care or capitation. What will be done with the rest who already have privileges and have been bringing patients for years? Medical staff integration and collaboration is the single most difficult step to take in creating an integrated system.

MECHANISMS FOR ACHIEVING INTEGRATION

One of the ways to integrate is to bring about a reduction of multiple medical staff memberships when those other hospitals are not part of the system. A monogamous system relationship will be essential in developing loyalties and incentives. As long as doctors can continue to play the old whipsaw game, it will be impossible to create practice patterns and agreed-upon clinical guidelines that can enable success with utilization rates and economic success with negotiating and performing contracts.

Another way to integrate hospital medical staffs into integrated system staffs will be to break away from the medical school faculty-style departmental groupings toward product or service lines that more nearly reflect patient and disease flow. Chasing to and from multiple medical specialists by patients was one of the more unlovely features of the fee-for-service system. Imagine how awful that could become when those specialists are scattered all across a system. Integrating specialists who have spent an entire career competing against and bad-mouthing other specialists in their field will be some trick, but it can be done by careful and knowledgeable leadership who communicate well and offer good financial data that will persuade the recalcitrant that there is actually no other equally good choice that has any real chance for success.

Because integrated systems will care for defined populations brought to them by contracts that feature risk sharing through capitation, systems must be able to offer services everywhere throughout their area. That requires physician integration, not a continuation of the medical arms race of recent decades. Each service point throughout the system must offer the same good quality but of a different service mix depending on need. Quality continues to be the responsibility of the medical staff, no matter what model is being used. Peer review, to see whether the doctor is performing well, will always be a crucial part of any delivery system, and it will not be the corporate office that performs peer review. The hospital might not even be the center of attention for all these services being delivered in patient-friendly settings.

MOVING TO SYSTEM SURVEYS

A necessary requirement of this next world of integrated system hospital medical staffs will be for the Joint Commission to add to its single hospital focus of surveys an ability to perform system surveys. System surveys must be built on the same attention to carefully developed standards that guided medical staff models to the present level of success and good performance. In those instances where there was not success and good performance, having a set of standards that could be applied almost uniformly (allowing for variances among surveyors), there were demonstrable examples to offer that would lead to remediation and correction. JCAHO will change, also, or become obsolete and replaced by another vehicle for accomplishing the same mission, to ensure the public that someone is paying attention to what doctors and hospitals are doing.

Individual physicians, in this vision of an integrated multihospital regional system surveyed by someone, will still retain their duty and responsibility as patient advocates, maintaining their professional ethic of service to patients. They will keep that ethic but will add another duty and responsibility, that of managers of care for those patients. Being a manager of care is intended to mean a more coherent, less splintered pattern for the patient that ensures more quality, while at the same time allowing the doctor and the corporation to be financially successful. If all integrated regional systems are ensuring high-quality care, achieving financial success, and practicing cost containment, then the larger social goal of reducing objectionable rates of increase in health care spending will also be met. At least, that is the way the theory works.

What Will Not Work

Cost containment *will not* occur in a fee-for-service system with a traditional Joint Commission model of a medical staff. High quality *can* occur, though, and there are many examples of positive results in the form of good outcomes to show for it. Financial success for doctors and hospitals *can* occur also, and the health care delivery system people think is the best in the world is the result. But only a competitive model can promise cost containment.

SUMMARY

The Joint Commission model that has evolved during the past decades would undoubtedly be different had there beeen some other form of health care delivery and payment system in place. There are a number of characteristics of the open model that allow any physician with appropriate training to enter the staff without regard for the number of doctors already on the staff in that specialty. The chapter lists those features, which include participatory democracy discussed in an earlier section, typical voluntary leadership, short-term focus, and inefficient committee system. Beneficial results from this structure include attention to credentialing, peer review, and maintenance of predictability.

In a competition model medical staff, there are package prices for clinical services, high-risk leadership, resource management, strategic plans, and the ability to decide faster and delegated decision making. If a hospital medical staff were formed this way, and resembled more closely a closed-panel medical group, there still would be needed the essential functions of credentialing, reappointment, privileging, and peer review, but with fewer committees and more paid executive leadership. The emphasis would be on competing successfully and encouraging integrated health care systems. The movement toward systems comes as a strategy to combine the organization, financing, and delivery of care responsive to demographics and economics in today's environment.

How these systems are able to integrate clinical services will be a measure of their success, but the real key is physician integration. How doctors identify with the system, use its services and facilities, and participate in its planning, management, and governance defines true integration. The chapter offers some suggestions for ways to improve integration, including system surveys by the Joint Commission if, indeed, JCAHO is to survive or be replaced. Perhaps the most profound conclusion yet reached in the book is that the Joint Commission model will not contain costs but can produce high quality and financial success.

REFERENCES

Gillies, R. R., Shortell, S. M., & Anderson, D. A. (1993). Conceptualizing and measuring integration: Findings from the health systems integration study. *Hospital and Health Services Administration, Winter,* 467–489.

Shortell, S. M., Gillies, R. R., & Anderson, D. A. (1994). The new world of managed care: Creating organized delivery systems. *Health Affairs, 13(5, Winter),* 46–64.

Shortell, S. M., Gillies, R. R., & Anderson, D. A. (1993). Creating organized delivery systems: The barriers and facilitators. *Hospital and Health Services Administration, Winter,* 447–466.

CHAPTER

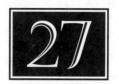

Alternative Models

Throughout this discussion, the catch phrase *Joint Commission model of a hospital medical staff* has been used to surround and include several concepts:

- Any physician could join by presenting proof of training and experience.
- No physician could be denied entrance for anticompetitive reasons.
- Certain functions should be performed.
- An organization and structure must be in place and functioning.
- There will be certain officers in place, usually elected.
- Economic performance is not a criteria for initial credentialing or for reappointment.
- There could be exclusive contracts for certain in-hospital specialty services.
- There will be requirements for how many delinquent medical records can be tolerated.
- There will be the trappings of organization, including agendas, minutes, and paper trails of actions considered and taken.

- There will be files maintained and notebooks or logbooks showing how the medical staff performed its self-governance duties.
- There will be a trained and certified medical staff services director or manager or coordinator to carry out all of the necessary medical staff clerical and operational functions.
- There will be leaders who understand how the peer review process works and can explain that process to a surveyor.
- There is sufficient administrative support for the medical staff functions, including enough staff to do the work.
- All of the Joint Commission standards are in compliance all of the time instead of a last minute effort just before a survey.
- The surgery department has a way to know immediately whether a surgeon has been granted the privileges to perform the procedure that has been scheduled.
- There is a way to make sure new procedures are not being performed without evidence of training and experience being provided in advance.

FIVE MODELS OF MEDICAL STAFF ORGANIZATION

All of these and doubtless other assumptions underlie the generalized references to the Joint Commission model. But there are other models beside that traditional one, which has evolved over time through many iterations of the *Manual for Accreditation.* There have been other local variations of the standards that have been recognized and allowed by individual surveyors if some idiosyncratic approach seemed to be working and accomplishing the main purposes of accreditation. Most of the list are commonsense provisions and should be done by an organized medical staff whether or not there even exists a Joint Commission. But there are a few important differences that can be identified and a few other alternative models to look at (Gill, 1993).

In the model shown in Figure 27–1, the hospital board acting through the administration, has created a medical staff development plan that specifies appointing individual physicians. These members have exclusive privileges, meaning that no others can apply or be accepted. On what basis or according to which criteria the members have been selected would need to be described in the development plan. The main difference between this model and the Joint Commission is that any doctor who applies will not be admitted. In actuality, this model of a staff would probably be formed by invitation only, according to how many practitioners would be needed to serve the expected patient base.

As soon as it was decided who would be the members of the staff, then the remainder of the list of Joint Commission characteristics would apply. There would still be medical staff services personnel to process the paperwork, there would still be medical records completion requirements, there would still be credentialing, reappointment, and

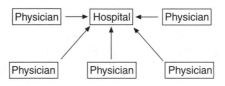

FIGURE 27–1   The hospital or integrated health care system has an individual contract with each member of the medical staff.

peer review processes that examined current clinical competence and provided for remedial action.

Why would anyone want to use this model? Probably for a specialty hospital that did not need or want applications from a broad spectrum of doctors. Or, perhaps, for a new hospital in the first phase of organization. But the essential point is that there is still self-governance and triennial surveys if there are to be public funds paid for services rendered.

In the model shown in Figure 27–2, a closed panel corporation of physicians enters into a contract with a hospital, a group of hospitals, or an integrated health care system to perform as the medical staff. As in Figure 27–1, this form also means that there is an exclusive grouping of members that does not allow for other doctors to apply or join, except by invitation. The group would manage itself and its business affairs and would need expert business management. But it would still perform all of the same functions mentioned in this chapter, except that there would not be elected officers. Instead, there would be a president of the group or a medical director instead of a chief of staff. There would still be department chairs, but they would be appointed instead of elected.

Medical groups using this model have a number of advantages over the traditional model, the principal one being very clear incentives. Performance goals for quality of care and financial targets offer a clear understanding of the interrelationships among the members of the group and how each can help or hurt colleagues. Utilization rates and practice patterns become group norms and goals instead of hateful interferences in practice judgment. There are also several other benefits. Doctors practice medicine on regular hours, are compensated at regular intervals, take regular vacations, and participate in CME. Closed panel groups are accused of earning less income than fee-for-service physicians, but there are some trade-offs that are attractive. When the entire benefits package

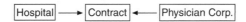

FIGURE 27–2   Physicians form a corporation that contracts with the hospital or integrated health care system for all patient medical services.

is put together, there may be some question whether, in fact, it is true that total compensation is really less, as charged, or whether that accusation is only sour grapes.

From the standpoint of the health care corporation that wants to participate in the managed care environment in a major way, this model offers some intriguing possibilities and may be the easiest to put together, when some subgroup of the entire staff is involved in forming the physician contracting group. For example, why could not the corporation simply put out a request for proposal and entertain bids from competing closed panel medical groups based on indicators of price and quality? That offers promise for being able to affect positively the overall cost of health care and affect absolutely the cost of care to the purchasers involved in that plan.

What if a hospital with a traditional model medical staff that has allowed all applicants to become members now wants to move toward this competitive model of an exclusive, closed panel contracted group? That would mean abolishing the previous staff and entering the bidding process. That is a tricky maneuver with a lot of pitfalls built in. It would require lots of help from legal counsel. The financial rewards of a medical staff development plan may be worth the effort for some hospitals as the managed care noose continues to tighten. This could mean dealing with 1 contractor instead of 500 individual independent contractors. HMOs could do it; community hospitals probably cannot.

The model in Figure 27–3, is a variation of Figure 27–1, in which the medical staff is chosen and appointed to salaried positions. Already in use in many places—such as military facilities, state or county hospitals, and some university medical schools—this model as shown in Figure 27–3 would not be possible in most community nonprofit hospitals. Specialty facilities such as psychiatric or other limited-purpose uses can and have used the salaried model very well. There are still a few states in which it is not possible for hospitals to directly employ physicians, but that can be handled by using the contract model shown previously. The salary model is of limited utility to nearly all of the hospitals currently using the traditional Joint Commission style. Even if it is used, there will still be the need to perform the functions of self-governance.

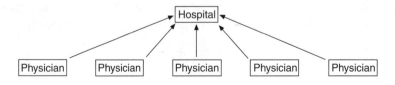

FIGURE 27–3   All physicians are salaried by the hospital or integrated health care delivery system.

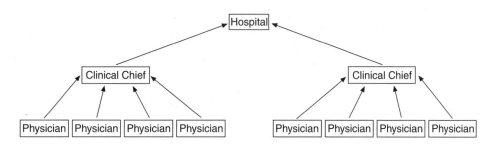

FIGURE 27–4 The hospital or integrated health care system pays clinical chiefs to supervise independent physicians.

In the model shown in Figure 27–4, there is a mix of permanent full-time medical directors who are contracted or employed on a salary or stipend basis to oversee the clinical work of otherwise independent community physicians who could be compensated on fee-for-service, hourly rate, or some other negotiated basis. There are some public facilities using this model as well as some medical school teaching hospitals where the faculty supervises local attending physicians. This is obviously not the sort of arrangement that will appeal to a local community hospital that has gone along in the traditional mode. This model is also not the first choice of an integrated health care corporation trying to move from a traditional open staff to a better vehicle for contracting and delivering managed care. Wherever it is used, there will still be Joint Commission functions, although this mixed model presents some real hardships in trying to carry out the staff work of credentialing, granting privileges, and doing reappointment. The mixed and crossing lines of authority and loyalty create conflicting incentives and eliminate many of the necessary accountabilities.

The model shown in Figure 27–5 would be interesting to those who wish to move in increments toward the managed care world from the foundation of a single hospital or a hospital chain. Boards may be consolidated to provide better governance; administrations may be merged and reduced in size to provide better management leadership, but until the physicians are integrated, there is still not a completed system. Both boards and management can be changed almost overnight, but integration of hospital medical staffs is a long, slow, careful process. However, it can be done, and this is probably the method of choice for most who might wish to proceed in that direction.

This product-line or service-line model builds on an existing characteristic of almost all Joint Commission hospitals. This characteristic of exclusive contracts for in-house hospital services by some specialty groups has been tried in court and its validity has consistently been upheld. A hospital can sign a contract with a group, such as imaging, pathology, emergency services, or others to perform the terms of the contract. That also means the partners in the group determine who will be members and, thus, who can

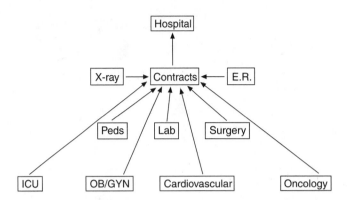

FIGURE 27–5 The hospital or health care corporation contracts with groups of physicians service by service.

practice in the hospital with exclusive rights. These new partners must pass through the usual process of credentialing and granting of privileges, but exclusivity means no other doctor in that specialty can service the particular contract in question or admit patients to the hospital. Carried to its extreme, this model could also mean that no other doctor in one of the contract specialties could even apply to the staff. Truly, that would be the direct opposite of the traditional Joint Commission model.

How to Do It

A not-for-profit hospital must serve public rather than private interests. Therefore, medical staff privileges must be generally available to all qualified physicians in the hospital's service area, consistent with the size and nature of its facilities (Rev. Rul. 69-545; *IRS Audit Guidelines for Hospitals,* March 27, 1992). Exceptions to the open staff principle are permitted if they are primarily related to improving patient care.

However, exclusive contracts have been challenged on other grounds, such as:

- unlawful restraint on the right to practice medicine;
- against public policy;
- hospital's decision is arbitrary, capricious, or lacking in evidentiary support or procedurally unfair;
- unlawful tying arrangement;
- conspiracy to monopolize;
- conspiracy in restraint of trade.

Nevertheless, court decisions have upheld exclusive contracts between hospitals and physicians, such as contracts for radiology, emergency room, anesthesiology, chronic hemodialysis, nuclear medicine, heart surgery, and cardiac catheterization laboratory services. In doing so, the courts have usually applied a balancing test to the particular facts and circumstances of each exclusive contract. The potential adverse effects on individual physicians are weighed against the importance of improving patient care at the hospital. Hospital proceedings leading to the adoption of an exclusive contract (closed staff) policy applicable to a department or service must provide an opportunity for interested parties to express their opinions.

Techniques for minimizing exposure to antitrust liability are beyond the scope of this volume, but they need to be melded into the decision-making process.

Although it would be a major cultural jump, it would be just as possible to contract for all cardiovascular services as it has been to contract for x-ray; for oncology as easily as pathology. There are no theoretical differences, except the tradition that all specialties except those under contract must accept all comers. The operational problem for a community hospital will be in the transition from tradition to a service-line model. What will be done with all those other doctors who will not be included in the contract group? The halfway step in moving toward this model is to put together contract groups to serve particular managed care contracts without doing anything about the other physicians on the staff who are not contracted for that particular health plan. Don't drop anyone from the staff, but become more selective about who services a contract. That approach will eliminate the major drawback to using any other model except the prevailing Joint Commission model. The drawback would be the upheaval in eliminating the present medical staff and replacing it with some other arrangement. That replacing can be done, but most boards do not have the stomach for that kind of tension. The turmoil in the doctors' lounge now is minor compared to after an announcement that all doctors are off the staff and only certain ones will be invited back!

MOVING TOWARD AN INTEGRATED STAFF

A partially integrated health care system, which means a system with executives who are integrated at the corporate level but without having yet achieved an equal level of integration with the doctors, could also use the same approach to reducing duplication. Each hospital in a system located in the same city does not need any longer to have one of everything. There are some economies of scale that can be achieved. There are some consolidations and mergers that can be affected. There are some managers that can be fired. There can be some flattening of the organization. There can be some downsizing or right-sizing or whatever is the latest jargon word, but until there is physician integration that matches the incentives of the corporate organization and buys into its mission, there is not an integrated system. The service-line model offers the easiest and quickest way to accomplish that integration without fighting the battle of eliminating all the doctors on the staff. Let those who want to try to continue in a fee-for-service mode stay on the staff, but they will not benefit from managed care contracts. If they can continue to bring in private pay patients to help with hospital census, let them continue, but it will be necessary to make sure that segment of the hospital medical staff does not make policy that interferes with or endangers survival success in a managed care world (White, 1991–1994).

Remember, no matter which model of membership is used, the remainder of the Joint Commission functions must still be carried on, and the medical staff will still practice credentialing, reappointment, and peer review.

SUMMARY

In previous chapters, there have been discussions and descriptions of the Joint Commission model of a hospital medical staff that has certain characteristics of organization and operating procedures. But, the Joint Commission model is not the only possibility, and alternative models are available. At least five others can be identified that may be useful in varying local circumstances and that depend upon what services are to be offered by the hospital or integrated health system.

There could be an arrangement where there is an individual contract with each member of the medical staff, which has been formed by invitation only. No other physicians can apply or be accepted except those that suit the development plan and the number and kind of patients expected. All of the Joint Commission requirements about credentialing, reappointment, privileges, and peer review would still apply. As a variation, all the physicians could be directly employed by the hospital or system in those states where there is no prohibition against the corporate practice of medicine.

A different form would see a contractual arrangement between a physician group and the hospital or health system. No doubt, in this model, there would be exclusive membership within the group, which would also perform the four traditional functions of self-governance. In a few instances, there could be an arrangement wherein the hospital or health system pays clinical chiefs to supervise independent practice physicians reimbursed on a fee-for-service basis without any other compensation from the hospital.

Finally, there is a model that simply extends the arrangements already in place, where the hospital or system contracts with groups of physicians service by service. This model might be interesting to those considering moving on an incremental basis from the open membership of a Joint Commission model to something more closed. The chapter offers some advice on how to move toward these alternative approaches or to an integrated system.

REFERENCES

Gill, S. (1993). [Faculty presentations]. Medical Staff Leadership Conferences, Sharp health care, San Diego, CA.

White, C. H. (1991–1994). [Faculty presentations]. Medical Staff Leadership Conferences, centralized credentialing conferences, Grossmont Hospital, La Mesa, CA, and Sharp Healthcare, San Diego, CA.

CHAPTER

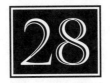

Staffs and Groups: Friends or Foes?

The solo practice of medicine has traditionally attracted the greatest number of practitioners. Indeed, it might be said that solo practice originated with the healing arts themselves. In primitive societies and for many years thereafter, until the advent of institutional care, all care was provided on an ambulatory basis by solo practitioners. Of course, the types of care given then have little resemblance to today's health care, but the history of civilization demonstrates a consistent commitment to caring for the sick, using whatever knowledge was available at the time. Remarkable forms of medical practice occurred in Greece, Rome, and other relatively sophisticated societies, most of it delivered by famous solo practitioners, including some who were slaves. Even most primitive societies and countries had or still have their own indigenous medicine men and religious healers (Williams, 1993).

ROLE OF THE PHYSICIAN

The role of physicians in relationship to organizations has changed dramatically in the last 50 years. Before World War II, most physicians were in solo general practice, with more or less organizational exposure to hospitals that served as their workshops. Over that 50-year period, physician practice moved steadily from the office and bedside to more and more complex organizational settings. Accordingly, relationships among and between doctors, health care organizations, and their managers have become increasingly interdependent. What has not changed is the physician's historic leadership role in diagnosis and treatment, even though patterns of medical practice and the role of physicians in hospitals have changed dramatically. The mission of physician services is best described by the oath most physicians take upon graduation from medical school. For many years, this was the Hippocratic oath, but the Declaration of Geneva was adopted by the General Assembly of the World Medical Association in 1948 and is now more frequently used (Schulz & Detmer, 1994). This pledge reads:

> At the time of being admitted as a member of the Medical Profession:
> * I solemnly pledge myself to consecrate my life to the service of humanity;
> * I will give my teachers the respect and gratitude that is their due;
> * I will practice my profession with conscience and dignity;
> * The health of my patient will be my first consideration;
> * I will respect the secrets which are confided in me;
> * I will maintain by all the means in my power the honor and the noble traditions of the medical profession;
> * My colleagues will be my brothers and sisters;
> * I will not permit considerations of religion, nationality, race, party politics or social standing to intervene between my duty and my patient;
> * I will maintain the utmost respect for human life, from the time of conception;
> * Even under threat, I will not use my medical knowledge contrary to the laws of humanity;
> * I make these promises solemnly, freely, and upon my honor.

THE BLACK BAG

In the early parts of this century, the physician could carry most of the standard medical equipment in a black leather bag and apply most of the accepted technologies of the time at the patient's bedside. The limited technological armament that physicians required allowed them to travel easily, carrying with them their principal equipment and supplies. Physicians' offices were frequently located in their homes or in other small buildings, as opposed to today's medical office buildings or large medical centers (Roemer, 1981). The general practitioner who made house calls, provided guidance, and offered available treatments was typical of the primary care offered before World War II (Williams, 1993).

Since that time, the explosion of medical knowledge has led to increased specialization, more complex technology, and rapid changes in the setting and nature of services. Fewer physicians are able or willing to travel to the patient's home, and many can no longer carry with them the equipment, supplies or specialized personnel available in an office. As Stephen Williams (1993) points out, a number of factors have led to the phasing out of the "traditional" general practitioner in the United States. Those factors include increased medical knowledge, technical specialization, social movements from small towns to cities and suburbs, and the desires of patients to have available all that medical science can offer.

Solo Practice

Use of the term *independent solo practice* is probably a misnomer. There are still many doctors who practice alone or practice with others but without pooling income or expenses, although that number is shrinking. The vision of the general practitioner of bygone days, traveling from house to house and ministering to the sick, represents the traditional role of primary care. The U.S. society has defined primary care as medicine that is oriented toward the daily, routine needs of patients, such as initial diagnosis and continuing treatment of common illness. This care is not highly complex and generally does not require sophisticated technology and personnel. While this historical vision of the past is lovable and nostalgic, it has been replaced in today's society by considerably better-skilled practitioners working in more modern, more scientific facilities.

Much of a modern, primary care practice has been centered around the hospital where the physician has membership and privileges. There are other health professionals involved, as well as peer review of hospital care. Solo practice has certain theoretical advantages for both the physician and the patient. The doctor has more independence than in other models of care and is a small business operator. The solo practitioner has more flexibility in referring fee-for-service patients to specialists or specialty groups. This may be a definite advantage to the patient, because referral can be to the most competent physician instead of being limited to the physician's group only. By dealing with only one physician in the practice, patients are likely to have more continuity in their relationship with their doctor.

Disadvantages of solo practice include less coverage for both the doctor (call and insurance coverage) and the patient, and less professional interaction and quality review (Schulz & Detmer, 1994). In the midst of the growing supply of doctors in the 1990s and the greater prevalence of managed care, it is becoming increasingly difficult, if not impossible, for new physicians to enter solo practice. There are the high costs of purchasing an established practice or establishing a new one, although some small or rural communities have supplied assistance in order to attract a town doctor. Then there are the mountainous debts incurred during medical school and residency. Given those, it is not surprising that so many new graduates choose instead to join groups in order to avoid the administrative burdens of trying to manage the many complexities of insurance, fiscal, and regulatory matters (particularly OSHA), all the while trying to be price competitive. Referring to Williams (1993) again, he has pointed out very well that, in addition to providing services directly, the primary care professional, whether in solo practice any longer or not, should serve the role of patient advisor, advocate, and system gatekeeper. In this coordinating role, the doctor refers patients to sources of specialized care, gives advice regarding various diagnoses and therapies, and provides continuing care for chronic conditions. In the solo practice model of the past, it was not the role of the solo practitioner to control overall health care costs, reduce utilization, or be concerned with the rational allocation of resources. Now, in the managed care era of organized systems, those factors are controlling.

The sociology of solo practice has often been associated with an increased feeling that the provider cares about the welfare of the patient, possibly resulting in a stronger bonding relationship of provider-patient than occurs in other settings. There is some evidence that this situation, when it occurs, is a result of the lower level of bureaucracy or organizational complexity in solo practice (Mechanic, 1976). Since there is also some evidence that the relationship between doctor and patient is related to patient compliance with the doctor's instructions, patients who perceive that they are receiving more personalized care may be, in fact, responding to the care process more positively (Williams, 1993). Solo practitioners are not as restricted in referrals to specialists as are providers in some other settings, such as group practice, where organizational loyalties may intervene.

There may also be a greater sense of identification with the community being served by the solo practitioner, since there can be many more direct social relationships of daily living between doctor and patients. Organizational forms, especially managed care, that incorporate solo practitioners into larger systems of care, with more organization and more bureaucracy, may be decreasing some of this doctor-patient bond. There will likely be fewer community interactions as friends and neighbors in the personal realm, while there will be more client interactions brought on by the bureaucracy such as waiting lines, increased productivity, and focus on the cost-effectiveness of the overall practice. Old-time solo doctors thought and acted in terms of units. Each patient was a unit. Now, the pressures of managed care and the allocation of resources try to bend both doctor and patient toward more global and large-scale multiple unit considerations. Think for a minute about the sheer unbelieveability of the idea that doctors and patients should consider, before beginning care, what the overall effect of that care will be on the federal share of total health care costs.

It must be kept in mind that all solo practitioners are not only primary care physicians. Some specialists have always had separate offices, where the content of their practices has been more narrowly defined than that of the primary care physician. These offices may also require more complex equipment and more highly trained support personnel. Services can be provided in the office, in outpatient departments, as well as in the hospital, usually on referral from the primaries. From the physician's perspective, whether primary or secondary, solo practice offers an opportunity to avoid organizational dependence and to be self-employed. There is also no necessity to share resources or income with other providers and be forced to work with other doctors who might not be liked very much. Solo practice has the same philosophical alignment of traditional economic and political orientations that have characterized the practice of medicine through the ages. Younger physicians now faced with discounting, contracting, and trying to fit into networks for care may no longer be able to, or may not want to, identify with these traditional perspectives any longer. The solo practice doctor must do everything necessary to run the business. The practice has distinct opportunities, it has emotional and philosophical appeal, but it also has problems and constraints.

Group Practice

As the organizational landscape of health care delivery is being rearranged, there are various partnerships or groups or professional corporations of physicians who have entered into some sort of business arrangement. Shortell estimates that more than 40 percent of the physicians are now practicing in groups, and even the groups are coming together to form larger structures (Shortell, Gillies, & Anderson, 1994). Groups can be single specialty, where the solo practice model is extended to include more physicians in the same specialty who pool their expenses, income, facilities, equipment, medical records, and support personnel in the provision of services through a formal, legally constituted organization. That was Rufus Rorem's definition in 1931, and it still is true. Another advantage is that the members can take call for each other and at least have informal quality reviews and interaction (Schulz & Detmer, 1994).

Groups can also be multispecialty, a model that provides for more professional interaction, which can support quality assurance and has the potential for skilled management. A disadvantage is less independence, less freedom to refer to physicians outside the group, and higher costs and revenues because of greater use of ancillary services. The formal definition of group practice, developed by the American Medical Association and the Medical Group Management Association, is three or more physicians formally organized to provide medical care, consultation, diagnosis, and/or treatment through the joint use of equipment and personnel and with income from medical practice distributed in accordance with methods determined by members of the group. There could be variance in the methods used to accomplish these aims, but the essential elements are formal sharing of resources and distribution of income (Williams, 1993). Traditionally, these definitions of group practices meant participation and ownership by physicians, but newer and more diversified models include other practitioners and extenders with doctors; and there are now more group practices of other practitioners such as nurses, dentists, optometrists, podiatrists, and others.

The development of group practices was stimulated by the increasing specialization of medicine and the rapid expansion of technology. No longer could the black bag of a single doctor accommodate all of the equipment and supplies that might be needed. No single practitioner could any longer afford or provide all of the medical care required by patients, such as personnel, equipment, and complex, expensive facilities. Groups offered economies of scale and the sharing of costs. The ability to treat patients under one roof thus reduced problems of physical access to care and coordination of services. Members of group practices are convinced that higher-quality of care will result because most of the different specialists that a patient requires are practicing together in close proximity and thus have the opportunity to discuss patient problems among themselves, share a common medical record, and be more able to ensure the quality and continuity of care. Those are the advantages for the patients. For the physicians, there are the added opportunities for easily developed referral arrangements, after-hours coverage, greater flexibility in working hours, relief from personal payment of liability insurance premiums, and less personal financial risk. Detractors from group practice have cited those same reasons in opposition, that quality was lower, the doctors were less well trained and skilled, and that patients would not receive the same level of personal attention as in solo practice.

EFFECT ON THE MEDICAL STAFF

Those group practice relationships described here are for office practice and are not subject to the accreditation standards of the Joint Commission. Nor are they covered by the bylaws and other self-governance activities of hospital medical staffs. One of the sacred truisms of medical staff peer review is that it is not possible to review office records or patterns of office practice when considering the current clinical competence of a doctor. Neither is it usually the case that office records can be presented as full or partial fulfillment of requirements for credentialing. Offices and clinics are not a part of medical staff evaluation.

However, when the physician(s) want to practice in the hospital, then those requirements apply. Where this issue comes into focus is the habit for many medical groups to depend upon the hospital medical staff to perform credentialing for them. Many independent practice associations (IPAs) state as a prerequisite for membership in the group that the physician must be a member in good standing of the medical staff of a certain hospital. Increasingly, this arrangement becomes important to health plans or insurers as they include a hospital staff membership requirement.

The doctor applies to the medical staff and wants instant approval in order to qualify for the plan so that patients may be immediately seen and payments made. But the credentialing process does not work that quickly and all the verifications must be made in writing. In some cases, the applicant is not able to present all of the necessary materials that will fit the customary complete application. The health plan wants the doctor to be able to show temporary privileges before seeing patients. The doctor wants the temporary privileges only in order to qualify to see patients, not caring how long it will take to complete the credentialing process.

Both of them are depending on the accuracy and credibility of the hospital medical staff process and the good work of the medical staff services personnel. On the other hand, the organized medical staff is reluctant to change its process, especially for these new physicians who may not be known in the community. The rallying cry will be: "we didn't give anyone else a break, why should we give one to these guys?" The point is well taken, because the hospital process is being asked to grant a seal of approval to doctors who will probably not practice in the hospital at all. What causes these tempests is usually that the corporate office has signed a contract with a new medical group and the contract officer blithely promised that it would be easy to get privileges. The contract officer never asked anyone from the medical staff, like a chief or department chair whether it would be easy or even possible to accomplish and how long it would take.

Hold on to Good Staff Work

So now there are more angry doctors, new ones this time, who in their eyes are being prohibited from making a living by the clerical staff at the hospital who are being too bureaucratic. The medical staff services staff who succeed in their professional life by being painstakingly careful and accurate, are now being asked to depart from their procedures to grant a phony or hasty temporary privileges just so someone can put in an insurance brochure that the doctor is a member of the medical staff of that hospital.

The chief of staff receives phone calls from the business manager of the medical group complaining about delays and doctors being harassed. The administrator is being pressured by the corporate office about why patients covered by that new plan not being admitted and treated since the revenue is desperately needed. In turn, the administrator calls the chief to complain about how tedious is the medical staff bureaucracy (which is the best protection the hospital has against liability cases). The administrator may descend on the medical staff services office to remind them that they are hospital employees and they are not being very loyal. Of course, if they violate their standard procedures they will be fired anyway for not doing what the medical staff wants them to do.

A fictional scenario? Not at all in these days of negotiated contracts and managed care health plans that are causing dislocations or relocation of doctors and hospitals and patients. The real point is that the Joint Commission model of a medical staff has succeeded so well and is widely recognized as the only existing mechanism that can assure that physicians are who they claim to be, that the doctor is adequately and appropriately trained for the medical practice to be carried on, and that the practice is being carried on according to community standards. There is no other mechanism available to replace it, even though the model is showing signs of being obsolete in some regards, particularly concerning incentives.

EFFECT ON THE MEDICAL GROUP

Medical groups are coming from a different place. Joint Commission hospitals must admit to the medical staff any candidate who has the proper credentials and who practices without errors of omission or commission regarding patient safety and appropriate care. Everyone who applies and qualifies must be accepted. Medical groups are put together on the grounds of similar specialties, similar practice styles, friendship, or convenience. Some groups simply lease contiguous office space, some share receptionists and records storage, some are full-fledged corporate partnerships and some are fully organized closed panel HMOs or health plan providers.

But they all have one thing in common. They all depend on the hospital medical staff to credential and grant privileges for specialty care in the hospital, which is where specialists do what they do. Primaries may or may not have privileges in the hospital, but if they do, then they will have passed through the same hurdles that everyone else did, and they are notably resistant about the new business of merely granting temporary privileges for brochure purposes. Most of the time, the specialists look to the hospital for their continuing medical education, not to the medical group. Primaries probably look more to their professional societies, since hospital CME is overwhelmingly targeted toward the specialists. So there is a strong bond interlocking groups and staffs.

Sometimes, there is another similarity. Depending upon structure, it may be necessary for the physicians in a medical group to also be reappointed in two-year cycles, just like the hospital staffs. For some groups, it is a matter of recontracting, but the principle is the same. The doctor is looked at, further training is taken into account, examples of successful as well as questionable practice are evaluated, and, in groups, utilization data are used more heavily in the reconsideration process. A hospital medical staff has a number of persuasions available to try to encourage a member to reduce excessive utilization, but discharge from the staff is rarely one of those. Appeals to change practice to fit the patterns of colleagues based on trustworthy data is a resort to the scientific method that has worked frequently. But any closed panel medical group that does not maintain careful utilization records and does not make recontracts based on practice comparisons is not long for this world. In fact, the best utilization records in the country are proudly exhibited by the closed panel groups to show that it is possible to practice the best quality medicine as well as the best quality and quantity utilization.

Where there are medical groups that perform their own reappointment or recontracting, there will be staff doing the work. Those staff employees are similar if not identical to the medical staff services personnel in hospitals. They have received similar training. They belong to the same local, state, and national organizations formed to advance their profession. They could be interchangeable and probably were, in fact, hired away from a hospital. They perform the work with the same dedication to professional performance and are the best friends that chiefs, chairs, and medical directors have when it comes to carrying out this process. The Joint Commission model has resulted in the creation and improvement of this profession that serves in either groups or hospitals.

Then there are the loosely organized "groups" that formed in the 1980s and early 1990s to combat the growth and success of closed panel groups by allowing each physician member to maintain the same office and practice style. Anyone who wanted to could join, and there was little more than token lip service to utilization controls. Most of those are gone now, bankrupt, leaving a legacy of anger and financial loss of initial capital stock as well as unpaid claims. To some people, the reason to put together such an organization was to prove that doctors could do it better than the business and administration types. To others, the disastrous result was to prove conclusively that they were not able to do it at all, much less better. Out of the ashes is rising a generation of business-trained and skilled physicians who are busy creating the next world of medical care and practice instead of trying to resist and prevent it from happening.

THE INTERSECTION WHERE THEY MEET

In the meantime, medical groups and hospital staffs can and must work together. For each it is a matter of developing and maintaining individual local habits and traditions. But the task at hand is to keep what is valuable about those habits and traditions each in its own place. Medical groups can and must pay strict attention to the economic credentialing of its members for mutual financial success. Hospital staffs can and must preserve the rule of treating each member fairly and consistently. When a member of a medical group practices in a hospital, the standards and patterns of the hospital apply. It is not all right for a member of a group to join a hospital staff and then try to refuse to do the same backup duties performed by all other members of the department on the grounds that the medical group does not do backup. Doctors cannot join partway.

For years, hospital staffs in some areas have bad-mouthed and resisted members of some closed panel groups. Now the exigencies brought on by managed care contracting have thrown some of these strange bedfellows together. And while it is funny to watch them trying to accommodate each other very carefully, nevertheless they must now discard the excess baggage and meaningless turf guarding of the past if there is to be an integrated health care system in a managed care environment. The real secret of forming successful integrated systems is physician integration, an art form that almost no one yet knows how to do.

It may come to pass in the managed care world that medical groups will become the medical staffs of hospitals, thus aligning incentives for mutual benefit. But what will be done with the doctors who are not part of the group? That is the question not yet answered for most hospital staffs. It is clear that fee-for-service practice styles in hospitals where anyone can be on the medical staff is incompatible with the vision of system integration of doctors serving patients with managed care coverage. The job of the next decade is to resolve these mutually incompatible situations.

SUMMARY

Medical groups may become the medical staffs of hospitals in the future so as to align incentives for mutual benefit. The perplexing dilemma of the next decades will be how to resolve the mutually incompatible situations of an open practice style where anyone can join the medical staff with system integration because of managed care coverage. Visible evidence of the problem and its beginning evolution can be seen in the movement from solo practice toward medical groups.

Since the end of World War II, physician practice has moved steadily from the general practice office and bedside toward more and more complex organizational settings, not always with happy acceptance by the practitioners. From the days of the doctor's black bag, which could carry practically everything medicine had to offer, the explosion of medical knowledge has led to increased specialization, more complex technology, and rapid changes in the setting and nature of services. The sociology of solo practice, which offered the feeling that the doctor cared about the welfare of the patient, may have been replaced by the production line techniques of managed care HMOs, and there may not be any longer as much doctor-patient relationship.

Now, nearly half of all physicians are practicing in groups of some sort, reaping the business advantages that can come from shared resources and medical skills. Group practices appear to be the way of the present and seem destined to grow larger in the future. Groups and their practice arrangements may mean another set of forces bearing down on the hospital medical staff, which could be expected to do the credentialing for the group. Groups are increasingly under the scrutiny of insurers and payers that want to balance quality and cost, and they may expect the hospital medical staff to help them do that.

REFERENCES

Mechanic, D. (1976). *The Growth of Bureaucratic Medicine.* New York: Wiley.

Roemer, M. (1981). *Ambulatory Health Services in America.* Rockville, MD: Aspen Systems Corporation.

Shortell, S. M., Gillies, R. R., & Anderson, D. A. (1994). The new world of managed care: Creating organized systems. *Health Affairs, Winter,* 46–64.

Schulz, R., & Detmer, D. E. (1994). Physician organization and management. In Taylor, R. J., & Taylor, S. B. (Eds.), *The AUPHA Manual of Health Services Management.* Gaithersburg, MD: Aspen Publishers.

Williams, S. J. (1993). Ambulatory health care services. In Williams, S. J., & Torrens, P. R. (Eds.), *Introduction to Health Services, (4th ed.).* Albany: Delmar Publishers.

CHAPTER

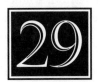

Supporting or Assisting Members

More attention has been paid in recent years to those few members of the medical staff who need particular assistance with their personal and professional lives at a time when they are vulnerable. What may not have been stated as frequently is the role of the medical staff in providing support and assistance to its members who need help. The exact number of physicians impaired by alcohol or substance abuse and mental disorders is unknown, according to the AMA, but is, perhaps, in the 10 to 14 percent range (Steindler, 1975). Whether that estimate is accurate or whether those data are dated is not the point. What does matter is that it is almost a certainty that any medical staff has some (hopefully few) members who fit the definition. Rather than argue about the actual number, start now to deal with the real problems of real people.

Called by various names, a larger number of medical staffs now have a committee or program to help physicians who fit into the category of "impaired." Impairment may only mean recuperation from a broken leg suffered on a CME-sponsored ski trip. But that is not really what is meant here by the use of "impaired." As a euphemism, that word is blank verse for substance abuse, whether drugs or alcohol, when that abuse grows to the point of affecting medical practice. When closet drunks spend time out on their boats, or on weekend binges, the medical staff may not know or have the need to care as long as that behavior is not carried over to the hospital. Impairment may also mean a condition of senile dementia or other illness that is progressively debilitating.

Partners need to know if one of their number is not functioning at a high level and is affecting their joint practice. Hospital medical staffs need to know if the habits of one or more of their members are being carried over into the facility where patient safety can be a concern, as well as the welfare and safety of hospital employees. The role of the medical staff is not only one of vigilance and detection but the larger and more difficult work of trying to assist and support. When a doctor is so far out of control that entry into the criminal justice system has occurred, the medical staff probably no longer has anything to say about subsequent events. The issue at that point is one of deciding whether membership on the staff and privileges have been compromised and whether corrective action must be taken. The medical staff organization, as has been described consistently during this book, is not "self-governing" in the sense of being completely autonomous from the hospital governing board. But the staff organization should be self-governing in the sense of maintaining self-control and self-discipline (Thompson, 1990).

COMMITTEE TO SUPPORT, NOT POLICE

Hospitals have certain legal responsibilities to take action against an incompetent physician who is exhibiting deficiencies in clinical work. Responsibility and liability to take action against an impaired physician are not as well defined. The examples are well known in any medical staff when it was easier to ignore or overlook signs of developing impairment in the hope that it, or the doctor, will just go away. Sometimes, when impairment is so blatant that it can no longer be overlooked, medical staffs then make up for lost time and attention and react in an overkill or punitive manner.

Hospital medical staffs need to have a mechanism to find out about and respond to those instances when a doctor can be observed to be acting under the influence. There should be an interview process for new applicants by one or more members of the particular specialty to identify physicians in need of aid. A doctor already on the staff whose professional demeanor has changed, whose attention to details of cases seems different or erratic, or whose behavior is not within usual patterns: All of these indicators or symptoms are warnings. Many of the existing medical mechanisms are readily available to serve for case finding, if only anyone will pay attention to the signs or symptoms.

Every hospital needs a sympathetic listener on the medical staff who can somehow relate to those very few colleagues who have a problem they can no longer control. The medical staff needs a committee that can offer assistance, support, and counseling. The committee acts as an advocate for the physician, not as a police officer. Every hospital should consider the problem as a possibility, if not an immediate emergency. Increasing tension and changes in practice brought about by advancing managed care may very well bring about an increase in troubled physicians who can then be classified as "impaired." Promote the concept of an organized physicians' aid committee and call it the advisory committee, assistance, or support. Stay away from the label of "impaired" in the name of the committee, which should be made a part of the bylaws as a standing committee, by whatever name. Call it an advisory committee, a support committee, or any other name that sounds helpful and not insulting or degrading. But the point is to develop a nonpunitive approach in which the hospital and the medical staff act as an advocate for the physician, rather than as an avenging angel. Of course, patients need to be protected from harm, but the purpose of this program is to detect emerging impairment, offer support to the physician and family, and encourage appropriate early treatment (Orsund-Gassiot, 1990).

The chief of staff, the VPMA, or both should see that an appropriate committee chair be appointed. The chair must be a person, no matter what specialty, who has a supportive personality and an earnest desire to help save the troubled doctor and to face problems realistically but without a punitive or policing attitude. Lots of times there is a jump to the conclusion that only a psychiatrist is appropriate for this position. Sometimes that is true and sometimes not. Skill and interest are preferable to any particular label. These special people are rare and can be single-handedly responsible for establishing and maintaining useful rapport and a relationship. The medical leadership must assist the committee to develop policies regarding identification, surveillance, consultation, confrontation, and, above all else, confidentiality.

The role of the committee is to provide support and counseling to individual physicians on the staff who have been identified, or who identify themselves. This may be the most important but most difficult part of the whole process. When a doctor's whole professional career and public image is at stake, extreme caution and denial are normal behaviors. That should also be the attitude of the committee and the medical staff leadership. As healers, they deal every day with people suffering through illnesses and injuries. So it is with colleagues who have put themselves or have been thrust against their will into an illness or injury situation that cannot fail to endanger or destroy their persons and their careers. The first concern is to save good doctors, even from themselves, and restore those professionals to more normal lives and productive careers. It won't be easy.

How the Committee Functions

Whatever it is or was that brought on the drinking problem or substance abuse, these are very smart people and they have learned to conceal or deny with highly developed skills. The chair and the committee should expect to be regarded with suspicion or distrust that may never quite go away. But it is a guarantee that if there are leaks in security or gossip by people who know but shouldn't talk, then the committee and its good intentions are useless. There should be no minutes kept of the meetings, and no agendas prepared to show who will be present. The committee chair should meet with the executive committee at least quarterly to give a general report on the work in progress by the committee, but without naming names that could be revealed. There have been too many instances of hearing members of the executive committee standing in a hallway or on a nursing unit discussing in loud voices things that should have remained back in the peer review session.

The committee and chair must develop and implement contracts with identified physicians that cite the terms of performance, peer support groups, diversion programs to be entered, clinical and chemical monitoring programs, as well as penalties for noncompliance. Frequently it is necessary for the troubled physician to be assigned to enter therapy. The chair or the committee must choose or at least approve the therapist. Do not allow the physician to alone choose the therapist. Then as part of the contract, the physician must give up the doctor/patient confidentiality arrangement so that the therapist can give regular reports to the chief of staff concerning progress and compliance. Therapy ends when the chief or the chair or the committee says it does, not when the physician chooses. Furthermore, all therapy is at the physician's expense. Never use medical staff or hospital funds for that purpose.

Many states, cities, or counties have established physicians aid organizations or networks that are dedicated to the same principles of help and support. But this is not just some do-gooder idea being discussed here. The doctor must be sincere and must act accordingly. The committee and the medical staff leadership must be timely and firm in dealing with compliance and contract observance in the monitoring program. The purpose of monitoring is to assure patients, the hospital, and the medical staff that a recovering physician can now practice medicine safely after treatment (*Guidelines,* 1988). Failure to cooperate or to progress with the contract program becomes instant grounds for initiating corrective action. Patient safety and good quality of care still ranks higher than the desire to not take away physician privileges or damage a reputation when it really becomes necessary.

ASSIGN BEHAVIORAL PROBLEMS TO A COMMITTEE

A lengthy diatribe about abusive or misbehaving physicians was presented in Chapter 7, in the context of peer review. Some medical staffs have found it to be helpful to delegate supervision and monitoring of those problems to the support committee. All of the mechanisms developed for use with substance abuse cases also apply to behavioral problems. There are differences between the approach to alcohol/substance abuse physicians and behavior problem physicians; namely, the former involve an intervention process that tries to persuade the physician to seek or accept help. There needs to be conveyed the hope that treatment can be accepted and effective. In the latter case, abusive behavior has been identified and brought into the peer review process, where there will be insistence, not just hope, that things will change. Responsibility for oversight by the support committee is assigned or delegated only by the executive committee, which will have a requirement for regular reporting back.

Either way, there will be counseling and gestures of support. There will be monitoring against a contract or "sentence" by the executive committee through the probationary or reentry phase. There should be treatment, required CME as appropriate, and a formal plan for both types of physician in recovery. The recovery plan for breaches of behavior will probably be more well known, since it is more likely to involve public apologies and sensitivity training with the hospital staff involved. One of the most important but frequently overlooked aspect of the recovery program for physicians recovering from abusive behavior, such as striking, cursing, or other verbal assaults on patients, families, or staff, is the need for the medical staff to satisfy itself that the physician's clinical skills and performance is still intact. There must also be a waiver of privilege allowing disclosure of the monitoring program with other hospital medical staffs where the physician has privileges. Any person forced to seek help in this way is long since past the point of being protected from "embarrassment" or "professional courtesy."

Try It—You'll Like It

Sometime, ask someone who has served on a committee like this or has been involved with trying to salvage a career and return a productive physician to society. They will express that nothing they have done in the hospital staff was so important and rewarding as to see an impaired physician put all of those troubles behind and go on to treat patients in a professional and caring manner once again.

SUMMARY

Trying to salvage a medical career and return a productive physician to practice and society is not only a noble goal but is an obligation on the part of the medical staff. Each self-governance program should have a committee or program to help and support members of the staff who can be considered to be "impaired" in some manner because of substance abuse. The medical staff is obligated to pay attention and notice whether the habits of a doctor are threatening patient safety and to do something about that situation. Going past vigilance and detection frequently means taking corrective action that may involve counseling, assistance, support, and appropriate treatment, as necessary. Entering into contracts with troubled physicians is one mechanism that has been useful, as described in the chapter.

REFERENCES

Guidelines for Physician Aid Committees of Hospital Medical Staffs (1988). San Francisco: California Medical Association.

Orsund-Gassiot, C. A. (1990). Dealing with the impaired physician. In Orsund-Gassiot, C. A., & Lindsey, S. (Eds.), *Handbook of Medical Staff Management*. Gaithersburg, MD: Aspen Publishers.

Steindler, E. M. (1975). *The Impaired Physician, American Medical Association Department of Mental Health Bulletin*. Chicago: AMA.

Thompson, R. E. (1990). The medical staff organization. In Orsund-Gassiot, C. A., & Lindsey, S. (Eds.), *Handbook of Medical Staff Management*. Gaithersburg, MD: Aspen Publishers.

CHAPTER
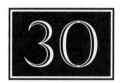

What Does It All Mean?

Earlier chapters have described many of the rapid changes affecting the U.S. health care system and the effect of those on the hospital medical staff. What further changes will affect the health care system—doctors and hospitals—between now and the year 2000? It is possible to construct at least two plausible scenarios, each involving changes having dramatic effects on patients and providers alike, changes caused and controlled by factors not in the grip of doctors and hospitals nor their integrated networks or systems. The methodology was first constructed years ago but can be updated and pushed forward now, with an updated set of predictions (White, 1988).

The world economic picture, the U.S. economy, demographics, and the mood of the electorate: all of these will have much more impact than health provider behavior. Hospitals and doctors themselves will not cause any of these broad-scale social developments, and doctors and hospitals will not, acting alone, alleviate their effects, good or bad. The first scenario can be called "Things Get Worse before They Get Better." In this scenario, the economy remains essentially stagnant and the share of gross national product devoted to health care is reduced. The other scenario can be called "Things Get Better before They Get Worse." In this scenario, the economy improves and the share of gross national product devoted to health care increases. Each has an effect on the hospital medical staff.

SCENARIO I: WORSE BEFORE BETTER

Things get worse: cost-containment pressures on hospitals and doctors in effect during the early to mid-1990s will remain the guiding principle for the remainder of the century. Public policy and health politics will be dictated less by the remainder of the World War II generation and more by what has become the largest segment of the U.S. population: the baby boom generation that now to a great extent composes the middle class. Still relatively young and with much greater education than their parents, this middle-age and middle-class group primarily value concerns for themselves and their families, even though a greater number of them are now single parents. More of them are financially secure than any previous generation in U.S. history, because of increasing education levels, more two-income families, and a greater interest in entrepreneurship. They are more sophisticated about consumer products and more skeptical about the value of major health care expenditures unless there is clear evidence that longevity will be increased and quality of life will not be threatened. Health is not their major concern, ranking behind crime, safety, education for their children, and their economic well-being. They are skeptical about politics and have developed a deep and abiding distrust of politicians and the media alike.

In this scenario, the U.S. economy averages 2 to 3 percent real growth per year, with an accompanying annual inflation rate of 4 percent or less (White & Lewis, 1986). The nation continues to experience a baby bust that reduces the supply of entry-level workers, which leads to continued immigration (legal or illegal) of persons from other countries who are willing to assume these lowest-wage positions. Competition among baby boomers for midlevel positions dampens income in what would otherwise be their peak years, with particular impact from corporate downsizing. Demand continues to be depressed for expensive items such as autos, the housing industry remains stagnant, international competition remains tight, world consumers find U.S. goods too expensive, and foreign loans are not repaid.

New trade agreements by the United States and neighboring countries have not yet had time to produce real results. World commodity and energy prices remain low, major smokestack industries continue to decline, the defense sector continues to slide, and the armed forces remain at their personnel levels of the early 1990s. The business climate remains competitive, government is concerned with budget deficits, and capital for renovation, remodeling, or upgrading is somewhat available but difficult to amortize

(White & Lewis, 1985). The social infrastructure of roads, bridges, and transportation systems are only partially replaced and repaired as a result of natural disasters. Interest rates remain fairly constant, adjusted by the Federal Reserve to control inflation, but at the price of stock market constraints.

Middle-Class Concerns

The middle-class consumers, in this scenario, are trapped in their debtor position, paying off 30-year mortgages on single family homes and paying installments for cars, clothes, vacations, and so on. Their prime concerns are family needs (house, education, child care, careers) and establishing professional and community roles and personal financial position. Local concerns predominate (parks, recreation, job safety, the environment, police and fire protection). One major goal is keeping government spending constant and predictable. Getting ahead for these college-educated families does occur, but only gradually and over a spread of more years than they thought it would take. Meanwhile, the number of homeless living on the streets in cities continues to grow without any solution being found for what to do with them. In a depressed economy, not enough people care what happens to the homeless. Health concerns will be minimal for those in the middle group, but paramount for the senior citizens. One dramatic change over previous generations is the inability and unwillingness of baby boomers to care for elderly parents in their own homes. When the issue is between college for kids or care for parents, the parents will generally lose out.

In this scenario, government cannot escape its vicious cycle of stagnation and deficit. Consumers unable to break free of financial constraints resist any major expansion of government activities. Baby boomers are aware that social systems are inadequate, but being cash poor, they are unwilling and unable to pay additional taxes. Neither social programs nor defense can grow. The GNP for health care declines from its previous highs; no new taxes and less government is the overwhelming national consensus, with the family-related issues of education, child care, and safety protection dominating. No effective plan can be found to stop the increased use of drugs with an accompanying growth in the expenditure of health care dollars in treating drug-related problems. Similarly, the march of AIDS continues, with no large-scale prevention program in place and without an effective cure being developed.

System Changes

As social program funding drops, means testing for benefits eligibility will increase, as will co-payments and deductibles. Health insurance becomes taxable and first-dollar coverage is finally completely unavailable. Direct control on physicians' fees, caps on liability claims and lawyers' contingency fees, elimination of joint and several liability, shrinking of the liability insurance industry: all of these result from stubborn pressure on profits. Business concerns now control health policy, and employers continue to push for more managed care systems and fixed prices on health care. Business is preoccupied with keeping health benefit costs as low as possible, further stimulating interest of the human resources professionals in delivering employee groups to prepaid capitation systems for more competitive process: the more managed, the better. Employers want workers to pay ever larger shares and up-front costs. They also insist on monitoring more closely the cost patterns of individual providers and storing up much more information on quality and satisfaction with care as well as outcomes to help both the company and the consumers make more efficient choices. All of these effects will have a negative impact on the hospital medical staff by reducing morale and weakening any collegial feelings that might remain.

Even more trust is placed in gatekeeper-dominated systems to reduce the cost of subspecialty services, but there are not enough primary care physicians to staff the integrated systems that emerge. The gatekeeper's function is to minimize the cost of the medical care delivered to the patient by seeing to it that only essential care is available. But what is essential is determined by the gatekeeper. This reduces both the *supply* of care by other providers and the effective *demand* for care by patients. If the patient really wants more care, then that person must go outside the managed care system and try to find available services in the private market and pay for them out-of-pocket. In this capitated system, the incentives are no longer to please the patient but to please the payer. There is greater financial discipline for physicians to order fewer tests, use fewer referral specialists, and have lower rates of hospitalization. The formerly high level of trust in physicians is reduced to the levels of other professionals—educators, clergy, judges, the military—but not as low as lawyers and politicians. Funding for medical education and research is not a high priority, and the overall number of physicians practicing health care begins to decline, as does annual income.

In this scenario, there is a pronounced change in attitudes about the right of people to refuse use of extreme measures to prolong life. Demands will increase for better information about costs and the relationship between extension and the quality of life. A consensus will build in many communities, and patients, families, doctors, and the clergy will agree that individuals have a right to refuse heroic measures to prolong life. The public will favor allowing patients the right to die when faced with incurable diseases or coma. Medical practice is then forced to adapt to both constraints on resources and the public's attitude to focus on early detection, prevention, and functional remedies in both research and care, shifting away from heroic measures in the last months and days of life.

Down the road it becomes clear that direct governmental controls such as DRGs or physician fee schedules can work reasonably well in the short run to control costs. But such controls eventually become political, substituting bureaucratic maneuvering for market systems (White, 1986). Eventually cost-control systems begin to concentrate on the wrong things, retard innovation, are carried on by newly formed constituencies, destroy much-needed but unprofitable products (e.g., hospitals serving the indigent), and gradually erode ethical standards. Implementers down the line always have trouble doing what was intended for them to do because of the difficulty of keeping competent staff and because of the changes in the political agendas every time a new president or governor is elected.

The kinds of care most likely to be affected in a cost-containment scenario are those that depend on dedicated capital equipment and highly specialized staff, far more than services that can be provided by regular hospital personnel and ordinary drugs and supplies. Decisions on more routine services will require individual physicians to deny individual care to specific patients. Long-term cost containment will require hard choices about who gets what—in short, rationing. How budget constraints are imposed will determine how much the income of individual physicians is affected and, thus, the level and degree of intrahospital conflict that will ensue. Those physicians who perform procedures involving substantial use of hospital resources are likely to be significantly affected by almost every payment methodology adopted. By contrast, physicians who perform procedures involving little capital, equipment, or personnel should be affected least.

Slight Constraints, Slight Effects

If there are only slight constraints, there will be only slight effects (White & Lewis, 1985). In the early stages of slowing growth of hospital expenditures, few changes occur in medical practice. Hospitals curtail purchases and replacement of equipment, economize on heating and lighting, delay replacement of linen, reduce quality of food, and defer maintenance. Nursing and other staff vacancies will be filled at slower rates; workloads will increase, with accompanying loss of staff morale but increased productivity. In short, mild budget limits only subject hospitals and their medical staffs to cost disciplines that competitive businesses routinely face but that hospitals and doctors were sheltered from by reimbursement based on costs and charges. All of these effects were detailed in Chapter 24.

Severe Limits, Severe Effects

More severe limits would have more severe effects, and the days of easy adjustment would end. Decisions will have to be made on what services are to be available to whom. Because public expectations remain high, these restrictions are perceived as painful (Aaron & Schwartz, 1985). As constraints increase, the effect on patient care becomes greater, because few options remain for reducing expenditures without appreciably changing patterns of medical practice. Diagnostic radiology and lab tests are among the most likely choices for reductions. Benefits lost with these reductions are less visible; the potential savings are large. The introduction of costly new treatments and diagnostic procedures is slowed, occurring only when, or even after, their effectiveness is clearly demonstrated.

Physicians on hospital medical staffs are forced to redefine what care constitutes standard medical practice and what care exceeds that standard. Acute illness and traumatic injuries continue to be diagnosed and treated with the best each hospital has to offer, so long as the victim has even a small chance to recover and achieve a normal life. Small and rural hospitals cannot survive under this overwhelming combination of pressures, and most of them close, leaving those patients at long distances from even the most rudimentary care.

Most illnesses of children and young adults continue to be treated aggressively, but serious ethical and legal questions arise in treating the badly impaired and unborn. Treatment of cancer probably continues to command nearly all the resources required to provide whatever benefit is available. Terminal care, on the other hand, is much reduced. Severe limits means less consumption of goods and services for terminal care than for medical care. Less intensive care and limitations on other specialized technologies curtail the provision of aggressive care for dying patients. In a world of resource constraints, the rules inevitably change. Using resources on the terminally ill may mean death, disability, and pain for those nonterminally ill patients denied care. When resources are too few to take care of all, care is provided to those who stand to benefit the most. This becomes the new ethic under the resource limits imposed by budget constraints.

Changes in Medical Practice

What changes in medical practice would occur in this scenario, which describes a gradually shrinking health care system that reduces both the supply and demand for care? It seems obvious that budget limits would gradually cause accepted standards of care to change. Good medicine would then call for fewer tests and imaging studies when the gain in information is slight, and for less surgery and less use of costly drugs when the advantage of expensive over inexpensive therapies is small. Physicians in U.S. hospitals would build into their practices a sense of the relation between the costs of care and the value of benefits from it. They would, that is, if they thought the period of tighter constraints was going to last for the foreseeable future. If, on the other hand, there was light at the end of the tunnel, so to speak, they would be inclined to just tough it out and maintain traditional standards of care.

Doctors would weigh not only the medical aspects of diagnosis and treatment but also the personal characteristics of each patient: age, underlying health, family responsibilities, and the patient's chance of recovering sufficiently to resume a normal life in a diminished society that was suffering from chronic underfunding. This would be a far-reaching change in attitude for many American doctors who practice in hospitals and who have been accustomed to more available payments. Physicians would then have redefined what care is "appropriate." Such rationalization is probably essential to the morale of the physician who finds that it is not Congress, not rate-setting agencies, not the utilization review nurses from the insurance companies, but the physician alone who must say no to the patient who wants more care but cannot have it. The task of saying no will become increasingly difficult as constraints become tighter and doctors must allocate existing capacity to the patients who will benefit most from care, which means denying it to others.

Patient Responses

As budget restraints become tighter, patients would seek safety valves that allow them to obtain care they would otherwise be denied (Aaron & Schwartz, 1985). But since most patients would be in managed care plans, without the ability to visit any other physicians, there are fewer opportunities for doctor shopping. Trying to cajole, browbeat, or bribe doctors to provide "full" care might be tried increasingly but without general success, since plans or medical groups would not allow such deviations from the standard benefits. Consequently, aggressive and influential patients would probably seek to obtain care superior to that offered by the benefit plan for employees. Besides putting more pressure on the physicians, patients would likely try to seek care outside the severely constricted hospital system. As constraints become more severe, a central question would be whether care could be obtained from providers not subject to budget limits. Could there be a system outside the system? Money always seems to buy everything.

Getting care outside the system would also create political, administrative, and economic problems, stemming from the desire of people to buy insurance to protect themselves from the risk that a certain type of care may be too expensive for the managed care system. Insurance of that kind passed into history in the early to mid-1990s and inevitably short circuits the incentives of the market-regulated effort to balance costs against benefits. Dissatisfied patients will appeal to their legislators. Media headlines and congressional mails will probably abound with horror stories about withholding or withdrawing care. Providers and insurers will be required to abide by the unseen hand of the market, but politicians are not bound by the same restraints and will have no compunction about blaming the doctors and hospitals.

Patients and families will turn to the media, which will highlight the effects of the budget shortfall by featuring heart-rending stories about patients that were not saved through heroic measures with heroic costs. Constituent pressure could become so widespread and tense that Congress and some state legislatures might begin to mandate specific exceptions to the budget constraints, which would make the decisions of doctors and hospitals even more difficult and more subject to second-guessing. The system of control would slowly become porous because of too many loopholes at state and federal levels, some of them contradictory. Finally, slowly growing public pressure would build up in favor of larger investments in health care than the severely limited budgets permitted, and another era of expansion might begin. Or it might not, even with public pressure, if the economic condition of the country would not permit any increases.

The Downward Spiral

The unresolved issue of access to care would be the key, in this scenario, to ending any cost-containment policy. The number of people with no coverage would gradually increase from 10 percent to 20 percent or more of the population, including temporarily unemployed people who are the victims of downsizing, part-time workers, unmarried partners and their children, and low-income workers in small businesses (the underemployed and underinsured). As the funding crunch, both public and private, continues year after year, this uncovered population's access to health care—access previously provided in large measure by county or teaching hospitals and clinics—will be reduced, and they will suffer further indignities of long waiting lines, busy telephones, extensive delays, and spotty geographic coverage. There will be more uncompensated care for doctors and hospitals to swallow.

With no remaining first-dollar coverage and mandatory participation in managed care plans, consumers will become more hesitant to use routine services because of the out-of-pocket charges for co-payments and deductibles. They will be especially hesitant to choose more expensive initial procedures. Employer-sponsored plans act as barriers to access for certain providers or certain services, payment mechanisms such as DRGs and physician fee schedules provide limited funds per episode of illness, and some patients receive less treatment than their condition might warrant. As the cost-containment spiral circles ever downward, there is increased "tiering" of the health care system. Care becomes more sporadic as most insurance rules grow more strict, and access to long-term care becomes even more problematic as state Medicaid funds dry up in the face of reduced appropriations. No meaningful health care reform legislation can be passed at either federal or state levels. Serious political tensions in the health care system will manifest themselves as a result of access problems disturbing the public. There will be growing concern about the lack of progress in medical research, the failure to find cures for cancer and AIDS, the decreasing pace of innovation, the lack of physicians entering research, and increased difficulties with medical education.

However, history will show that the cost-containment movement, which began in the late 1980s and continued in the 1990s in the form of managed care plans and capitation, did succeed in reversing the trend toward major increases in cost rates that occurred during the preceding decades (White & Morse, 1985). Quality of care and access for most people—those middle aged and middle class—remains essentially uncompromised, even though people on the margins suffer some dislocations. The consensus of the public after years in this scenario is that the health care system served them pretty well when they needed to concentrate on other things. But the question is whether the health care system that evolved during this scenario will serve as well the baby boom generation when they become aged during the twenty-first century. Will there be enough remaining capacity and enough quality and quantity? Will there be enough supply to meet the inevitable demand? Will things be as bad for them as for their parents who grew old during the scenario and found shortages all around them?

Effect on the Medical Staff

In reality, this scenario is an extension and extrapolation of the beginning of the managed care era that began in the early 1990s. All of the economic and social conditions of that time have been carried further, with predictions of the effect on the health care system, on doctors and hospitals. Managed care itself is the enemy of the harmonious and cooperative working relationships visualized in the Joint Commission model of a hospital medical staff performing self-governance. All of the incentives that would cause individual physicians to work voluntarily, out of a sense of professionalism and service, to perform credentialing, reappointment, and peer review would be severely impacted by the forces described in scenario one. Nothing but bitterness and hostility by the doctors against everyone and everything would be the legacy of that imaginary scenario. Truly, that would not be the kind of medical practice they were taught in medical school. The most necessary action of self-governance that would be effective in that scenario would be utilization review, which is the most despised and hated of the duties and responsibilities, as described in Part 1 of this book.

SCENARIO II: BETTER BEFORE WORSE

What changes will affect health and hospital care and the medical staff that delivers that care from now until the year 2000? The introduction to the first scenario pointed to the controlling influence on health policy, health politics, and health care financing of some larger social forces. With a different set of assumptions about the world and national environment, the second scenario predicts a very different picture. In this scenario, the cost-containment enthusiasm of the 1980s and 1990s subsides as the economy improves. The historic growth pattern of the health care delivery system resumes its upward path after what appears in retrospect to have been only a temporary glitch from managed care plans, DRGs, per-diem contracts, and a short-lived boom in HMOs and PPOs.

The driving force in this renewed expansion is the overwhelming pressure to provide a wider range of health services to an aging (and voting) population. Although nearly as numerous as the middle-aged baby boom generation, aged people hold the balance of political power and are very eager to use that leverage (Institute for the Future, 1986). While the baby boomers are more concerned with family and career matters, aged people discover access problems and threats of denial of service in the erstwhile cost-containment philosophies and practices. Fortunately for them, the stimulated economy will allow growth in the health sector to resume.

Clear-cut distinctions emerge between the wants and needs of population subgroups. The effects of diet, exercise, health care, less smoking, pollution cleanup, and environmental safety produce a larger group of "young old" (age 65 to 75) people (Institute for the Future, 1986). Still largely employed, young old people need health benefit plans that offer acute care services, transplants, and rehabilitation not based on means testing. They want private insurance coverage that looks very much like the commercial indemnity plans of the 1970s, with first-dollar benefits.

"Middle old" (75 to 85) people includes some workers. This age group wants acute care services as well as long-term care, aid to daily living, home care, and rehabilitation. Their children do not want to care for aging parents and cannot afford to. An improved economy based on growing productivity, higher oil and energy costs, and the rebuilding of the infrastructure also brings renewed inflation and a shortage of affordable housing, hence a shortage of space at home for parents.

Expanded numbers of "very old" (over 85) people create special demands for elderly housing, including both custodial care and life care projects (White & Lewis, 1985). As the market improves, pension and retirement systems are worth more. Thus, more seniors will qualify as income increases. The fastest growing subgroup of aged people consists of those over 100, and there is a resulting need for assisted-living units. Particularly in need for both living arrangements and health care will be the low-income group living on Social Security and limited retirement income. Some of them will be the formerly homeless, for whom assistance is now available due to larger budgets. Few of these patients will appear now at the large, complex, tertiary care, private hospitals. The burden of unfunded care for these facilities will largely be an artifact of the brief periods in history when those patients did not have access to care at public facilities.

A middle segment will include those citizens with owned but modest housing. These patients are somewhat mobile and have a wider access to care in a manner similar to the mid-1990s, when there were HMOs and PPOs, with reasonable access to primary and specialty care. Then there are upscale retirees with large pensions, investment income, and the fruits of matured IRAs. This high-end group is able to take advantage of the complete array of everything medical science has to offer, since there are no budget restraints. The training of subspecialty physicians is greater than it has ever been, and so are incomes for doctors. The gap widens between earnings of primaries versus specialties. Greater attention and public support of the identification and treatment of mental illness further reduces the number of homeless people, with an attendant reduction in morbidity, mortality, and uncompensated care for private doctors and hospitals.

Progress does not produce cures, necessarily, but does show measurable benefits that are clear and well understood by the public. Pressure builds to make interventions more available as the public accepts them. There is still some residual skepticism about the long-term benefits of medical technology—its uses and benefits in general and heroic medicine in particular—are still prevalent with regard to care for the terminally ill. But, in general, the prevailing mood of the country is to try everything that can be done, if it offers some hope for longer life in a society that reveres longevity. The elderly are particularly attracted to interventions aimed at chronic or debilitating diseases such as arthritis, Alzheimer's, or Parkinson's disease. Public funds are poured into extending the range of chronic and rehabilitative services. Acute care hospitals, improved by the shock therapy of competitive market economies in the early 1990s, are more trim and efficient, since unnecessary costs were eliminated. Surplus beds remain out of the system and historical trends toward full-service hospitals are reversed. The hospice movement continues to grow, because there are still many illnesses where the limits of medical science are obvious to the public, and bioethical attitudes that first arose in the 1980s remain in force.

The long-announced service economy arrives, just when there is a large number of aging workers who are not technologically adept. Providing full health benefits even in a booming economy becomes more difficult for the private sector as Medicare is denied to workers under 67 and the Social Security threshold moves to age 72. Growth in the labor force participation among those over 60 poses a higher risk for those businesses that self-insured in the late 1980s, particularly when the risk group is small. Fewer young people enter the labor market as the country grows increasingly older. Many of the entry-level workers not receiving full health coverage are immigrants, whether legal or illegal. Business expenses and health insurance benefits will be taxed as a result of congressional deficit-reducing measures in the mid- to late 1990s.

States with greater numbers of resident working elderly force employers to restore health benefits that were cut back or co-paid during the cost-containment years. States with higher proportions of younger workers enable business to offer either take-home pay or cost-shared benefits. With changes largely forced through by older workers, health plans offer more and cost more. Businesses have not completely forgotten their hard-learned lessons from the cost-containment years and continue to monitor health care delivery, maintain profiles of providers, and keep faith in review systems as the secret of success in retaining utilization. They still want managed systems and fixed prices whenever available and impose structural controls, such as the bulk purchasing of supplies and services. But the continuing aging of the workforce, which increases the volume of care, along with easier access to care and the adoption of new technology, all have the same effect: cost increases.

Economic growth after the mid-1990s shifts emphasis firmly toward a new growth cycle and stamps out sympathy for cost containment in the health sector, although these effects are dampened again by the actions of the Federal Reserve to maintain high interest rates as an anti-inflation tactic. DRG systems, after endless tinkering and adjustments to fit transient political agendas of first one party and then the other, become totally discredited. By now, that mechanism has become too complex, too unwieldy, too unfair, and too unpopular with providers, consumers, and payers alike. All support has been lost, if there ever was any. Business responds to a tight labor market at the lower end of the wage scale. There are too few workers for entry-level jobs, and those available lack education and skills necessary in a service economy.

High-paid older workers want better health care coverage, particularly insurance that can be portable from job to job, a fear that was created by the downsizing of the 1990s. Hospitals complain that physicians were never subjected to the same extremes of DRG pressures that resulted in reduced size of facilities and loss of executive positions. Doctors complain that reduced incomes from pressures on specialty services have changed medical practice and make it less attractive. Governments have tried to patch the system with bandage approaches, because comprehensive health reform was never passed by Congress after its high-water mark of 1993 to 1994. Private insurers have enjoyed several years without cost shifting and forget how much they disliked it. Everyone wants more access to more high-quality care at whatever the cost to government or payers but at a more reasonable personal out-of-pocket cost. If it requires more tax money to pay for more health care, then that is acceptable in the last few years of the century, because the country and the middle class are prospering.

The public's agenda is now very clear, but the federal government's dilemma is growing increasingly acute. Although the president made her campaign promises in 2000 that Medicare would be reviewed and access would be increased for the growing number of older baby boomers, it is clear that the real crisis will recur after the turn of the century when those baby boomers begin to pass retirement age. The president must figure out a way to offer a federal health system that will work in the short- and medium-term to hold off political pressure from seniors and fulfill political commitments to them but will also anticipate the need to control massive expenditures when the time comes. Costs of health care are increasing rapidly enough even without the additional volume expected by 2020, when the last of the baby boom generation reaches 65 (White & Lewis, 1985). A control mechanism seems inevitable to government planners, who devise a new proposed policy called "cost containment." However, that approach is not politically popular enough to be acceptable in the current boom times, and since the system is not broke, why fix it?

As the system becomes less constrained, it can accept increases in benefits, and services can now be offered to the unsponsored and the underinsured. Medicare, which merged with Medicaid, combines a more generous voucher system with stop-loss provisions of catastrophic insurance, much like an earlier plan a decade before that the seniors of that day hated and caused to be repealed. As the medical liability crisis that occurred between 1975 and 1985 becomes ancient history, the insurance industry has more flexibility, but both public and private payers want control of postacute care, better discharge planning, and continuity of care, particularly long-term care. There are fewer insurance companies in the health market now, since many left the field during the shakeout in the 1990s managed care era. Insurance and tax benefits for long-term care and rehabilitation are provided and health benefits show lower rates of taxation.

Assumptions Underlying Expansion

The developments in this scenario of growth and increase are based on four assumptions that underlie the expansion in volume and cost. The first assumption is that the economy will remain strong after the brief recession in the early to mid-1990s that aggravated all the negative effects of managed care, DRGs, cost outliers, and cost containment.

The second assumption is that there will be strong political support for growth in the health care portion of the gross national product by seniors, especially in the East and Midwest. That strength will control elections. Aged voters in the Sun Belt states also support the idea of expansion in health care but will not share as much in its beneficial effect, because of the inability of their states to participate in paying its costs.

The third assumption is that those middle-aged and middle-class workers will prefer to pay increased taxes to care for aging parents. They are unwilling to take care of parents in their homes and are too financially committed to stop working or pay long-term care bills. They are beginning to look forward to their need for increased health care and want to ensure that some kind of appropriate system will be in place when it is their turn to receive.

Hope springs eternal, though, and the fourth assumption is that there will be enough progress in medical technology, gene therapy, and monoclonal antibody research achievements to offer the promise of even more advances if more research funding is made available.

The economy cooperates, to go along with the four planning assumptions. Real estate growth creates real gain for households, businesses, and government. Inflation stays low enough as a partial result of recession. The balance of trade improves, international tensions improve and ease enough for some repayments of international loans, and the U.S. deficit becomes manageable. Assistance to Mexico is rewarded by greater trade in both directions, and the pressures of illegal immigration slow to the point that political relationships between the two neighbors reaches an all-time high. Russia is able to move forward slowly toward the stage of being self-sufficient, with an unmistakable trend toward a private market economy, democratic processes, and an interest in the concepts of a private health care delivery system. American consumers favor fiscal conservatism and vote for politicians who promise to achieve those goals. If short-term results are not apparent, then incumbents are voted out in favor of newer candidates, regardless of party. There is still a willingness to spend for those things people want to have or do. As affluence increases, it becomes clear that health care is one of those things.

As the flow of medical technology increases rapidly with its release from cost containment, a wide range of diagnosis and treatment improvements appear. The shift of diagnostic functions to physicians' offices and the home, spurred on by the managed care period, becomes permanent, and hospitals do not regain their former preeminent position. Steady improvement creates benefits that do not particularly increase but also do not substantially reduce costs. Progress in cancer therapy and AIDS detection (but not immunization) fuels public demand for access to highly publicized technologies.

Other technologies that ameliorate (at high cost) but do not cure include those for diagnosis of coronary artery disease, dietary links to arteriosclerosis, Alzheimer's disease, and management of patients in drug therapy. Public realization of the destructive effects of substance abuse, developments in fertility diagnosis and therapy, microsurgery, and neonatal care open a wide range of new possibilities in enhancing reproduction and sustaining low–birth weight infants. As progress is made in providing better birth control information to teenagers, better prenatal care reduces the number of expensive cases and liability claims. OB/GYN physicians reenter practice in large numbers, creating better access and availability of care as the birth rate begins to climb again among the baby bust generation now becoming middle aged and middle class.

In scenario two, there are no strong brakes being applied to increases in health care spending. Each sector of the industry, acting in its own best interest, does not yet see the danger signals that brought on the cost-containment movement in the first place, although some economists are aware of them but cannot get anyone to listen. Predictions of future spending crises fall on deaf ears, as presidents, governors, and legislators keep busy balancing their own short-run political interests. Business, government, doctors, hospitals, and consumers push for increases in both supply and demand for more health care at ever greater costs. The leveling off or modest decreases of the middle 1990s in health spending prove to have been an aberration.

Sympathy for alternative delivery systems was motivated by economic constraints, but this sympathy is now reduced since money is plentifully available. Pluralistic responses of market competition (HMOs, PPOs, contracting, discounting, prepayment, capitation) continue to coexist with regulation (DRGs, fee schedules, fixed-price payments), but fee-for-service plans make a comeback to a joyous reception by specialist physicians (those who are left). Applications to the reduced number of medical schools increases, as do residency programs in integrated health care systems. Public hospitals have largely fallen by the wayside during managed care, so now there is no place else to train subspecialists.

By the early twenty-first century few people see any problems of access to the health care delivery system. All but the most serious care has been shifted to outpatient settings, where there are nearly enough primary care doctors, while many new and exciting diagnostic and therapeutic modalities are being used in physicians' offices and ambulatory settings. Nationalized health care systems, such as Canada or Britain, seem so remote as not to be written about in any of the journals any more. In fact, those systems are seriously considering moving in the direction of the revitalized U.S. style.

Hospital buildings have been adapted to a wide range of uses, with remodeling or renovation costs paid mostly by philanthropy, including some of the doctors who have no place else to practice. Once managed care and other public and private funding restrictions removed operating funds as a capital source, and the loss of tax-exempt bond funding removed another traditional source, most nonprofit hospitals found it advisable to become publicly traded. Additional court rulings placed in doubt the tax-exempt status of many hospitals for not offering uncompensated care during the depths of the cost-containment period. When the economy revived, there seemed to be no reason to depart from investor-owned status.

Outpatient technology is cheap and effective, mental health care is benefited by breakthroughs in diagnosis and therapy, and custodial support for the elderly is included in third-party payment. All of these are welcome to providers and patients alike. All of these help to increase costs of the total system. There are no remaining controls on technology, and providers duplicate costly facilities and services in order to compete for paying patients. Clinically inappropriate but available technologies are often used.

After declaring a physician shortage in 1965 and a surplus in 1985, the federal government repeats history and declares another shortage in 2005 to begin gearing up for the baby boom generation volume. Incentive structures change once again to favor treatment rather than prevention. Expanded use of technologies are not seen to yield significant improvements in health status. The realization occurs that costs and expenditures, both absolutely and proportionally, are growing rapidly. And all of this is happening before the real increase in the elderly population has begun to take place.

Effect on the Medical Staff

In this scenario, the expansion of services and the availability of money to pay for more care parallels, in general, the history of the U.S. health care delivery system in recent decades, during the period when the Joint Commission model was being developed and refined, in fact. Conditions as laid out in the expansion mode lessen tension between the hospitals and the doctors (but only to a certain point) and would favor the revival of interest in self-governance. A Joint Commission model would flourish in these circumstances, because the hospital-based specialists are not so dependent upon primary care gatekeepers for referrals and capitation payments. If there is a rosy future for the model discussed through most of this book, that future should be scenario two.

In scenario one, short-run cost containment grew worse, constrained the system, and resulted in a political backlash demanding new expansion. In scenario two, the more favorable short-run environment eventually leads to the same excesses that caused cost containment in the first place. It all means that there will be a hospital medical staff in either scenario. Incentives will be very different, thus controlling behavior and attitudes. Life in the medical groups will be different in each scenario, but there will still be doctors chosen to belong to the groups, and attention paid to how they perform. In scenario one, much of that self-governance would take place outside the hospital, which might include one or more of the alternative models of a medical staff presented and discussed in Chapter 27.

MOTION TO ADJOURN THE MEETING

The preface began this volume by describing the many faces and roles of the doctors on hospital medical staffs. It all means that doctors have a private life that is, hopefully, pleasurable and rewarding, away from the practice of medicine. They also have a practice life devoted to patient care and advocacy that is, hopefully, pleasurable and rewarding. They also have an organizational life in the hospital as an organized medical staff, having been delegated tasks and functions of self-governance by the governing body that they might perform anyway as a professional obligation. No matter what the payment system or the delivery system, there will still be the need to make sure that doctors are *who they say they are* (credentialing), that they were *trained to do what they want to do* (privileging), of *how well they do it* (peer review), and that *should they be allowed to continue doing it* (reappointment). It would be better if making sure of those things were pleasurable and rewarding also, but it has always been a mixed process, at best.

How those functions are performed is the work program of the organized medical staff and its elected leaders. How that work is organized and documented has been the work program of the Joint Commission and its survey efforts.

All doctors on the medical staff, as members of the participatory democracy of the self-governance program, bear an equal responsibility for carrying out Joint Commission standards. However, only some members of the hospital medical staff actually carry out that work program of complying with standards, preparing and carrying out surveys, including sitting through unpaid meetings and occasionally being forced to take corrective or disciplinary action against a colleague. But that is the way it is in a democracy; some people do the work, some do not, some do the policing and judging, while a few others commit the crimes.

To their everlasting credit, enough cooperative physicians have done enough of a good job that the overall national system has worked well enough so that achieving Joint Commission accreditation has been a worthwhile goal and has been a worthwhile effort to protect patient safety. Like all other democratic systems, some have excelled and perfected the Joint Commission model to an exemplary level of accomplishment. Some others have not excelled but did well enough to get by with a tolerable survey result that enabled them to forget the whole thing for another three years, at which time they can get frantic again at the last minute in hopes of just scraping by again.

Then, there are a very few who did not pass at all, but they managed to fix enough things to be able to save their accreditation on the focused survey and thus get off probation. Most of the time, being burned once and reading their name in the paper as a hospital of low quality that could not comply with some unknown but very ominous-sounding requirements was enough to bring about a level of improvement that was all that was needed in the first place. In those hospitals that form the lower quartile, lots of the doctors on the medical staff predictably resented the whole event and did not understand or accept that someone also had the effrontery to question them or their judgment about anything. The whole Joint Commission thing is a big bother, anyway.

Bother or not, it is there until it is changed or replaced. This book has been dedicated to those who have performed the duty even when they were not enthusiastic but did a competent enough job, even if excruciatingly slowly. And then there are those good souls who understood the delegation, accepted the assignment, and carried it out with grace and style, even through those times when they had to stand fast in the face of punishing a colleague and friend who needed sanction or punishment. It would have been so much easier to just ignore it or let it slide, particularly since the meetings were all in executive session where no one else knew what was being said. That is called doing your duty. If it had been a general, there would have been a statue erected in the park. There are no statues in the medical staff for doing your duty. In fact, in the doctor's lounge there are very few heroes and being a peer review enthusiast is not one of them.

There should be a special place somewhere for chiefs of staff who accepted their elected positions knowing full well that they could not possibly come out of it with any dignity or respect. All politicians know that going in, but chiefs do not get any of the fringe benefits that a politician gets or steals. New business comes to people in politics in hopes that they will be favorably impressed to do what the petitioner wants. In the medical staff, new business does not come to the chief in the form of new referrals, because the chief made an unpopular decision and someone must get revenge for that without worrying whether there will be a next time, when another decision might go the other way. And yet perfectly sensible, good doctors keep on becoming chief in spite of it all, and do remarkably good jobs. Everyone is better off because they did, even if they never knew anything about it because of the secrecy.

Chiefs can function best, and so can the Joint Commission model or any of its alternatives as presented in Chapter 27, when there is unity among the medical staff members. In the 1990s, reform is in the air again. Instead of fostering unity in the medical profession, managed care incites conflicts of interest among the specialties, and each pursues its own policies and special interests. It can be seen on every side that managed care greatly magnifies the role of the primary care physician as the case manager, as the first stage of treatment, and referral gatekeeper for every patient. Specialty societies in family practice, internal medicine, and pediatrics endorse reform proposals and the advent of managed care. Societies in surgery and other technically advanced invasive fields oppose reform proposals and extensions of managed care. The national, state, and county medical associations and societies cannot participate in managed care at all, except to try to give information and advice to their members. No matter what advice they give, it will help some doctors and hurt others.

Proposed legislative reforms have fragmented the medical profession, preventing it from developing coordinated reform strategies. This frustrates a unified approach. Glaser (1994) notes that other industrialized and developed countries have learned that health care systems must minimize costs in trouble as well as in money. As described in Chapter 2, the medical profession always presents special problems of relationships and authority. Doctors prefer individualism in judgments, bilateral relationships with patients, independence from controls by laypeople in governments and in payer organizations, and restrictions and guidelines (if any) only from their peers in the professional community. Other countries enacted universal payment systems long ago, and relations between doctors and public authorities passed through stages, Glaser (1994) relates, of professional organization, disputes, negotiations to resolve each dispute, and standing decision-making machinery. Some large scale national health care systems have moved from the point where physicians exercised authority over patients to the stage where physicians in many countries share responsibility for the management of the system with public authorities.

Next Steps in Professional Development

The American medical profession at the macrolevel, and the hospital medical staff at the microlevel, have evolved only partially through these stages. The absence of a national health insurance system and the recurrent faith in private-sector solutions has led to little experience in bargaining and collaboration with governments and united fronts of payer organizations. Can doctors and hospitals in the form of integrated systems move past the era of individualistic and competitive behavior that continues to be hostile to government? Tom Weil (1994) has offered the opinion that "managed care may only be a transitory solution for reforming our health system with a three-to five-year window." He goes on to predict that a likely scenario is that managed care networks will ultimately become such massive alliances that public-utility-type regulation will be required. Within five years, there could be only one regional network in some urban areas of the country, while in others, there could be only a few operating as oligopolies.

In that case, the public would become disenchanted with such concentrated regional systems because of their bureaucratic manner, the quality and access to care offered, and their cost. Then public pressure for cost containment and better quality of care will force a type of public-utility regulation on these oligopolistic systems, in the form of a backlash against the very characteristics that have led to the rise of managed care. Weil (1994) says that a "fundamental issue for regulators under such a public utility model will be effecting an appropriate balance between the rights of consumers and providers, and the need for public controls." That assumption could form the basis for a third scenario describing an inevitable drift into a regulated U.S. health care system.

Can the medical staff move on past self-centered individualism and interest-group aspirations, or will managed care only, in the end, increase the problems of the status quo, not solve them? Is the hospital really the enemy of the doctors? Can there ever be a truly integrated system until the doctors are integrated, and the nonbelievers, the non-cooperative, the nonparticipators are practicing somewhere else? Or, will the society continue to run parallel systems that utilize the self-governing principles of the Joint Commission model with doctors on the medical staff who do not believe in either the Joint Commission or the local/regional integrated health care system? Yet, somehow in spite of this dissonance, there are still competent processes of credentialing, privileging, reappointment, and peer review going on at this very moment.

SUMMARY

It is possible to construct at least two plausible scenarios involving further changes in the U.S. health care system between now and the year 2000 or beyond. Earlier chapters have described the past and present, leaving the opportunity now to predict possible futures that have dramatic effects on patients and providers. In each case, it is necessary to estimate the effect, if any, of the hospital medical staff that has been the subject of this book.

In the first scenario, the present movement toward a constrained system that features managed care is extended forward with estimated results. Though fictitious, the scenario is a bad news version that sees the nation's economy remain stagnant and the portion of the gross national product devoted to health care reduced. Cost-containment pressures dominate behavior, and neither government nor its citizens are able to break out of the cycle of stagnation and deficit. The health care system will change accordingly to reduce both access to care and quality.

In the second scenario, a different set of assumptions about the world lead to a different outcome. In this case, larger social forces not under the control of doctors and hospitals help shape a health care system that benefits from national prosperity and the steady growth of a productive economy. An increasing supply of new money in the economy and in governmental tax revenues leads to a new growth cycle that stamps out the iron grip of the cost-containment sympathy that came earlier. However, there are still some bitter memories of the previous cycles of boom or bust in health care, and this time there is not a complete return to the fee-for-service and cost-based reimbursement patterns. The medical staff is affected once again.

REFERENCES

Aaron, H. J., & Schwartz, W. B. (1985). *The Painful Prescription—Rationing Health Care.* Washington, D.C.: Brookings Institution.

Glaser, W. A. (1994). Doctors and public authorities: The trend toward collaboration. *Journal of Health Politics, Policy, and Law, 19(4),* 705–727.

Institute for the Future (1986). *Looking Ahead at American Health Care.* Menlo Park, CA.

Weil, T. (1994). *Rate Controls.* Reprinted in *Healthcare Trends Report, 8(12, Dec.),* 7.

White, C. H. (1986). Smaller carrot—bigger stick. *Western Journal of Medicine, 145,* 535.

White, C. H. (1988). Changes affecting health care: Two possible scenarios. Monagle, J. F., & Thomasma, D. C. (Eds.), *Medical Ethics.* Rockville, MD: Aspen Publishers.

White, C. H., & Lewis, S. (1985). *Strategic Planning Assumptions for Hospitals, 1985–1987.* Sacramento, CA: California Hospital Association.

White, C. H., & Lewis, S. (1986). *Strategic Planning Assumptions for Hospitals, 1986–1988.* Sacramento, CA: California Hospital Association.

White, C. H., & Morse, L. E. (1985). *Hospital Fact Book (10th Ed.).* Sacramento, CA: California Hospital Association.

INDEX